Energy Metabolism and Obesity

Contemporary Endocrinology

P. Michael Conn, *Series Editor*

Energy Metabolism and Obesity: Research and Clinical Applications, edited by *Patricia A. Donohoue*, 2008

Polycystic Ovary Syndrome: Current Controversies, from the Ovary to the Pancreas, edited by *Andrea Dunaif, Jeffrey R. Chang, Stephen Franks, and Richard S. Legro*, 2008

The Metabolic Syndrome: Epidemiology, Clinical Treatment, and Underlying Mechanisms, edited by *Barbara C. Hansen and George A. Bray*, 2008

Genomics in Endocrinology: DNA Microarray Analysis in Endocrine Health and Disease, edited by *Stuart Handwerger and Bruce Aronow*, 2007

Controversies in Treating Diabetes: Clinical and Research Aspects, edited by *Derek LeRoith and Aaron I. Vinik*, 2007

Autoimmune Diseases in Endocrinology, edited by *Anthony P. Weetman*, 2007

When Puberty is Precocious: Scientific and Clinical Aspects, edited by *Ora H. Pescovitz and Emily C. Walvoord*, 2007

Insulin Resistance and Polycystic Ovarian Syndrome: Pathogenesis, Evaluation and Treatment, edited by *John E. Nestler, Evanthia Diamanti-Kandarakis, Renato Pasquali, and D. Pandis*, 2007

Hypertension and Hormone Mechanisms, edited by *Robert M. Carey*, 2007

The Leydig Cell in Health and Disease, edited by *Anita H. Payne and Matthew Phillip Hardy*, 2007

Treatment of the Obese Patient, edited by *Robert F. Kushner and Daniel H. Bessesen*, 2007

Androgen Excess Disorders in Women: Polycystic Ovary Syndrome and Other Disorders, Second Edition, edited by *Ricardo Azzis, John E. Nestler, and Didier Dewailly*, 2006

Evidence-Based Endocrinology, edited by *Victor M. Montori*, 2006

Stem Cells in Endocrinology, edited by *Linda B. Lester*, 2005

Office Andrology, edited by *Phillip E. Pantton and David E. Battaglia*, 2005

Male Hypogonadism: Basic, Clinical, and Therapeutic Principles, edited by *Stephen J. Winters*, 2004

Androgens in Health and Disease, edited by *Carrie Bagatell and William J. Bremner*, 2003

Endocrine Replacement Therapy in Clinical Practice, edited by *A. Wayne Meikle*, 2003

Early Diagnosis of Endocrine Diseases, edited by *Robert S. Bar*, 2003

Type I Diabetes: Etiology and Treatment, edited by *Mark A. Sperling*, 2003

Handbook of Diagnostic Endocrinology, edited by *Janet E. Hall and Lynnette K. Nieman*, 2003

Pediatric Endocrinology: A Practical Clinical Guide, edited by *Sally Radovick and Margaret H. MacGillivray*, 2003

Diseases of the Thyroid, Second Edition, edited by *Lewis E. Braverman*, 2003

Developmental Endocrinology: From Research to Clinical Practice, edited by *Erica A. Eugster and Ora Hirsch Pescovitz*, 2002

Osteoporosis: Pathophysiology and Clinical Management, edited by *Eric S. Orwoll and Michael Bliziotes*, 2002

Challenging Cases in Endocrinology, edited by *Mark E. Molitch*, 2002

Selective Estrogen Receptor Modulators: Research and Clinical Applications, edited by *Andrea Manni and Michael F. Verderame*, 2002

Transgenics in Endocrinology, edited by *Martin Matzuk, Chester W. Brown, and T. Rajendra Kumar*, 2001

Assisted Fertilization and Nuclear Transfer in Mammals, edited by *Don P. Wolf and Mary Zelinski-Wooten*, 2001

Adrenal Disorders, edited by *Andrew N. Margioris and George P. Chrousos*, 2001

Endocrine Oncology, edited by *Stephen P. Ethier*, 2000

Endocrinology of the Lung: Development and Surfactant Synthesis, edited by *Carole R. Mendelson*, 2000

Sports Endocrinology, edited by *Michelle P. Warren and Naama W. Constantini*, 2000

Gene Engineering in Endocrinology, edited by *Margaret A. Shupnik*, 2000

Endocrinology of Aging, edited by *John E. Morley and Lucretia van den Berg*, 2000

Human Growth Hormone: Research and Clinical Practice, edited by *Roy G. Smith and Michael O. Thorner*, 2000

Hormones and the Heart in Health and Disease, edited by *Leonard Share*, 1999

Energy Metabolism and Obesity

Research and Clinical Applications

Edited by

Patricia A. Donohoue, MD

University of Iowa, Iowa City, IA

Humana Press Totowa, New Jersey

999 Riverview Drive, Suite 208
Totowa, New Jersey 07512
www.humanapress.com

This publication is printed on acid-free paper. ∞

ANSI Z39.48-1984 (American National Standards Institute) Permanence of Paper for Printed Library Materials.

Cover Illustration: Fig. 1 of Chapter 1 (Molecular control of energy homeostasis) by Wendy K. Chung and Rudolph L. Leibel

Cover design by Karen Schulz

For additional copies, pricing for bulk purchases, and/or information about other Humana titles, contact Humana at the above address or at any of the following numbers: Tel: 973-256-1699; Fax: 973-256-8341; E-mail: humana@humanapr.com or visit our website at http://humanapress.com

eISBN 978-1-60327-139-4

Library of Congress Control Number: 2007931071

Printed in the United States of America. 10 9 8 7 6 5 4 3 2 1

Preface

This new volume, Energy Metabolism and Obesity: *Research and Clinical Applications*, is a compilation of highly informative reviews, written by undisputed leaders in the field. These authors elucidate the most important aspects of genetic background, neuropeptide secretion and action, neuronal pathways, adipokines, gut hormones, and environmental influences (physical activity, pharmacologic agents, and surgical alteration of the gastrointestinal tract), as well as the complex interactions among them. Understanding the physiology of energy storage and partitioning has become quite a daunting task, as a huge amount of information has flooded the biomedical literature in the past decade. As researchers and clinicians, we face the challenge of understanding this information and applying it to the practice of obesity prevention and treatment. This challenge is, and will remain for some time, one of our greatest public health priorities. The excellent overviews in this book will undoubtedly provide us with a better understanding of the multifaceted entity of obesity.

Patricia A. Donohoue, MD
Volume Editor

Contents

Contributors

STEPHEN C. BENOIT, PhD, *Department of Psychiatry, Genome Research Institute, Obesity Research Center, University of Cincinnati, Cincinnati, Ohio, USA*

CYRIL Y. BOWERS, MD, *Department of Endocrinology, Tulane University Health Sciences Center, New Orleans, Louisiana, USA*

WENDY K. CHUNG, MD, PhD, *Division of Molecular Genetics and the Naomi Berrie Diabetes Center, Columbia University Medical Center, New York, New York, USA*

KRISTEN J. CLARKE, PhD, *Department of Biochemistry, Scripps Florida, and Division of the Scripps Research Institute, Jupiter, Florida, USA*

DEBORAH J. CLEGG, PhD, *Department of Psychiatry, Genome Research Institute, Obesity Research Center, University of Cincinnati, Cincinnati, Ohio, USA*

MOLLY EMOTT, MD, *Department of Pediatrics, Duke University Medical Center, Durham, North Carolina, USA*

PAUL W. FRANKS, PhD, MPH, MSc, *Genetic Epidemiology and Clinical Research Group, Division of Medicine Department of Public Health and Clinical Medicine, Umeå University Hospital, Umeå, Sweden*

MICHAEL FREEMARK, MD, *Department of Pediatrics, Duke University Medical Center, Durham, North Carolina, USA*

ANDREA HAQQ, MD, *Department of Pediatrics, Duke University Medical Center, Durham, North Carolina, USA*

DAVID L. HURLEY, PhD, *Department of Biochemistry, Tulane University Health Sciences Center, New Orleans, Louisiana, USA*

MOHAMMAD K. JAMAL, MD, *Department of Surgery, The University of Iowa Carver College of Medicine, University of Iowa Hospitals and Clinics, Iowa, City, Iowa, USA*

ROBERT L. JUDD, PhD, *Department of Anatomy, Physiology and Pharmacology, College of Veterinary Medicine, Auburn University, Auburn, Alabama, USA*

BLANDINE LAFERRÈRE, MD, *New York Obesity Research Center, St. Luke's Roosevelt Hospital Center, Columbia University, New York, New York, USA*

RUDOLPH L. LEIBEL, MD, *Division of Molecular Genetics and the Naomi Berrie Diabetes Center, Columbia University Medical Center, New York, New York, USA*

ROBERT H. LUSTIG, MD, *Department of Pediatrics, University of California, San Francisco, San Francisco, California, USA*

DANIEL L. MARKS, MD, PhD, *Department of Pediatrics, Center for the Study of Weight Regulation, Oregon Health and Sciences University, Portland, Oregon, USA*

EDWARD E. MASON, MD, PhD, *Department of Surgery, The University of Iowa Carver College of Medicine, University of Iowa Hospitals and Clinics, Iowa, City, Iowa, USA*

JOHN W. NEWCOMER, MD, *Department of Psychiatry, Washington University School of Medicine, St. Louis, Missouri, USA*

Ruben Nogueiras, PhD, *Department of Psychiatry, Genome Research Institute, Obesity Research Center, University of Cincinnati College of Medicine, Cincinnati, Ohio, USA*

Thomas M. O'Dorisio, MD, *Department of Internal Medicine, The University of Iowa Carver College of Medicine, University of Iowa Hospitals and Clinics, Iowa, City, IA, USA*

Diego Perez-Tilve, PhD, *Department of Psychiatry, Genome Research Institute, Obesity Research Center, University of Cincinnati College of Medicine, Cincinnati, Ohio, USA*

Ofer Reizes, PhD, *Procter and Gamble Pharmaceuticals, Cincinnati, Ohio, USA*

Stephen M. Roth, PhD, *Department of Kinesiology, University of Maryland, College Park, Maryland, USA*

Roland H. Stimson, PhD, *Endocrinology Unit, Queen's Medical Research Institute, University of Edinburgh, Edinburgh, Scotland, UK*

Ya-Xiong Tao, PhD, *Department of Anatomy, Physiology and Pharmacology, College of Veterinary Medicine, Auburn University, Auburn, Alabama, USA*

Matthias H. Tschöp, MD, PhD, *Department of Psychiatry, Genome Research Institute, Obesity Research Center, University of Cincinnati College of Medicine, Cincinnati, Ohio, USA*

Johannes D. Veldhuis, MD, *Mayo Medical and Graduate Schools, Mayo Clinics, Rochester, Minnesota, USA*

Brian R. Walker, PhD, *Endocrinology Unit, Queen's Medical Research Institute, University of Edinburgh, Edinburgh, Scotland, UK*

Hilary Wilson, *Department of Psychiatry, Genome Research Institute, Obesity Research Center, University of Cincinnati College of Medicine, Cincinnati, Ohio, USA*

Color Plates

Color Plates follow p. 68

1 Molecular Physiology of Monogenic and Syndromic Obesities in Humans

Wendy K. Chung and Rudolph L. Leibel

CONTENTS

Abstract

Obesity has become an increasingly prevalent public health problem and represents the complex interaction of genetic, developmental, behavioral, and environmental influences. Although rare, the study of monogenic forms of obesity provides insight into underlying molecular and physiologic mechanisms by which adiposity is regulated through food intake, energy expenditure, and partitioning of stored calories. The identification of the genetic basis for many forms of monogenic obesity has provided a group of candidate genes and molecular pathways for study of the genetic control of energy homeostasis. Many of the genes identified relate to the development and function of the hypothalamus and central control of food intake and energy homeostasis. Allelic variations in these genes could contribute to nonsyndromic forms of obesity.

Key Words: Alstrom syndrome, Bardet-Biedl syndrome, Borjeson-Forssman-Lehmann syndrome, Cohen syndrome, genetic, leptin, leptin receptor, mahoganoid, mahogany, melanocortin 4 receptor, monogenic, obesity, Prader-Willi syndrome, prohormone convertase 1, pro-opiomelanocortin, SIM1, TUB

INTRODUCTION

Obesity or increased adiposity is primarily the result of a net imbalance of caloric intake over energy expenditure over time. Even small differences resulting in positive energy balance—when integrated over long periods of time—can produce increased adiposity. In some instances, preferential partitioning of excess calories toward fat can exacerbate the process. With the increasing availability of highly palatable, calorically

From: *Contemporary Endocrinology: Energy Metabolism and Obesity: Research and Clinical Applications*
Edited by: P. A. Donohoue © Humana Press Inc., Totowa, NJ

dense food, as well as increased mechanization and an increasingly sedentary lifestyle, net positive energy imbalance in many individuals has resulted in alarming increases in obesity worldwide. In the United States, 65% of adults are considered overweight (body mass index [BMI] 25.0–29.9), and more than 30% of the adult population is now considered obese (BMI >30) *(1)*. The problem also affects children in whom the percentage with BMI >95th percentile between the ages of 6 and 19 years is now 16% *(2)*. The burden of obesity falls disproportionately on African Americans and Hispanics. Although these trends are most pronounced in the United States, European and Asian countries have noted similar trends in adults and children. Increasing in parallel with these trends in obesity are the frequently associated comorbidities of diabetes, hypertension, and cardiovascular disease *(3, 4)*.

MOLECULAR ELEMENTS IN THE CONTROL OF BODY WEIGHT

Body weight and fat stores are determined by the net excess or deficit of food intake over energy expenditure. The hypothalamus acts centrally to integrate redundant signaling pathways involving the neuroendocrine and autonomic nervous systems to determine food intake, energy expenditure, and nutrient partitioning. Leptin and insulin are secreted in proportion to peripheral fat mass and signal the hypothalamus regarding the state of long-term energy stores (Fig. 1.1) *(5)*. Leptin appears to act primarily to signal critical minimal energy (triglyceride) reserves for functions such as reproduction *(6)*. Low concentrations of leptin and insulin generate an anabolic signal to increase food intake and reduce energy expenditure *(7)*. Leptin and insulin bind to receptors on neurons in the arcuate nucleus, which is partially outside of the blood-brain barrier. The arcuate nucleus contains two discrete neuronal populations producing either agouti-related protein (AgRP) and neuropeptide Y (NPY) or pro-opiomelanocortin (POMC) and cocaine and amphetamine regulated transcript (CART) that act reciprocally to increase and decrease food intake, respectively, and to transduce outflow signals regulating body fat stores *(5)*. Leptin and insulin inhibit the NPY/AgRP neurons and reciprocally stimulate the POMC/CART neurons. AgRP is the naturally occurring inverse agonist of melanocortin 3 and 4 receptors (MC3R and MC4R) and is expressed in cell bodies in the arcuate that coexpress NPY and that project to "second order" nuclei expressing MC3R and MC4R to stimulate food intake. The "default" action of this neural system is to generate a net anabolic signal unless leptin and insulin signal sufficient energy stores. Both sets of neurons respond vigorously to starvation, but only the POMC/CART neurons respond to excess energy intake in part explaining why it is easier for individuals to gain rather than lose weight. Energy expenditure is then coordinated through the autonomic nervous system and hypothalamic control of thyroid function.

Human adiposity resolves complex interactions among genetic, developmental, behavioral, and environmental influences. Evidence for potent genetic contributions to human obesity is provided by familial clustering of increased adiposity, including a three- to sevenfold increased relative risk (λs) among siblings *(8)* as well as estimates of heritability (the fraction of the total phenotypic variance of a quantitative trait caused by genes in a specified environment) for fat mass between 40% and 70% in twin studies *(9, 10)*. Clearly, genetic change cannot account for the recent trends toward increased adiposity. However, what is likely genetically determined is the relative rank

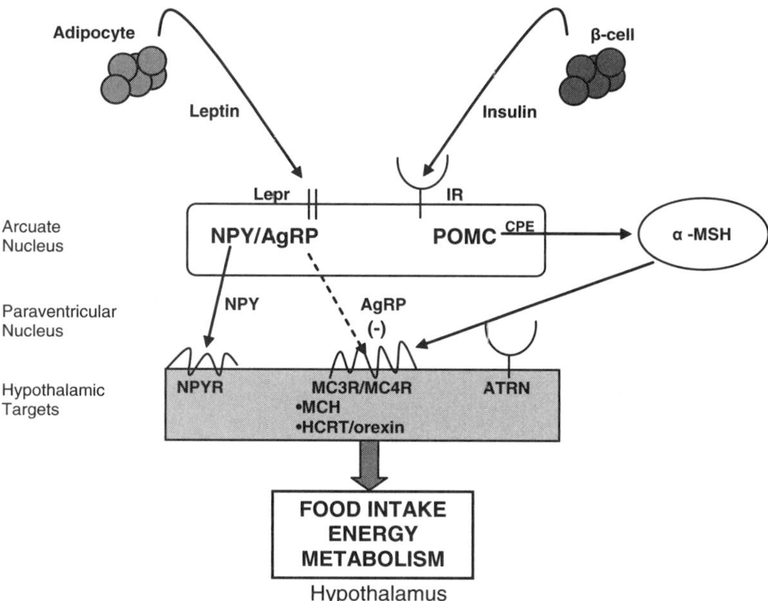

Fig. 1.1 Molecular control of energy homeostasis. Peripheral signals including leptin and insulin bind to receptors on cell bodies in the arcuate nucleus of the hypothalamus. Neuropeptide Y (NPY)/agouti-related protein (AgRP) and pro-opiomelanocortin (POMC)/cocaine and amphetamine regulated transcript (CART) neurons in the arcuate nucleus project onto cell bodies in other hypothalamic nuclei to affect energy balance through food intake, energy expenditure, and nutrient partitioning. The melanocortin pathway is an integral part of the control of energy homeostasis. α-MSH (α-melanocortin stimulating hormone) is derived from proteolytic processing of POMC and is an agonist (*solid arrow*) for melanocortin receptor 3 (MC3R)/melanocortin receptor 4 (MC4R) centrally producing catabolic effects on energy homeostasis. AgRP is an inverse agonist (*dashed arrow*) at MC3R/MC4R, producing anabolic effects on energy balance. LEPR, leptin receptor; IR, insulin receptor; CPE, carboxypeptidase E; ATRN, attractin; MCH, melanin concentrating hormone; HCRT, hypocretin/orexin.

of adiposity of an individual within a population living in a specific environment. As the environment becomes more, or less, conducive to the development of obesity (ease of access to food, need for physical exertion to obtain it, putative intrauterine and perinatal influences), the median adiposity of the population shifts accordingly. The distribution of adiposities representing the population would not be expected to shift in perfect Gaussian symmetry around this median *(1)*. That is, as a population is exposed to these environmental "pressures," the tails of the distribution may not change in proportion. Those who are thinnest may show disproportionate resistance to upward pressure by the environment, whereas those who are fattest may show greater sensitivity to the upward bias imposed by the environment. The opposite responses would characterize these "tails" in the context of environmentally mediated restriction of access to food. There are reasonable evolutionary arguments for such asymmetries in response, based on the likelihood that strong selective pressure in favor of energy efficiency and proclivity in the acquisition and storage of calories has prevailed. The phenotypic differences among individuals at these extremes of adiposity presumably reflect allelic variation at genes that affect energy intake, expenditure, and the chemical form in which excess calories are stored ("partitioning"). The nature of these genes is of obvious interest. The number of "candidate genes"—based on spontaneous and induced genetic variation in model organisms and molecular physiology—is now well over 50 *(11)*. Although a growing number of association studies have indirectly implicated some of these genes, the molecular genetic basis for human susceptibility to obesity is not well understood.

Genetic factors are currently estimated to account for 40% to 70% of the variance in human adiposity *(8)*. In most individuals, the genetic basis for obesity is complex and likely to involve the interaction of multiple genes as well as gene-by-environment interactions. As with other complex phenotypes, there are rare examples of mono/oligogenic causes for obesity that serve as models for understanding the complex hormonal and neural networks that regulate adiposity and provide insight to pathways that may account for more common causes of obesity as well as provide targets for therapeutic intervention. In this chapter, we review the important genetic and physiologic insights provided by the study of these relatively rare forms of obesity.

NONSYNDROMIC MONOGENIC OBESITY

The understanding of body weight regulation in humans has been tremendously aided by the study of monogenic rodent models of obesity (Table 1.1). For most of the genes causing obesity in murine models, human counterparts have been identified with generally similar physiology.

Leptin Deficiency

Leptin was identified as a cytokine-like hormone secreted almost exclusively by adipocytes and deficient in the *obese* (Lep^{ob}/Lep^{ob}) mouse *(12)*. Two alleles of *Lep* have been identified in the mouse both of which result in no detectable leptin production. Lep^{ob} is due to a nonsense mutation that results in the synthesis of a truncated protein that is apparently degraded in the adipocyte *(12)*, while Lep^{ob2j} is due to an insertion of a retroviral-like transposon in the first intron of *Lep* that leads to the production of chimeric RNAs in which the first exon is spliced to sequences in the transposon *(13)*. By screening obese subjects for serum leptin concentrations, Montague et al. were able to identify a single family with two children with undetectable levels of leptin in plasma *(14)*. As in the mouse, human congenital leptin deficiency is inherited in an autosomal recessive manner and produces extreme, early-onset obesity associated with intense hyperphagia *(14)*. Five individuals, all members of consanguineous Pakistani families, were found to be homozygous for the frameshift mutation ΔG133, producing a truncated protein that is not secreted *(15)*. In addition, a large consanguineous Turkish family has been identified with three family members who are homozygous for the missense Arg105Trp mutation that is associated with low levels of circulating leptin *(16)*. Congenital leptin deficiency in humans is associated with hyperphagia but normal resting and free living energy expenditure, hypogonadotrophic hypogonadism with delayed but spontaneous pubertal development, and abnormalities of T-cell number and function *(17)* similar to findings in *obese* mice. Unlike the phenotype in mice, human leptin deficiency is not associated with somatic growth retardation (growth hormone and thyroid hormone axes are normal) or elevated plasma cortisol. Injected

Table 1.1
Nonsyndromic monogenic forms of obesity in rodents and humans

Gene	*Murine mutation*	*Murine phenotype*	*Human mutation*	*Human phenotype*
Leptin	*obese* Lep^{ob} Lep^{ob2j}	Extreme, early-onset obesity, decreased length, hyperphagia, hypogonadotrophic hypogonadism, cold intolerance, hypercorticosteronemia, T-cell abnormalities	ΔG133 Arg105Trp	Extreme, early-onset obesity, hyperphagia, delayed puberty, T-cell abnormalities
Leptin receptor	*diabetes* $Lepr^{db}$	Extreme, early-onset obesity, decreased length, hyperphagia, hypogonadotrophic hypogonadism, cold intolerance, hypercortisolemia, T-cell abnormalities	Exon 16 splice donor G→A	Extreme, early-onset obesity, short stature, hyperphagia, delayed puberty
Pro-opiomelanocortin	Induced deletion of *Pomc*	Later-onset obesity, slightly increased length, adrenal agenesis, yellow coat color	G7013T, 7133delC, C3804A A6851T 6996del 7100insGG 7134delG	Early-onset obesity, adrenal insufficiency, red hair
Agouti signaling peptide	A^y	Later-onset obesity, increased length, yellow coat color	None	
Carboxypeptidase E	Cpe^{fat}	Late-onset obesity, hyperproinsulinemia	None	
Proconvertase 1	Induced deletion of *Pc1*	Dwarf with low GHRH, normal weight, elevated proinsulin, normal corticosterone	Gly483Arg, A→C+4 intron 5 donor splice site, Glu250Stop, Del213Ala	Childhood onset obesity, elevated proinsulin, hypocortisolemia, depressed POMC, reactive hypoglycemia, hypogonadotrophic hypogonadism
Tubby	*tub*	Late-onset obesity, retinal degeneration, sensorineural hearing loss	None	
Melanocortin 4 receptor	Induced deletion of *Mc4r*	Early-onset obesity, hyperphagia, increased fat mass, increased lean mass, increased linear growth, hyperinsulinemia	Numerous	Early-onset obesity, hyperphagia, increased fat mass, increased lean mass, increased bone mineral density and bone mineral content, increased linear growth, and hyperinsulinemia

leptin replacement in three of these children produced normalization of hyperphagia without demonstrable effects on basal metabolic rate or free living energy expenditure even within the setting of weight loss *(17)*, suggesting that the greatest effect of leptin deficiency is on food intake, but that energy expenditure was raised above that expected in a weight-losing subject. Earlier studies in *obese* mice by Coleman demonstrated that the greatest metabolic effect of the mutation was on food intake *(18)*.

Although obesity is clearly most marked in mice homozygous for the Lep^{ob} mutation, we found a 27% increase in fat mass and 23% increase in percentage body fat in heterozygous $Lep^{ob}/+$ mice *(19)*. Heterozygous leptin-deficient humans also have a higher prevalence of obesity and increased percentage body fat than predicted for height and weight and have lower levels of serum leptin than would be predicted for percentage body fat *(20)*. These data suggest that the leptin-related regulatory system is sensitive to haploinsufficiency or decreased production of leptin and can respond by increasing adiposity to achieve a critical lower threshold for circulating leptin. Teleologically, this response may be a safeguard against starvation and loss of reproductive integrity. This observation is consistent with the hypothesis that fat mass is more critically regulated at the low end than at the high end and that counterregulatory measures are stronger to protect against starvation than against excessive adiposity *(21,22)*. Although clearly homozygous loss of function *LEP* mutations are rare in the general population, heterozygous mutations, or more subtle regulatory variants, may contribute to more common forms of obesity. Mice that are heterozygous for both Lep^{ob} and $Lepr^{db}$ mutations demonstrate increased adiposity versus single heterozygotes at Lep^{ob} or $Lepr^{db}$, suggesting that there are additive interactions on adiposity within this pathway *(19)*.

Leptin plays an important role in reproduction by signaling the availability of minimal fat stores necessary for reproductive success. Leptin-deficient C57BL/6J mice generally display hypogonadotrophic hypogonadism although this phenotype is clearly dependent upon modifier genes as evidenced by the reduced obesity and increased fertility of Lep^{ob}/Lep^{ob} mice on a Balb/cJ genetic background in contrast with the extreme obesity and infertility on a C57BL/6J background *(23)*. Leptin-deficient humans do progress through spontaneous yet delayed puberty, but no leptin-deficient human has yet demonstrated fertility *(17)*.

Leptin Receptor Deficiency

Based on the early parabiosis experiments by Coleman, the *obese* mouse was predicted to produce a circulating factor to which the *diabetes* mouse was unable to respond *(24)*. *Diabetes* mice have a phenotype virtually indistinguishable from *obese* mice when maintained on the same genetic background. Like *obese* mice, *diabetes* mice are characterized by extreme, early-onset obesity with hyperphagia, reduced body length, cold intolerance, infertility, hypercorticosteronemia, and T-cell abnormalities *(25)*. Soon after *Lep* was identified, the leptin receptor (*Lepr*) was discovered, and loss of function mutations were identified in the *diabetes* mouse allelic series (*26–28*) as well as the *fatty* rat *(29,30)*. *Lepr* is a member of the cytokine receptor family and mediates leptin signaling through phosphatidylinositol 3-kinase and signal transducer and activator of transcription-3 (STAT3), predominately in hypothalamic neurons *(31)*. STAT3 signaling is crucial for the regulation of food intake but not critical for the regulation of reproduction and growth. By screening obese human subjects for elevated serum leptin concentrations, a consanguineous family was identified in which three members showed extreme early-onset obesity associated with statural growth retardation caused by impaired growth hormone secretion *(32)*. All three subjects were homozygous for a splice site mutation in exon 16 that truncates the receptor before the transmembrane domain, rendering all cells incapable of transmitting an intracellular signal. Similar to the *diabetes* mouse, human leptin receptor deficiency produces extreme obesity in an autosomal recessive manner. Human leptin receptor–deficient subjects have normal basal temperature, resting metabolic rates, spontaneous but delayed puberty, and normal plasma cortisol concentrations *(32)*. Although *obese* and *diabetes* mice on the same genetic background are phenotypically indistinguishable, there are some important phenotypic differences between human leptin-deficient and leptin receptor–deficient subjects. Leptin receptor–deficient subjects have unique neuroendocrine features including mild growth retardation in early childhood, impaired basal and stimulated growth hormone secretion, and hypothalamic hypothyroidism. These data suggest that the leptin receptor has some leptin-independent effects on neuroendocrine function. However, the number of subjects is quite small and could also be related to the effects of other modifying genes.

Pro-opiomelanocortin Deficiency

Agouti (*Yellow*) was the first murine gene related to monogenic obesity to be positionally cloned *(33)*. The autosomal dominant agouti promoter mutation A^y results in ubiquitous ectopic overexpression of agouti signaling protein (ASP) throughout the body, producing the characteristic yellow coat color when it antagonizes the binding of α-melanocortin stimulating hormone (α-MSH) at melanocortin 1 receptors (MC1R) in the skin and producing increased length as well as body mass through antagonism of the melanocortin 3 and 4 receptors (MC3R and MC4R) in the hypothalamus *(34)*. The natural agonist of the melanocortin receptors, α-MSH, suppresses food intake and increases energy expenditure by actions at MC4R. The physiologic antagonist (and inverse agonist) at MC4R was later identified as agouti related protein (AgRP). α-MSH and adreno-corticotropic hormone are both derived from pro-opiomelanocortin (POMC) bysequential cleavage by prohormone convertases (see discussion of *PC1* mutation below) and other processing enzymes in the arcuate nucleus of the hypothalamus. Many of the POMC neurons in the arcuate nucleus also express the leptin receptor, and POMC expression is positively correlated with ambient leptin *(35)*. Targeted disruption of *Mc4r* and to a lesser extent *Mc3r* in mice produces obesity and increased linear growth similar to the A^y mice except for the expected lack of effect on coat color *(36)*. Mice deficient in AgRP have no discernible abnormalities of body weight or composition in the basal state, with food deprivation, or with overfeeding *(37)*, suggesting that there are powerfully redundant mechanisms for orexigenic signaling.

Autosomal recessive *POMC* deficiency due to compound heterozygosity or homozygosity for loss-of-function mutations in five human subjects produces severe, early-onset obesity associated with hyperphagia *(38,39)* due to lack of α-MSH acting centrally at MC3R and MC4R. Because of a lack of peripheral α-MSH action, the children also demonstrated pale skin color and red hair due to lack of peripheral agonism at MC1R. The five children initially presented with undetectable levels of cortisol and ACTH early in infancy, consistent with the absence of ACTH ligand for the adrenal cortical MC2R. Heterozygous parents were found to have intermediate increases in body weight, suggesting a gene dosage effect for *POMC (39)*. Mice with an induced deletion for the coding regions of all the POMC-derived peptides segregate autosomal recessive, later-onset obesity associated with slightly increased length, adrenal agenesis with undetectable corticosterone and aldosterone, and yellow pelage *(40)* similar to the human counterparts. Recently, a heterozygous missense mutation (Arg236Gly) in *POMC* has been reported that disrupts the dibasic cleavage of β-MSH and β-endorphin *(41)*. In vitro studies indicate that this mutation produces an aberrant fusion protein of β-MSH and β-endorphin that binds to MC4R but has reduced ability to activate the receptor. This Arg236Gly missense mutation has been identified in the heterozygous state in 0.9% of patients with severe early-onset obesity with normal adrenal function and hair and skin pigmentation *(41)*. Mutations of this sort may constitute a mechanism whereby variation in this gene contributes to more common, isolated obesity.

Mahogany and Mahoganoid

Mahogany ($Atrn^{mg}$) and *mahoganoid* ($Mgrn1^{md}$) are mutations in unlinked genes that have similar pleiotropic effects on coat color and energy expenditure in A^y mice. Both mutations are uniquely able to act epistatically to A^y to suppress both the yellow coat color and obese phenotypes caused by ectopic overexpression of *ASP*. Both mutations also cause variable degrees of spongiform degeneration of the brain *(42,43)*. The $Atrn^{mg}$ mutation does not suppress the obesity caused by other rodent genetic models of obesity including *Mc4r*, $Lepr^{db}$, Lep^{ob}, *tub*, or Cpe^{fat} *(44,45)*. *Attractin (Atrn)* encodes a single-pass transmembrane protein. Binding of ASP, but not AgRP, to ATRN in transgenic, biochemical, and genetic-interaction experiments demonstrates that attractin is a low-affinity receptor for ASP, but not for AgRP, in vitro and in vivo *(42,43)*. These experiments support the hypothesis that ATRN acts as a low-affinity receptor for ASP to colocalize ASP to MC1R and to thereby inversely agonize MC1R in the hair follicle, producing a darker coat color. Only under circumstances of *Asp* overexpression in the A^y mouse does ATRN act to colocalize ASP (which is not normally expressed in the brain) to MC3R/MC4R in the hypothalamus. ATRN does not similarly bind AgRP to bring AgRP in proximity to MC3R/MC4R. Therefore, $Atrn^{mg}/Atrn^{mg}\ A^y$ mice lacking ATRN are unable to colocalize the overexpressed ASP to MC3R/MC4R and consequently are not obese *(46)*.

The mouse coat color mutant *mahoganoid* ($Mgrn1^{md}$) has effects on pigmentation and energy metabolism that are similar to *mahogany* ($Atrn^{mg}$) in that *mahoganoid* specifically suppresses A^y-induced yellow pigmentation and obesity *(47)*. The gene mutated in *mahoganoid* mice, named *Mahogunin* (*Mgrn1*), encodes an intracellular protein with a C3HC4 RING domain that functions as an E3 ubiquitin ligase *(43,48)*. Mahogunin may ubiquitinate MC3R/MC4R or a MC3R/MC4R-associated protein (e.g., POMC, α-MSH) to influence the physical proximity or binding of ASP or AgRP to their melanocortin receptors, increase binding of ATRN to ASP, or decrease the amount of α-MSH available to MC1R or MC3R/MC4R through sequestration or turnover of α-MSH. Inactivating mutations of this gene would be expected to increase access of α-MSH to its receptors, darkening coat and reducing food intake. Identification of the molecular targets of MGRN1 should further elucidate the mechanism of action.

Mutations in *ATRN* and *MGRN1* have not yet been identified in humans either in lean individuals or in subjects with neurodegenerative conditions, but neither of these genes has been studied extensively in humans. However, the interactions of these genes within a single pathway demonstrates the complex epistatic interactions that may similarly underlie the genetics of obesity in humans.

Prohormone Convertase 1 Deficiency

Like the *Pomc* knockout mouse, the *fat* mouse is an example of autosomal recessive obesity of later onset and reduced severity relative to the *obese* and *diabetes* mice. Observation of increased levels of circulating proinsulin in these mice led to the identification of the Ser202Pro mutation in the positional candidate gene carboxypeptidase E (*Cpe*) that is responsible for prohormone cleavage of C-terminal basic residues from prohormones and proneuropeptides such as proinsulin, proneuropeptide Y, progonadotropin, and POMC *(49)*. Realizing that aberrant prohormone processing could produce obesity, Jackson et al. identified two subjects with compound heterozygous mutations in *Prohormone Convertase 1 (PC1)*, an enzyme that cleaves prohormones at dibasic amino acids in the step immediately prior to CPE processing *(50)*. Both subjects have been described as having childhood-onset obesity, elevated proinsulin, hypocortisolemia with elevated POMC, reactive hypoglycemia, and hypogonadotropic hypogonadism *(50, 51)*. The subjects' obesity phenotype is likely due to aberrant POMC and other prohormone processing, and the phenotype of the human subjects recapitulates that of the *fat* mouse. However, unlike the *fat* mouse, the second PC1-deficient subject described also had severe, malabsorptive diarrhea as a neonate, and the first PC1-deficient subject, in retrospect, also had clinically asymptomatic intestinal malabsorption *(50)*. Therefore, PC1 may also have a role in prohormone processing in enteroendocrine cells that is essential for normal gastrointestinal function, including absorption. Interestingly, the induced homologous recombinant mouse that is deficient for *Pc1* is growth retarded due to impaired processing of growth hormone releasing hormone *(52)* and not obese or adrenally insufficient even though POMC processing is impaired *(52)*. This animal highlights one of the few examples of a striking divergence in phenotypes between human and murine mutations.

Melanocortin 4 Receptor Deficiency

Perhaps the most common monogenic form of obesity in humans is due to mutations in *MC4R*. The mutations are generally inherited in a codominant manner, and homozygous loss of function mutations have been identified and result in more severe obesity in the homozygous state than in the heterozygous state *(53)*. The penetrance of heterozygous *MC4R* mutations is, however, incomplete for both partially active and inactive *MC4R* mutations, especially in males *(53, 54)*. The prevalence of mutations in *MC4R* appears to vary between 1% and 6% of cases of severe obesity (*53–56*) depending on the age of onset and severity of obesity in each study population. Notably, most of the 50 mutations identified have been missense mutations and almost all are unique and found in single families *(53, 57)*. There is no evidence to date of common founder mutations that would account for a significant fraction of the variance in obesity. If this distribution of mutations is representative of genetic variation in other genes increasing adiposity, it will be difficult to identify genes for obesity by traditional association methods unless highly inbred or isolated populations are used. Phenotypically, carriers of *MC4R* mutations have early-onset hyperphagia, increased fat mass, increased lean mass, increased bone mineral density and bone mineral content, increased linear growth, and hyperinsulinemia relative to fat mass *(53)*, findings similar to those of the *Mc4r* knockout mouse. Unlike subjects with mutations in *LEP* or *LEPR*, carriers of *MC4R* mutations tend to have amelioration of their obesity and hyperinsulinemia over time *(58)*. Binge eating has not been consistently demonstrated to be associated with mutations in *MC4R* (*59–63*).

TUB

A final example of monogenic obesity in the mouse is the autosomal recessive *tubby* mutation that produces mild, late-onset obesity in association with cochlear and retinal degeneration due to deficiency of one of a family of tubby-like proteins (TULPs) that encode heterotrimeric-G-protein-responsive intracellular signaling molecules important in neuronal preservation (*64–66*). Although the phenotype of the mice resembles both Bardet-Biedl syndrome and Alstrom syndrome (see discussion below), mutations in *TUB* have not yet been identified in humans. However, *tubby* mice may indicate that loss of specific populations of neurons, possibly in the hypothalamus, can lead to altered energy homeostasis and that loss of these neurons by other mechanisms could also lead to altered weight regulation. Mutations in a related gene, *TULP1,* have been associated with nonsyndromic autosomal recessive retinitis pigmentosa (RP14) without obesity in humans *(67, 68)*.

Lessons to Be Learned from Nonsyndromic Obesity

Monogenic forms of nonsyndromic obesity have elegantly demonstrated the utility of animal models in identifying key molecular components in the control of food intake and energy expenditure. Most of the recent advances in this field have been based on the identification of genes and metabolic pathways originally detected and elucidated in rodent models. Furthermore, with the exception of mutations in *MC4R*, humans with other monogenic forms of nonsyndromic obesity were identified only after defining a specific subphenotype (high or low leptin, hyperproinsulinemia, hypocortisolemia, unusual skin and hair pigmentation) implicating a defect in a particular molecular pathway. This experience underscores the need—when possible—to collect subphenotypic data when attempting to determine the genetic basis for nonsyndromic obesity. Additionally, it should be noted that in most cases of nonsyndromic obesity in humans, the largest contribution to positive energy balance is, apparently, excess caloric intake. This characteristic may also be more generally applicable to common forms of obesity and suggests that a significant portion of intervention and prevention strategies should be focused on controlling food intake. We are also beginning to appreciate the complex metabolic and neural pathways in which the genes controlling adiposity interact. It is becoming increasingly apparent that in many cases there are gene dosage effects in heterozygotes. In addition, there are interactions of different genes within the same pathway. It is, therefore, possible that quantitative differences in expression or function of these same genes, either alone or in combination with one another, may underlie the more common and genetically complex forms of human obesity. However, to detect genes of small effect size—or that require interactions with other genes—will require much larger study populations than have been previously examined. Again, access to detailed characterization of subphenotypes (energy expenditure, appetitive behaviors, body composition, endocrine, neuroendocrine and autonomic phenotypes that may contribute to or reflect special aspects of obesity as a convergent phenotype) may be helpful in identifying subgroups of human subjects in whom to analyze specific genes.

SYNDROMIC OBESITY

Syndromic obesity is obesity occurring in the clinical context of a distinct set of associated clinical phenotypes (Table 1.2). More than 25 syndromic forms of obesity have been identified. Recently, the genetic bases for some of these syndromes have been elucidated and are beginning to provide insights into the pathogenesis of the derangements of energy homeostasis. Interestingly, although clinically well-defined, there is increasing evidence of genetic heterogeneity for some of these conditions with multiple genes within the same pathway producing identical phenotypes. This finding suggests that for more common polygenetic forms of nonsyndromic obesity, multiple allelic variants within the same molecular pathway may interact in either additive or synergistic ways to produce increasing adiposity. Presented below are a few of the most common syndromic forms of obesity for which the genetic basis has been partially or completely elucidated.

Prader-Willi Syndrome

Prader-Willi syndrome (PWS) is the most common syndromic form of obesity, with an incidence of approximately 1 in 15,000 to 25,000 live births. PWS is the result of loss of expression of paternal genes on the imprinted region of 15q11–13. Loss of maternal expression of genes in the same region produces Angelman syndrome, a very different symptom complex characterized by severe mental retardation, ataxia, and epilepsy. PWS is characterized by intrauterine and neonatal hypotonia, poor feeding, and failure to thrive that evolves into extreme hyperphagia and central obesity at 1 to 6 years of age if caloric restriction is not imposed. PWS is associated with decreased lean body mass, increased adiposity, short stature, and growth hormone deficiency, all of which are partially corrected by growth hormone replacement. Total energy expenditure was 47% lower in subjects with PWS compared with obese counterparts, and 14% lower when normalized to lean body mass *(69)*. Physical activity is reduced and associated with hypotonia *(70)*. There is also reduced resting metabolic rate, even when corrected for the smaller fat-free mass, which further reduces energy requirements *(69, 71)*. Hypothalamic hypogonadism and hypogenitalism are both characteristic, although there have been instances of successful pregnancies in females with PWS that can give rise to children with Angelman syndrome (due to maternally transmitted deletions of 15q11–13) *(72)*. In addition to the endocrinologic abnormalities, there are specific dysmorphisms including almond-shaped palpebral fissures and small hands and feet. Individuals with PWS characteristically show mild-to-moderate mental retardation with a mean IQ of 60 accompanied by specific obsessive-compulsive and ritualistic behaviors (including severe skin picking) and an increased incidence of psychosis in individuals with maternal uniparental disomy *(73)*. Genetically, PWS can have several

Table 1.2
Syndromic forms of human obesity

Syndrome	*Gene*	*Mode of inheritance*	*Phenotype*
Prader-Willi syndrome	Contiguous gene disorder	Imprinting defect with loss of paternally expressed genes on 15q11-13	Neonatal hypotonia, poor feeding, evolving into extreme hyperphagia, central obesity, decreased lean body mass, short stature, hypothalamic hypogonadism, mild mental retardation, obsessive compulsive behavior
SIM1 deficiency	*SIM1*	Translocation of 1p22.1 and 6q16.2	Early-onset obesity associated with increased linear growth and hyperphagia
Bardet-Biedl syndrome	At least eight loci (BBS1–BBS8); seven genes identified	Oligogenic: either autosomal recessive or tri-tetra allelic	Progressive rod-cone dystrophy, postaxial polydactyly, renal cysts, progressive renal disease, dyslexia, learning disabilities, hypogonadism, occasional congenital heart disease, and progressive late-childhood obesity
Alstrom syndrome	*ALMS1*	Autosomal recessive	Mild truncal obesity, short stature, type 2 diabetes, retinopathy, sensorineural hearing loss, nephropathy, dilated cardiomyopathy
Cohen syndrome	*COH1*	Autosomal recessive	Mild truncal obesity, thin extremities, short stature, mild mental retardation, microcephaly, dysmorphic features, hypotonia, joint laxity, intermittent neutropenia, retinochoroidal dystrophy
Borjeson-Forssman-Lehmann syndrome	*PHF6*	X-linked dominant	Late-childhood truncal obesity, short stature, gynecomastia, hypotonia, poor feeding, large ears, small genitalia, mental retardation, microcephaly, epilepsy

etiologies but is always associated with loss of expression of paternally transmitted genes on 15q11–q13. Seventy-five percent of cases are due to paternal deletions of 15q11–q13, 22% are due to maternal uniparental disomy, less than 3% are due to imprinting errors caused by microdeletions of the imprinting center at the *SNURF-SNRPN* gene locus, and less than 1% are due to paternal translocations *(74)*. Regardless of the type of mutation, all patients with PWS share the same basic clinical features. Subjects with the paternal deletion have a higher frequency of hypopigmentation of the skin, hair, and eyes due to a contiguous deletion involving the *P* gene that causes oculocutaneous albinism *(75)*. Notably, there are no known cases of classic PWS or isolated obesity associated with aberrations in a single gene within the 15q11–q13 critical region *(74)*, suggesting that deficiencies of several genes may be necessary to produce the phenotype. Many of the genes in the PWS critical region are expressed within the hypothalamus *(76)* consistent with an obesity phenotype that appears to be central in origin. The heritable deletion of the mouse orthologous region on mouse chromosome 7 that is similarly imprinted has provided a useful mouse model for PWS *(77)*, although these studies have been hampered by early neonatal mortality due to respiratory distress and poor feeding *(78)* as often characterizes human neonates with PWS. Hopefully, these mouse models will provide further insight into the underlying molecular etiology in the future.

The molecular pathophysiology of PWS has not yet been completely elucidated. PWS clearly involves all three possible mechanisms for increased adiposity, but in most individuals hyperphagia apparently contributes more significantly than decreased energy expenditure or increased partitioning of calories to fat. Based on the associated growth hormone deficiency and hypogonadism and the pattern of expression of genes in the critical genetic interval, a hypothalamic defect is likely to be the primary etiology for the obesity associated with PWS. A defect in hypothalamic development could readily account for the characteristic derangements in energy balance, and there is evidence for reduction in the total number of cells in the paraventricular nucleus from five adults with PWS *(79)*. Additionally, peripheral factors may exacerbate the hyperphagia. Recently, PWS patients have been found to have increased circulating levels of ghrelin, an orexigenic hormone released from the stomach that serves as an endogenous ligand for the growth hormone secretagogue receptor *(80)*. Ghrelin stimulates food intake in humans *(81)*, and prolonged elevation may be the mechanism for reduced growth hormone secretion in PWS through desensitization of the growth hormone secretagogue receptor (GHRHR) in the pituitary gland *(82)*.

To date, no studies of nonsyndromic obesity have identified mutations in any of the genes in the PWS critical region, nor has linkage or association to obesity been demonstrated for genes on 15q11–13.

SIM1

A single case of early-onset obesity associated with increased linear growth and hyperphagia has been associated with a de novo balanced translocation between 1p22.1 and 6q16.2, disrupting the single-minded (*SIM1*) gene, separating the 5′ flanking promoter region from the rest of the downstream coding exons *(83)*. *SIM1* is a member of the bHLH-PAS (basic helix loop helix + period aryl hydrocarbon receptor single-minded) gene family that is expressed in the supraoptic and paraventricular nuclei of the hypothalamus and acts as a transcription factor involved in midline neurogenesis. Although the downstream targets of SIM1 have not yet been defined, it is intriguing that it is continually expressed in the paraventricular nucleus of the hypothalamus, which integrates food intake and energy expenditure and in which destructive lesions can cause obesity *(84)*. The phenotype of this child resembles closely the phenotype of the human subjects with *MC4R* mutations; and paraventricular neurons express MC4R as well neuropeptide Y receptors Y1 and Y5, orexin 2 receptors, and corticotrophin releasing factor and its receptors *(85)*. Interstitial deletions involving 6q16 are also associated with obesity and share some features of PWS including hypotonia, feeding problems in infancy, and hypogonadism *(86)* that may point to dysfunction of the paraventricular nucleus of the hypothalamus as part of the etiology for the obesity observed in PWS. Haploinsufficiency of *SIM1* can cause increased weight gain and linear growth, suggesting that transcription factors may play important roles in regulation of human adiposity in a manner analogous to the role of transcription factors for maturity-onset diabetes of youth (MODY) *(87)*. To date, no other subjects have been identified with mutations confined to *SIM1*, and no animal model of this mutation has been identified or produced.

Bardet-Biedl Syndrome

Bardet-Biedl syndrome (BBS) is a rare syndromic form of obesity with an estimated incidence of 1 in 150,000 live births in North America and Europe *(88)* and a higher incidence in isolated populations of Newfoundland *(89)* and Arab Bedouins *(90)*. Although the populations in Newfoundland and Kuwait are relatively small and isolated, surprisingly, multiple BBS genes contribute to the occurrence of the syndrome in both populations *(91)*. BBS is associated with progressive rod-cone dystrophy, postaxial polydactyly, renal cysts and progressive renal disease, dyslexia, learning disabilities, blunted affect, hypogonadism, occasional congenital heart disease; progressive late childhood obesity with a BMI >30 is observed in approximately half of subjects with BBS *(92)*. Obesity in BBS is associated with hyperphagia and reduced spontaneous physical activity beyond that of comparably obese individuals.

The genetics of BBS before the discovery of the underlying genes was thought to be classical autosomal recessive. Although the resulting phenotypes are essentially indistinguishable, seven different genes have now been identified as causing BBS, and at least one additional linkage group *(93)* has been established based on families in which the syndrome does not segregate with any of the eight known loci. The disease segregates in families as both a classical autosomal recessive trait as well as a digenetic trait in which three or even four alleles interact to determine the penetrance of BBS or to modify the severity and age of onset of disease manifestations *(94)*. All genetically distinct forms of BBS except the recently identified BBS8 locus (accounting for only three pedigrees to date) have been associated with tri- or tetra-allelic inheritance *(95)*. BBS2 and BBS6 are especially likely to show oligogenic inheritance *(92)*. Notably, all but one example of oligogenic inheritance have included missense alleles; ultimately, functional assays will be required to determine which of these alleles are pathogenic. Although great progress has been made in identifying the genes for BBS, in more than 50% of families the genetic basis has not yet been determined, leaving open the possibility of several additional BBS genes *(96)*. *BBS1* is the most common gene involved in BBS and accounts for approximately 20% to 25% of all cases; a common founder European/North American M390R allele accounts for 80% of all *BBS1* mutations *(97)*. The high prevalence of this ancient mutation could be due to a selective advantage for carriers. However, the M390R mutation has not been associated with nonsyndromic obesity in the general population of Newfoundland where it is common and implies that it causes only syndromic obesity and/or that studies have not had sufficient power to detect the effect in heterozygous carriers in whom it may interact with other unidentified genes *(98)*. Mutations in the gene for BBS1 also cause the McKusick-Kaufman syndrome, which consists of hydrometrocolpos, postaxial polydactyly, and congenital heart disease, and overlaps phenotypically with BBS. McKusick-Kaufman syndrome is found most commonly in the Amish population *(99)* and is not associated with obesity. The difference in the phenotypes is likely related to the specific mutation in *BBS1* and/or mutations at other interacting loci that produce BBS.

Recent identification of the *BBS8* gene encoding a protein involved in pilus formation and twitching mobility that localizes to the basal bodies and centrosome in physical juxtaposition to BBS4 suggests that these proteins play a role in the function of the pericentriolar region of ciliated cells *(95)*. It is, therefore, possible that the underlying pathogenic mechanism for BBS involves dysfunction of the basal body in ciliated cells *(95)*. *Caenorhabatis elegans* orthologues of BBS1, BBS2, BBS7, and BBS8 are also expressed in the ciliated dendritic endings of neurons. Developmental brain abnormalities resulting from aberrant basal body performance could account for the learning disabilities, behavioral problems, and hyperphagia seen in BBS patients. Defective protein transport across photoreceptor-connecting cilium can cause retinal dystrophy *(100)*, and aberrant mechanosensation at the primary cilium of renal tubular cells can lead to polycystic kidney disease *(101)*. Nodal cilium dysfunction can also cause situs inversus and associated congenital heart disease *(102)*, rare manifestations in some BBS families. Anosmia has also been demonstrated in subjects with BBS and is likely due to defects in the olfactory ciliary structure and function *(103)*. Therefore, the multiple genes causing BBS may be components of a molecular complex or act sequentially in the same cellular process(es) to cause progressively more severe dysfunction as mutations are added in genes in the same "pathway." This model of multiple "hits" within the same pathway may also be more broadly applicable to the much more common polygenic forms of common obesity. The genetic complexity of this very distinct phenotype of BBS may also be a clue to the genetic complexity of polygenic obesity and to strategies for unraveling it by close attention to gene-gene interactions in putative biochemical, structural, and functional "pathways."

Alstrom Syndrome

Alstrom syndrome is a rare autosomal recessive, genetically homogeneous disorder characterized by mild truncal obesity that usually begins within the first year of life and continues throughout life unless caloric restriction is imposed *(104)*. It is particularly common among the French Acadians in Nova Scotia and Louisiana, as well as other consanguineous populations. Alstrom syndrome is associated with short stature that is usually not apparent until after puberty *(105)*, hyperinsulinemia that is out of proportion to the degree of adiposity, and, ultimately, type 2 diabetes. Other consistently associated clinical findings are retinopathy with cone-rod degeneration often presenting as nystagmus and photodysphoria within the first year of life and ultimately resulting in blindness, progressive sensorineural hearing loss, and progressive chronic nephropathy in the second to third decade of life ultimately resulting in renal failure, which is the most frequent cause of death. Other more variable manifestations include dilated cardiomyopathy that may present in infancy and remit and recur with time, hepatic dysfunction secondary to hepatic fibrosis, hypothyroidism, primary gonadal failure, and psychomotor developmental delay. Unlike BBS, Alstrom syndrome is not associated with polydactyly *(105)*. The gene for Alstrom syndrome, *ALMS1*, was recently identified simultaneously by two groups and encodes a gene of unknown function expressed ubiquitously at low levels and containing a predicted leucine zipper motif, serine-rich region, potential nuclear localization signal, histidine-rich region, and large tandem repeat domain comprising 34 imperfect repetitions of 47 amino acids *(106, 107)*. Gene disruption due to a balanced translocation of 2p13 as well as small numbers of nonsense and frameshift mutations have been reported in Alstrom patients *(106, 107)*. Ubiquitous expression of the gene suggests a reason for the protean clinical manifestations. However, the mechanism by which loss-of -function mutations in this gene produce obesity or any of the other associated phenotypes is still unknown.

Cohen Syndrome

Cohen syndrome is a rare autosomal recessive condition overrepresented in the Finnish population. The syndrome is characterized by mild truncal obesity, thin extremities, and short stature starting in mid-childhood *(108)*. Cohen syndrome is associated with nonprogressive global developmental delay, mild-to-moderate mental retardation, microcephaly, characteristic facial features (downslanting and wave-shaped palpebral fissures, prominent nasal root, short philtrum, prominent central incisors, thick hair), hypotonia, joint laxity, intermittent neutropenia, and progressive myopia often associated with retinochoroidal dystrophy *(108, 109)*. The clinical findings are not all apparent within the first few years of life and can be variable among individuals of different ethnicities *(110)*. The gene for Cohen syndrome, *COH1*, was positionally identified, and 28 frameshift, premature termination, and missense mutations have been identified in this ubiquitously expressed putative transmembrane protein with a complex domain structure *(111)*. Homology to the *Saccharomyces cerevisiae* VPS13 proteins suggests that it may be involved in vesicle-mediated sorting and transport of proteins within the cell *(111)*. Which protein targets may be aberrantly sorted as a result of mutations in *COH1,* and how they relate to obesity, have not yet been identified.

Borjeson-Forssman-Lehmann Syndrome

Borjeson-Forssman-Lehmann syndrome is a rare X-linked dominant condition associated with late-childhood truncal obesity, short stature, and gynecomastia *(112, 113)*. Male infants generally display hypotonia, poor feeding, large ears, and small genitalia, similar to infants with PWS with the exception of the large ears. As males get older, they show moderate mental retardation, microcephaly, epilepsy, tapering fingers with lax interphalangeal joints, shortened toes, gynecomastia in adolescence, and progressively coarse facial features with deep-set eyes. Many carrier females have no clinical phenotype due to complete X inactivation skewing, although females with incomplete X inactivation skewing have a milder phenotype similar to males. The gene for Borjeson-Forssman-Lehmann syndrome is a novel, widely expressed zinc finger gene plant homeodomain (PHD)-like finger (*PHF6*) that accumulates in the nucleolus and may have a role in transcription *(114)*. The molecular targets of *PHF6* have not yet been identified nor has the metabolic basis for the obesity in subjects with Borjeson-Forssman-Lehmann syndrome been investigated due to the small number of subjects affected.

Lessons to Be Learned from Syndromic Obesity

Most syndromic forms of obesity are associated with mild to severe cognitive deficits and unusual behaviors. Although many other syndromes affecting cognition such as Down syndrome are also associated with a higher incidence of obesity *(115)*, the syndromic forms of obesity described above appear to have specific effects on food intake. These data suggest that there may be specific neuroanatomic or functional deficits, particularly in the hypothalamus, that lead to increased energy intake. The development of new techniques including functional imaging of the brain should permit noninvasive determination of which parts of the brain function aberrantly in the context of food intake in each of the syndromic forms of obesity. With few exceptions, although genes for several forms of syndromic obesity have been identified, their function, relevant cells, and their targets have yet to be identified. As additional genomic and informatics capabilities emerge, these questions should be more readily answered and should provide additional insight into the pathophysiology of obesity. To date, mutations in the genes causing syndromic obesity have not been shown to have mutations or to be linked or associated with nonsyndromic obesity; however, this point has not been fully investigated. Other molecules in the pathways identified for syndromic obesity may be more directly relevant to the more common forms of obesity.

CONCLUSION

Like the monogenic mouse obesities, the human syndromic obesities will probably have most heuristic significance for the new molecules and pathways that they reveal in the complex regulatory system that controls body weight. The relevance of these genes and pathways in the genetics that clearly underlies susceptibility to obesity in humans will require the same sort of large-scale analyses that will be needed for other putative molecular players in the relevant processes. Fundamentally, this will require the simultaneous consideration of several alleles of many genes in very large numbers of well-phenotyped subjects. Awareness of the relationships among specific candidate molecules—gleaned from model organisms and syndromic or sporadic severe obesities in humans—will help to rationalize the selection of genes for any specific analysis and permit explicit mechanistic hypothesis testing, thereby enhancing statistical power. Further refinement can be achieved by selection of subjects based on specific subphenotypes.

ACKNOWLEDGMENTS

We appreciate the assistance of Roberto Almazan with manuscript preparation. This work was supported in part by NIH DK52431.

REFERENCES

1. Flegal KM, Carroll MD, Ogden CL, et al. Prevalence and trends in obesity among US adults, 1999-2000. JAMA 2002;288:1723–1727.
2. Hedley, AA, Ogden CL, Johnson CL, et al. Prevalence of overweight and obesity among US children, adolescents, and adults, 1999-2002. JAMA 2004;291:2847–2850.
3. Calle EE, Thune MJ, Petrelli JM, et al. Body-mass index and mortality in a prospective cohort of U.S. adults. N Engl J Med 1999;341:1097–1105.
4. Must A, Spadano J, Coakley EH, et al. The disease burden associated with overweight and obesity. JAMA 1999;282:1523–1529.
5. Cummings DE, Clement K, Purnell JQ, et al. Elevated plasma ghrelin levels in Prader Willi syndrome. Nat Med 2002;8:643–644.
6. Rosenbaum M, Nicolson M, Hirsch J, et al. Effects of weight change on plasma leptin concentrations and energy expenditure. J Clin Endocrinol Metab 1997;82:3647–3654.
7. Woods SC, Seeley RJ, Porte D Jr, et al. Signals that regulate food intake and energy homeostasis. Science 1998;280:1378–1383.
8. Allison DB, Faith MS, Nathan JS. Risch's lambda values for human obesity. Int J Obes Relat Metab Disord 1996;20:990–999.
9. Stunkard AJ, Foch TT, Hrubec Z. A twin study of human obesity. JAMA 1986;256:51–54.
10. Stunkard AJ, Harris, JR, Pedersen, NL, et al. The body-mass index of twins who have been reared apart. N Engl J Med 1990;322:1483–1487.
11. Snyder EE, Walts B, Perusse L, et al. The human obesity gene map: the 2003 update. Obes Res 2004;12:369–439.
12. Zhang Y, Proenca R, Maffei M, et al. Positional cloning of the mouse obese gene and its human homologue. Nature 1994;372:425–432.
13. Moon BC, Friedman JM. The molecular basis of the obese mutation in ob2J mice. Genomics 1997;42:152–156.
14. Montague CT, Farooqi IS, Whitehead JP, et al. Congenital leptin deficiency is associated with severe early-onset obesity in humans. Nature 1997;387:903–908.
15. Rau H, Reaves BJ, O'Rahilly S, et al. Truncated human leptin (delta133) associated with extreme obesity undergoes proteasomal degradation after defective intracellular transport. Endocrinology 1999;140:1718–1723.
16. Strobel A, Isaad T, Camoin L, et al. A leptin missense mutation associated with hypogonadism and morbid obesity. Nat Genet 1998;18:213–215.
17. Farooqi IS, Matarese G, Lord GM, et al. Beneficial effects of leptin on obesity, T cell hyporesponsiveness, and neuroendocrine/metabolic dysfunction of human congenital leptin deficiency. J Clin Invest 2002;110:1093–1103.
18. Coleman DL. Increased metabolic efficiency in obese mutant mice. Int J Obes 1985;9:69–73.
19. Chung WK, Belfi K, Chua M, et al. Heterozygosity for Lep(ob) or Lepr(db) affects body composition and leptin homeostasis in adult mice. Am J Physiol 1998;274:R985–R990.
20. Farooqi IS, Keogh JM, Kamath S, et al. Partial leptin deficiency and human adiposity. Nature 2001;414:34–35.
21. Leibel RL. The role of leptin in the control of body weight. Nutr Rev 2002;60:S15–19.
22. Rosenbaum M, Murphy EM, Heymsfield SB, et al. Low dose leptin administration reverses effects of sustained weight-reduction on energy expenditure and circulating concentrations of thyroid hormones. J Clin Endocrinol Metab 2002;87:2391–2394.
23. Chehab FF, Qiu J, Mounzih K, et al. Leptin and reproduction. Nutr Rev 2002;60:S39–46.
24. Coleman DL. Effects of paraboisis of obese with diabetes and normal mice. Diabetologia 1973;9: 294–298.
25. Coleman DL. Diabetes-obesity syndromes in mice. Diabetes 1982;31, 1–6.

26. Wu-Peng XS, Chua SC Jr, Okada N, et al. Phenotypes of mouse diabetes and rat fatty due to mutations in the OB (leptin) receptor. Science 1996;271:994–996.
27. Lee GH, Proenca R, Montez JM, et al. Abnormal splicing of the leptin receptor in diabetic mice. Nature 1996;379:632–635.
28. Tartaglia LA, Dembski M, Weng X, et al. Identification and expression cloning of a leptin receptor, OB-R. Cell 1995;83:1263–1271.
29. Wu-Peng XS, Chua SC Jr, Okada N, et al. Phenotype of the obese Koletsky (f) rat due to Tyr763Stop mutation in the extracellular domain of the leptin receptor (Lepr): evidence for deficient plasma-to-CSF transport of leptin in both the Zucker and koletsky obese rat. Diabetes 1997;46:513–518.
30. Phillips MS, Liu Q, Hammond HA, et al. Leptin receptor missense mutation in the fatty Zucker rat. Nat Genet 1996;13:18–19.
31. Bates SH, Myers MG, Jr. The role of leptin receptor signaling in feeding and neuroendocrine function. Trends Endocrinol Metab 2003;14:447–452.
32. Clement K, Ferre P. Genetics and the pathophysiology of obesity. Pediatr Res 2003;53:721–725.
33. Bultman SJ, Michaud EJ, Woychik RP. Molecular characterization of the mouse agouti locus. Cell 1992;71:1195–1204.
34. Rossi M, Kim MS, Morgan DG, et al. A C-Terminal fragment of agouti-related protein increases feeding and antagonizes the effect of alpha-melanocyte stimulating hormone in vivo. Endocrinology 1998;139:4428–4431.
35. Cheung CC, Clifton DK, Steiner RA. Proopiomelanocortin neurons are direct targets for leptin in the hypothalamus. Endocrinology 1997;138:4489–4492.
36. Huszar D, Lynch CA, Fairchild-Huntress V, et al. Targeted disruption of the melanocortin-4 receptor results in obesity in mice. Cell 1997;88:131–141.
37. Qian S, Chen H, Weingarth D, et al. Neither agouti-related protein nor neuropeptide Y is critically required for the regulation of energy homeostasis in mice. Mol Cell Biol 2002;22:5027–5035.
38. Krude H, Beibermann H, Lucky W, et al. Severe early-onset obesity, adrenal insufficiency and red hair pigmentation caused by POMC mutations in humans. Nat Genet 1998;19:155–157.
39. Krude H, Biebermann H, Schnabel D, et al. obesity due to proopiomelanocortin deficiency: three new cases and treatment trials with thyroid hormone and ACTH 4-10. J Clin Endocrinol Metab 2003;88:4633–4640.
40. Yaswen L, Diehl N, Brennan MB, et al. Obesity in the mouse model of pro-opiomelanocortin deficiency responds to peripheral melanocortin. Nat Med 1999;5:1066–1070.
41. Challis BG, Pritchard LE, Creemers JW, et al. A missense mutation disrupting a dibasic prohormone processing site in pro-opiomelanocortin (POMC) increases susceptibility to early-onset obesity through a novel molecular mechanism. Hum Mol Genet 2002;11:1997–2004.
42. Gunn TM, Inui T, Kitada S, et al. Molecular and phenotypic analysis of attractin mutant mice. Genetics 2001;158:1683–1695.
43. He L, Lu XY, Jolly AF, et al. Spongiform degeneration in mahoganoid mutant mice. Science 2003;299:710–712.
44. Nagle DL, McGrail SH, Vitale J, et al. The mahogany protein is a receptor involved in suppression of obesity. Nature 1999;398:148–152.
45. Dinulescu DM, Fan W, Boston BA, et al. Mahogany (mg) stimulates feeding and increases basal metabolic rate independent of its suppression of agouti. Proc Natl Acad Sci USA 1998;95: 12707–12712.
46. He L, Gunn TM, Bouley DM, et al. A biochemical function for attractin in agouti-induced pigmentation and obesity. Nat Genet 2001;27:40–47.
47. Miller KA, Gunn TM, Carrasquillo MM, et al. Genetic studies of the mouse mutations mahogany and mahoganoid. Genetics 1997;146:1407–1415.

48. Phan LK, Lin F, LeDuc CA, et al. The mouse mahoganoid coat color mutation disrupts a novel C3HC4 RING domian protein. J Clin Invest 2002;110:1449–1459.
49. Naggert JK, Fricker LD, Varlamov O, et al. Hyperproinsulinaemia in obese fat/fat mice associated with a carboxypeptidase E mutation which reduces enzyme activity. Nat Genet 1995;10:135–142.
50. Jackson RS, Creemers JW, Farooqi IS, et al. Small-intestinal dysfunction accompanies the complex endocrinopathy of human proprotein convertase 1 deficiency. J Clin Invest 2003;112:1550–1560.
51. Jackson RS, Creemers JW, Ohagi S, et al. Obesity and impaired prohormone processing associated with mutations in the human prohormone convertase 1 gene. Nat Genet 1997;16:303–306.
52. Zhu X, Zhou A, Dey A, et al. Disruption of PC1/3 expression in mice causes dwarfism and multiple neuroendocrine peptide processing defects. Proc Natl Acac Sci USA 2002;99:10293–10298.
53. Farooqi IS, Keogh JM, Yeo GS, et al. Clinical spectrum of obesity and mutations in the melanocortin 4 receptor gene. N Engl J Med 2003;348:1085–1095.
54. Vaisse C, Clement K, Durand E, et al. Melanocortin-4 receptor mutations are a frequent and heterogeneous cause of morbid obesity. J Clin Invest 2000;106:253–262.
55. Farooqi IS, Yeo GS, Keogh JM, et al. Dominant and recessive inheritance of morbid obesity associated with melanocortin 4 receptor deficiency. J Clin Invest 2000;106:271–279.
56. Hinney A, Schmidt A, Nottebom K, et al. Several mutations in the melanocortin-4 receptor gene including a nonsense and a frameshift mutation associated with dominantly inherited obesity in humans. J Clin Endocrinol Metab 1999;84:1483–1486.
57. Lubrano-Berthelier C, Cavazos M, Dubem B, et al. Molecular genetics of human obesity-associated MC4R mutations. Ann NY Acad Sci 2003;1994:49–57.
58. O' Rahilly S, Farooqi IS, Yeo GS, et al. Minireview: Human obesity-lessons from monogenic disorders. Endocrinology 2003;144:3757–3764.
59. Branson R, Potoczna N, Kral JG, et al. Binge eating as a major phenotype of melanocortin 4 receptor gene mutations. N Engl J Med 2003;348:1096–1103.
60. Farooqi IS, Yeo GS, O'Rahilly S. Binge eating as a phenotype of melanocortin 4 receptor gene mutations. N Engl J Med 2003;349:606–609.
61. Gotoda T. Binge eating as a phenotype of melanocortin 4 receptor gene mutations. N Engl J Med 2003;349:606–609.
62. Herpertz S, Siffert W, Hebebrand J. Binge eating as a phenotype of melancortin 4 receptor gene mutations. N Engl J Med 2003;349:606–609.
63. List JF, Habener JF. Defective melanocortin 4 receptors in hyperphagia and morbid obesity. N Engl J Med 2003;348:1160–1163.
64. Santagata S, Boggon TJ, Baird CL, et al. G-Protein signaling through tubby proteins. Science 2001;292:2041–2050.
65. Noben-Trauth K, Naggert JK, North MA, et al. A candidate gene for the mouse mutation tubby. Nature 1996;380:534–538.
66. Kleyn PW, Fan W, Kovats SG, et al. Identification and characterization of the mouse obesity gene tubby: a member of a novel gene family. Cell 1996;85:281–190.
67. Banerjee P, Kleyn PW, Knowles JA, et al. TULP1 mutation in two extended Dominican kindreds with autosomal recessive Retinitis pigmentosa. Nature Genetics 1998;18:177–179.
68. Hagstrom SA, North MA, Nishina PL, et al. Recessive mutations in the gene encoding the tubby-like protein TULP1 in patients with retinitis pigmentosa. Nat Genet 1998;18:174–176.
69. Schoeller DA, Levitsky LL, Bandini LG, et al. Energy expenditure and body composition in Prader-Willi syndrome. Metabolism 1988;37:115–120.
70. van Mil EG, Westerterp KR, Kester AD, et al. Activity related energy expenditure in children and adolescents with Prader-Willi syndrome. Int J Obes Relat Metab Disord 2000;24:429–434.
71. Goldstone AP, Brynes AE, Thomas EL, et al. Resting metabolic rate, plasma leptin concentrations, leptin receptor expression, and adipose tissue measured by whole-body magnetic resonance imaging in women with Prader-Willi syndrome. Am J Clin Nutr 2002;75:468–475.

72. Schulze A, Mogensen H, Hamborg-Petersen B, et al. Fertility in Prader-Willi syndrome: a case report with Angelman syndrome in the offspring. Acta Pediatr 2001;90:455–459.
73. Boer H, Holland A, Whittington J, et al. Psychotic illness in people with Prader-Willi syndrome due to chromosome 15 maternal unipaternal disomy. Lancet 2002;359:135–136.
74. Nicholls RD, Knepper JL. Genome organization, function, and imprinting in Prader-Willi and Angelman syndrome. Annu Rev Genomics Hum Genet 2001,2:153–175.
75. Gillessen-Kaesbach G. Robinson W, Lohmann D, et al. Genotype-phenotype correlation in a series of 167 deletion and non-deletion patients with Prader-Willi syndrome. Hum Genet 1995;96:638–643.
76. Lee S, Walker CL, Wevrick R. Prader-Willi syndrome transcript are expressed in phenotypically significant regions of the developing mouse brain. Gene Expression Patterns 2003;3:599–609.
77. Gabriel JM, Merchant M, Ohta T, et al. A transgene insertion creating a heritable chromosome deletion mouse model of Prader-Willi and Angelman syndromes. Proc Natl Acac Sci USA 1999;96:9258–9263.
78. Nicholls RD, Stefan M, Ji H, et al. Mouse models for Prader-Willi and Angelman syndromes offer insights into novel obesity mechanisms. Prog Obes Res 2003;9:313–319.
79. Swaab DF, Purba JS, Hofman MA. Alterations in the hypothalamic paraventricular nucleus and its oxytocin neurons (putative satiety cells) in Prader-Willi syndrome: a study of five cases. J Clin Endocrinol Metab 1995;80:573–579.
80. Cummings DE, Clement K, Purnell JQ, et al. Elevated plasma ghrelin levels in Prader-Willi syndrome. Nat Med 2002;8:643–644.
81. Kojima M, Kanagwa K. Ghrelin, an orexigenic signaling molecule from the gastrointestinal tract. Curr Opin Pharmacol 2002;2:665–668.
82. Date Y, Murakami N, Kojima M, et al. Central effects of a novel acylated peptide, ghrelin, on growth hormone release in rats. Biochem Biophys Res Commun 2000;275:477–480.
83. Holder JL Jr, Butte NF, Zinn AR. Profound obesity associated with a balanced translocation that disrupts the SIM1 gene. Hum Mol Genet 2000;9:101–108.
84. Kirchgessner AL, Sclafani A. PVN-hindbrain pathway involved in the hypothalamic hyperphagia-obesity syndrome. Physiol Behav 1988;42:517–528.
85. Cummings DE, Clement K, Purnell JQ, et al. Elevated plasma ghrelin levels in Prader-Willi syndrome. Nat Med. 2002;8:643–644.
86. Faivre L, Cormier-Daire V, Lapierre JM, et al. Deletion of the SIM1 gene (6q16.2) in a patient with a Prader-Willi-like phenotype. J Med Genet 2002;39:594–596.
87. Yamagata K. Regulation of pancreatic beta-cell function by the HNF transcription network: lessons from maturity-onset diabetes of the young (MODY). Endocr J 2003;50:491–499.
88. Klein D, Ammann F. The syndrome of Laurence-Moon-Bardet-Biedl and allied diseases in Switzerland. Clinical, genetic and epidemiological studies. J. Neuro Sci 1969;9:479–513.
89. Green JS, Parfrey PS, Harnett JD, et al. The cardinal manifestations of Bardet-Biedl syndrome, a form of Laurence-Moon-Biedl syndrome. N Engl J Med 1989;321:1002–1009.
90. Farang TI, Teebi AS. High incidence of Bardet-Biedl syndrome among Bedouin. Clin Genet 1989;36:463–464.
91. Woods MO, Young TL, Parfrey PS, et al. Genetic heterogeneity of Bardet-Biedl Syndrome in a distinct Canadian population: Evidence for a fifth locus. Genomics 1999;55:2–9.
92. Beales PL, Badano JL, Ross AJ, et al. Genetic interaction of BBS1 mutations with alleles at other BBS loci can result in non-Mendelian Bardet-Biedl syndrome. Am J Hum Genet 2003;72:1187–1199.
93. Young TL, Penney L, Woods MO, et al. A fifth locus for Bardet-Biedl Syndrome maps to chromosome 2q31. Am. J. Hum. Genet 1999;64:900–904.
94. Badano JL, Kim JC, Hoskins BE, et al. Heterozygous mutations in BBS1, BBS2 and BBS6 have a potential epistatic effect on Bardet-Biedl patients with two mutations at a second BBS locus. Hum Mol Genet 2003;12:1651–1659.

95. Ansley SJ, Badano JL, Blacque OE, et al. Basal body dysfunction is a likely cause of pleiotropic Bardet-Biedl syndrome. Nature 2003;425:628–633.
96. Katsanis N. The oligogenic properties of Bardet-Biedl syndrome. Hum Mol Genet 2004;13:R65–R71.
97. Mykytyn K, Nishimura DY, Searby CC, et al. Evaluation of complex inheritance involving the most common Bardet-Biedl Syndrome Locus (BBS1). Am J Hum Genet 2003;72:429–437.
98. Fan Y, Rahman P, Peddle L, et al. Bardet-Biedl syndrome 1 genotype and obesity in the Newfoundland population. In J Obes 2004;28:680–684.
99. Stone DL, Slavotinek A, Bouffard GG, et al. Mutation of a gene encoding a putative chaperonin causes McKusick-Kaufman syndrome. Nat Genet 2000;25:79–82.
100. Pazour GJ, Baker SA, Deane JA, et al. The intraflagellar transport protein, IFT88, is essential for vertebrate photoreceptor assembly and maintenance. J Cell Biol 2002;157:103–114.
101. Nauli SM, Alenghat FJ, Luo Y, et al. Polycystins 1 and 2 mediate mechanosensation in the primary cilium of kidney cells. Nat Genet 2003;33:129–137.
102. Nonaka S, Tanaka Y, Okada Y, et al. Randomization of left-right asymmetry due to loss of nodal cilia generating leftward flow of extraembryonic fluid in mice lacking KIF3B motor protein. Cell 1998;95:829–837.
103. Kulaga HM, Leitch CC, Eichers ER, et al. Loss of BBS proteins causes anosmia in humans and defects in olfactory cilia structure and function in the mouse. Nat Genet 2004;36:994–998.
104. Alstrom CH, Hallgren B, Nilsson LB, et al. Retinal degeneration combined with obesity, diabetes mellitus and neurogenous deafness: a specific syndrome (not hitherto described) distinct from Laurence-Moon-Biedl syndrome. A clinical endocrinological and genetic examination based on large pedigree. Acta Psychiat 1959;34:1–35.
105. Marshall JD, Ludman MD, Shea SE, et al. Genealogy, natural history, and phenotype of Alström Syndrome in a large Acadian kindred and three additional families. Am J Med Genet 1997;73: 160–161.
106. Hearn T, Renforth, GL, Spalluto C, et al. Mutations of ALMS1, a large gene with tandem repeat encoding 47 amino acids, causes Alstrom syndrome. Nat Genet 2002;31:79–83.
107. Collin GB, Marshall JD, Ikeda A, et al. Mutations in ALMS1 cause obesity, type 2 diabetes and neurosensory degeneration in Alström syndrome. Nat Genet 2002;31:74–78.
108. Cohen MM, Jr, Hall BD, Smith DW, et al. A new syndrome with hypotonia, obesity, mental deficiency, and facial, oral, ocular, and limb anomalies. J Pediatr 1973;83:280–284.
109. Chandler KE, Kidd A, Al-Gazali L, et al. Diagnostic criteria, clinical characteristics and natural history of Cohen syndrome. J Med Genet 2003;40:233–241.
110. Hennies HC, Rauch A, Seifert W, et al. Allelic heterogeneity in the COH1 gene explains clinical variability in Cohen syndrome. Am J Hum Genet 2004;75:138–145.
111. Kolehmainen J, Black GC, Saarinen A, et al. Cohen syndrome is caused by mutations in a novel gene, COH1, encoding a transmembrane protein with a presumed role in vesicle-mediated sorting and intracellular protein transport. Am J Hum Genet 2003;72:1359–1369.
112. Börjeson M, Forssman H, Lehmann O. An X-linked recessively inherited syndrome characterised by grave mental deficiency, epilepsy and endocrine disorder. Acta Med Scand 1962;171:13–21.
113. Turner G, Lower KM, White SM, et al. The Clinical picture of the Börjeson-Forssman-Lehman syndrome in males and heterozygous females with PHF6 mutations. Clin Genet 2004;65: 226–232.
114. Lower KM, Turner G, Kerr BA, et al. Mutations in PHF6 are associated with Börjeson-Frossman-Lehman Syndromesyndrome. Nat Genet 2002;32:661–665.
115. Bell AJ, Bhate MS. Prevalence of overweight and obesity in Down syndrome and other mentally handicapped adults living in the community. J Intellect Disabil Res 1992;36:359–364.

2 Leptin Signaling In the Brain

Ofer Reizes, Stephen C. Benoit, and Deborah J. Clegg

CONTENTS

Abstract

This chapter reviews current literature on hormonal and neural signals critical for the regulation of individual meals and body fat. Body weight is regulated via an ongoing process called energy homeostasis, or the long-term matching of food intake to energy expenditure. Reductions from an individual's "normal" weight due to lack of sufficient food lowers levels of adiposity signals (leptin and insulin) reaching the brain from the blood, activates anabolic hormones that stimulate food intake, and decreases the efficacy of meal-generated signals (such as cholecystokinin, or CCK) that normally reduce meal size. A converse sequence of events happens when individuals gain weight: adiposity signals are increased, catabolic hormones are stimulated, and the consequence is a reduction in food intake and a normalization of body weight. The brain also functions as a "fuel sensor" and thereby senses nutrients and generates signals and activation of neuronal systems and circuits that regulate energy homeostasis. This chapter focuses on how these signals are received and integrated by the central nervous system.

From: *Contemporary Endocrinology: Energy Metabolism and Obesity: Research and Clinical Applications*
Edited by: P. A. Donohoue © Humana Press Inc., Totowa, NJ

Key Words: arcuate nucleus, body weight regulation, central nervous system (CNS), hypothalamus, neuropeptides, obesity.

INTRODUCTION

Body adiposity is a tightly regulated variable. To maintain fat stores over long periods of time, caloric intake must precisely match expenditure. Such a process relies on the complex interactions of many different physiologic systems. One negative feedback system is composed of hormonal signals derived from adipose tissue that inform the central nervous system (CNS) about the status of peripheral energy stores. These signals from peripheral fat stores comprise one side of the hypothesized feedback loop. The receiving side of this regulatory system includes multiple central effectors that translate this information into subsequent ingestive behavior. When the system detects low levels of adipose hormones, food intake is increased while energy expenditure is decreased. In the presence of high adiposity signals on the other hand, food intake is reduced and energy expenditure increased. In this way, the body's negative feedback system can maintain energy balance or body adiposity over long periods of time.

THE DUAL-CENTERS HYPOTHESIS

The conceptual framework that historically dominated thinking about hypothalamic control of food intake was the dual-centers hypothesis proposed by Elliot Stellar in a very influential article in *Psychological Review (1)*. Years later, coinciding with the discovery of leptin, *Psychological Review* honored this article as one of the 10 most influential articles it had published in a century of publications. Stellar argued that hypothalamic nuclei are the central neural structures involved in "motivation" generally and in the control of food intake more specifically. This control is divided into two conceptual categories controlled by two separate hypothalamic structures. The first category was "satiety" and was thought to be controlled by the ventromedial hypothalamus (VMH). The most important data supporting this hypothesis was that bilateral lesions of the VMH resulted in rats that ate more than controls and became obese. VMH-lesioned rats were thought to have a defect in satiety, and therefore the structure was termed the "satiety" center. Additionally, electrical stimulation of the VMH also caused the animals to stop eating. These experiments seemed to demonstrate a role for the VMH in enhancing satiety. In contrast with the VMH, the lateral hypothalamic area (LHA) was thought to be the "hunger" nucleus as lesions of the LHA resulted in rats that underate and lost body weight. Likewise, electrical stimulation of the LHA caused hyperphagia in sated animals. Based on data such as these, the VMH and LHA were respectively thought to be the satiety and hunger centers. This characterization, the dual-centers hypothesis, was the dominant conceptualization of CNS-controlled food intake for almost 30 years.

CHALLENGES TO THE HYPOTHESIS

As with all good theories however, challenges against the dual-centers idea emerged. The first was a realization that there were limitations to understanding of the neurocircuitry using the lesions as an experimental approach to understanding CNS function. Conclusions made about larger lesion studies were often difficult to interpret because lesions usually destroy all fibers and cell bodies in the nuclei, not just those of specific interest. Consistent with this observation was the occurrence of nonspecific effects of the lesions themselves. For example, although lesions of the VMH result in hyperphagic and obese rats, they also result in rapid and dramatic increases in insulin secretion from pancreatic β-cells *(2)*. Indeed, exogenous peripheral insulin administration results in increased food intake, and repeated administration can result in rapid weight gain *(3)*. Therefore, in addition to regulating food intake, the VMH also appeared to have an important role in the regulation of insulin secretion *(2)*. Disentangling the potential roles of the VMH from those of fibers of passage became key. In fact, subsequent data indicated that it was not cell bodies in the VMH but rather fibers from the paraventricular nucleus (PVN) to the brain stem that were critical for the effect of VMH lesions on insulin secretion *(4,5)*. So while the changes in insulin secretion were potentially responsible for the effects of VMH lesions on food intake and body weight, the control of insulin secretion may not be directly mediated by the VMH. Furthermore, the VMH contains multiple neurotransmitters and receptors and probably does not serve a single unified function related to the control of food intake. Therefore, one additional early criticism of the dual-centers hypothesis is that it labeled diverse nuclei like the VMH as the "satiety" center, and this seems to ignore many other potential functions of the cells located within it.

Another challenge to the dual-centers hypothesis came from the work of Grill and colleagues, which focused on transection of the neuraxis at different levels by utilizing the chronic decerebrate rat. This model has a complete transection of the neuraxis at the meso-diencephalic junction that completely isolates the caudal brain stem, severing all neural input from more rostral structures like the hypothalamus. Hence, neither the VMH nor LHA (nor any other hypothalamic nuclei for that matter) could exert direct influence on the motor neurons in the brain stem critical for executing ingestive behavior *(6)*. The basic premise of a lesion is to eliminate the contribution of a specific area of the brain and then to assess what an animal can no longer do. Presumably, the compromised area then subserves the function that is no longer present. Importantly, despite a complete loss of neural input from the hypothalamus, the chronic decerebrate animal will engage consummatory behavior and adjust that behavior in response to both external and internal stimuli. For example, chronic decerebrate rats respond appropriately to taste stimuli (*6–9*). This suggests that the integration of sensory taste information into ongoing motor behavior can be done within the caudal brain stem. More importantly, chronic decerebrate rats exhibit satiety, and meal size is regulated by factors that influence meal size in a normal rat *(6,8)*. Thus, the caudal brain stem is sufficient to integrate regulatory signals that limit meal size into ongoing ingestive behavior independent of the hypothalamus. These data strongly challenged the dual-centers hypothesis and indicated that a distributed neural network mediates the control of food intake as opposed to either a "hunger" or "satiety" center.

BEYOND THE HYPOTHESIS

These challenges led to new models for understanding the role of the hypothalamus in the control of food intake. Importantly, other research focused on factors and signaling pathways that control long-term energy balance. The reasoning for this was simple: Adult mammals typically match their caloric intake to their caloric expenditure in a remarkably accurate fashion. In the 1950s, Gordon Kennedy suggested animals could regulate their body weight by monitoring the predominate form of energy storage in the body—adipose mass *(10)*. When caloric intake exceeds expenditure, adipose stores are expanded. When expenditure exceeds caloric intake, these stores are reduced. The logic was, "If the size of these stores is monitored, energy intake and energy expenditure can be adjusted to keep adipose mass constant and thereby keep the energy equation balanced over long periods of time." Obviously, the hypothalamus was deemed critical for this regulation.

There are at least two peripheral hormones that provide afferent information to the CNS that could be used for body weight regulation. Leptin, a relatively recently discovered peptide hormone, is secreted from adipocytes in proportion to fat mass and has received tremendous attention during the past decade. Considerable evidence implicates leptin as one of the body's most important adiposity signals (*11–14*). Plasma leptin levels correlate directly with body fat, and peripheral or central administration of leptin reduces food intake and increases energy expenditure.

Importantly, the amount of leptin is better correlated with subcutaneous fat than with visceral fat in humans, such that the reliability of leptin as an adiposity signal varies with the distribution of body fat. In humans and rats, body fat is stored with a sexual dimorphism. Males tend to store fat in the visceral adipose depot, whereas females tend to deposit relatively more fat in the subcutaneous depot. Because females tend to have more subcutaneous fat than males, on the average, leptin is a better correlate of total adiposity in females than in males *(15)*. Further, when energy balance is suddenly altered (as occurs in fasting), leptin levels decrease at a faster rate than does body adiposity (*16–18*). Hence, although much has been suggested about leptin as an adiposity signal, it may not be ideal in and of itself, suggesting that other signals may exist. One obvious candidate is the pancreatic hormone insulin.

Insulin is well-known for its critical role in regulating glucose homeostasis. However, an often underappreciated role for insulin is as an adiposity signal. Insulin levels in the blood also directly correlate with body adiposity, and though leptin is a better correlate of subcutaneous adiposity, insulin is a stronger correlate of visceral adiposity (*19–22*). Moreover, when energy balance is disrupted, changes in plasma insulin closely follow changes in homeostasis *(23)*. Therefore, both leptin and insulin can be considered adiposity signals, each providing different information to the brain; insulin is a correlate of visceral adiposity and leptin is a correlate of subcutaneous adiposity and together or separately, they are markers of changes of metabolic status.

CNS CONTROL OF FOOD INTAKE

Caloric intake occurs in distinct bouts or meals, and the regular number and size of meals comprises a meal pattern. Within these patterns, ingestive behaviors are thought to be regulated by signals from the gut, brain stem, and hypothalamus. Indeed, most humans consume approximately the same number of meals, and at about the same time of day *(24, 25)*. Signals that control when meals occur are different than those that terminate a meal; that is, different factors control meal onset and meal size *(25, 26)*. Meal initiation was historically considered a reflexive response to a reduction in the availability of some critical parameter related to energy balance. One hypothetical mechanism was the availability of glucose, coined the "glucostatic theory." This theory posited that reduced glucose utilization by specialized hypothalamic sensing cells might give rise to the sensation of hunger and therefore meal initiation *(27,28)*. An alternative hypothesis was that hunger arose from changes in fuel utilization, likely in the periphery. These signals could arise from changes in body heat, upon fat utilization by the liver, or upon the generation of adenosine triphosphate (ATP) and other energy-rich molecules by cells in the liver and/or brain (*29–32*).

Importantly, however, ingestive behaviors may be stimulated by factors other than simple changes in energy substrates. One hypothesis for meal initiation is that most meals take place at times that are convenient or habitual and thus based on social or learned factors rather than fluxes of energy within the body *(33)*. In this conceptual framework, the physiologic regulation of food intake is exerted on how much food is consumed once a meal is started rather than on when the meal occurs *(34,35)*. Individuals have flexibility with respect to their respective meal patterns, which are influenced by their environment and lifestyle. Nonetheless, there are physiologic factors that can regulate and determine meal size, which is generally equated with the phenomenon of satiety or fullness *(26)*.

THE TERMINATION OF MEALS: SATIETY

Food intake can be considered to be regulated in that there are distinct cues that signal the completion of a meal. For this to be accomplished, the individual must have a means of measuring reliably how much food has been eaten; that is, the number of calories consumed, or perhaps the precise mix of carbohydrates, lipids, and proteins, and/or other food-related parameters. Additionally, consumption must be monitored during the progression of the meal so that the individual knows when to say "I'm full" and put down the fork *(26)*. A variety of parameters or signals can provide valuable feedback during an ongoing meal. Some of these signals can be perceptual, in the form of vision, smell, or taste to gauge the amount of energy consumed. However, several types of experiments have found that the regulatory control of these stimuli is minimal at best. Therefore, an obvious alternative method for gauging meal size is via signals arising from the gut.

To assess whether the gut provides a signal for meal termination, animals have been experimentally implanted with gastric fistula *(36)*. When the fistula is closed, swallowed food enters the stomach, is processed normally, and is moved into the duodenum. When the fistula is open, however, food enters the stomach and then rapidly exits the body through the open fistula in a process called termed "sham eating." In both instances, perceptual stimuli such as sight and smell are identical, but the amount eaten varies considerably. When the fistula is closed, animals eat normal-sized meals; when the fistula is open (representing the experimental condition, or sham eating), animals will continue eating for long intervals and consume very large meals (*36–38*). Hence, the signals that gauge how many calories have been consumed must arise no more proximally to the mouth than the distal stomach and/or small intestine.

Importantly, as food passes through the stomach and intestine, it elicits the secretion of numerous gut peptides and neural activity that may function to coordinate and optimize the digestive process. In a landmark 1973 study, Gibbs and Smith and their colleagues reported that the gut peptide cholecystokinin (CCK) acts as a satiety signal by regulating the size of meals. When purified or synthetic CCK was administered to rats or humans prior to a meal, it dose-dependently reduced the size of that meal *(39–43)*. Additional support for the role of endogenous CCK in eliciting satiety is found in the observation that administration of specific CCK-1 receptor antagonists prior to a meal causes increased meal size in animals and humans *(44–47)* and reduces the subjective feeling of satiety in humans *(44)*.

In addition to CCK, there are several other gut peptides that might normally contribute to reductions in meal size and number *(48,49)*. These include gastrin releasing peptide (GRP) *(50)*, neuromedin B *(51)*, enterostatin *(52,53)*, somatostatin *(54)*, glucagon-like peptide-1 (GLP-1) *(55,56)*, apolipoprotein A-IV *(57)*, and peptide YY(3-36) (PYY3-36) *(58)*. All are peptides secreted from the gastrointestinal system and have been reported to reduce meal size when administered systemically. Additionally, amylin *(59,60)* and glucagon *(61,62)*, both secreted from the pancreatic islets during meals, have this property.

All of these peptides likely signal the central nervous system via multiple mechanisms and all may contribute to the phenomenon of satiety. The principle mechanism thought to be used by most is the activation of receptors on vagal afferent fibers passing to the hindbrain [e.g., CCK *(63–65)*, glucagon *(66,67)*], or the direct stimulation of hindbrain at sites with a relaxed blood-brain barrier [e.g., amylin *(68,69)*]. Signals from this array of peptides are thought to be integrated either within the vagal fibers themselves or within the hindbrain, as they generate an overall signal that ultimately causes the individual to stop eating *(70–73)*.

In summary, consumed food interacts with receptors lining the stomach and intestine, initiating the release of peptides and other factors in a process to coordinate digestion of the food being consumed. Some of the peptides provide a signal to the nervous system, and as the integrated signal accumulates, it ultimately creates the sensation of fullness and contributes to cessation of eating.

An important but generally unanswered question is whether satiety signals have any therapeutic value to treat obesity. Obviously, they might be given prior to each meal in attempts to reduce meal side (e.g., by administering CCK prior to each meal). However, considerable data demonstrate that individuals simply adjust by increasing how often they eat, which unfortunately maintains total daily intake relatively constant *(74,75)*. Compounding this problem is that CCK and the other gut-derived satiety signals have very short half-lives, of the order one minute or a few minutes. Hence, long-acting analogues of the satiety signals may have efficacy in causing weight loss. This is an area of considerable research activity at present. As an important aside, rats with a genetic ablation of functional CCK-1 receptors gradually become obese over their lifetimes *(76)*, suggesting that the body relies on the CCK satiety cues to prevent obesity. This lack of satiety is not counterbalanced by the increase in leptin that would result from the higher fat mass in these animals.

LEPTIN: MOLECULAR SIGNALING PATHWAYS

The state of the adipose stores impacts a variety of physiologic functions including reproduction and growth, metabolic rate, immune functions, insulin sensitivity, as well as feeding behavior and energy expenditure *(77)*. Leptin is a hormone produced by adipocytes that signals the brain on the state of adipose tissue reserves *(78)*. Initially, leptin was considered a satiety signal, though subsequent studies revealed a more complex function for this hormone *(78)*. The effects of leptin on the hypothalamus are mediated via the long form of the leptin receptor, termed LRb, in nuclei within the hypothalamus *(79, 80)*. This receptor is a class I Jak/Stat cytokine receptor *(81)*. The leptin receptor appears to process the leptin signal and regulate these diverse functions *(77)*. A variety of studies have begun to address at the molecular level how the leptin receptor transduces these functions.

Leptin receptor signaling is mediated via tyrosine phosphorylation of the receptor and activation of distinct signaling pathways *(80, 81)*. The leptin receptor does not have intrinsic signaling activity but has an associated kinase that is activated by extracellular ligand binding. The receptor exists as a homodimer and upon leptin binding undergoes a conformational change that allows transphosphorylation of the receptor on unique tyrosine residues *(80, 82, 83)*. The phosphorylation of these unique tyrosines leads to the recruitment of a unique set of SH2 domain–containing adapter proteins that stimulate protein kinase and phosphatase cascades as well as activate transcription factors. These adapter proteins include the latent transcription factor Stat3, insulin receptor substrate (IRS)/phosphatidylinositol-3-OH kinase (PI-3) kinase, and the Src Homology Protein-2 (SHP-2) tyrosine phosphatase *(82, 84)*.

Leptin receptor activation leads to generation of three distinct signaling pathways *(80)*. Jak2 kinase activation occurs in response to leptin binding. Tyr-985 phosphorylation recruits and leads to activation of the SHP-2 tyrosine phosphatase. SHP-2 subsequently activates the ras p21/Extracellular Regulated Kinase (ERK) signaling pathway. Tyr-985 is also a site for suppressor of cytokine signaling (SOCS-3), an inhibitor of leptin receptor signaling. Finally, Tyr-1138 phosphorylation leads to recruitment of Stat3 and activation of transcription.

Jak2 activation mediates signal pathways independent of the direct tyrosine phosphorylation and adapter protein recruitment on the leptin receptor *(84, 85)*. Jak2 kinase initiates a signaling cascade that involves ERKs though in a SHP-2 phosphatase–independent manner. Jak2 signaling and the unique phosphorylation sites on the kinase are not well elucidated, though Jak2 appears to phosphorylate IRS proteins and leads to PI-3 kinase–mediated signals.

Tyr-985 phosphorylation leads to recruitment and activation of the SHP-2 tyrosine phosphatase *(86)*. SHP-2 null mice are hypometabolic and obese *(87)*. The SHP-2 gene was selectively ablated in the forebrain of mice using a flox construct and crossing with CaMKIIα-Cre transgenic mice *(87)*. The mice were normal but developed adult-onset obesity. Obesity was not due to hyperphagia, though their core body temperature was lower than their controls. The obese mice develop diabetes and fatty liver disease. Importantly, the mice exhibit defects in leptin signaling with reduced hypothalamic staining for phosphorylated-Erk in the hypothalamus. Additionally, leptin increases the expression of pro-opiomelanocortin (POMC) and represses the expression of agouti-related peptide (AgRP) as well as neuropeptide Y (NPY). Fasting in mice leads to reduced leptin and reduced expression of POMC and induction of AgRP and NPY. In the SHP-2 null mice, fasting did not lead to an increase in NPY expression, suggesting that leptin-induced inhibition of NPY is mediated by recruitment of the SHP-2 phosphatase *(87)*.

Tyr-1138 phosphorylation site leads to recruitment of Stat3 and regulation of transcription *(80)*. Stat3 regulates transcription of POMC, SOCS-3, and other genes.

SOCS-3 is an inhibitor of leptin signaling by binding to Tyr-985, as well as to separate sites on Jak2 and Stat3 *(88, 89)*. Leptin receptor signaling via the Stat3 pathway is critical for food intake and energy expenditure. Indeed, mutations in the Tyr-1138 phosphorylation site lead to hyperphagia and decreased energy expenditure *(90, 91)*. These mutants also show reduced POMC expression and increased AgRP but normal NPY expression indicating that the leptin- Stat3 signal is crucial for regulation of the melanocortin pathway. Thus, the leptin- Stat3 signal appears important for energy balance. NPY signaling appears to regulate gonadal growth effects including infertility and growth retardation.

IRS-2 deletion leads to obesity, and pharmacologic inhibition of PI3 kinase leads to suppression of feeding by leptin *(92)*. The role of leptin receptor Stat3 is well established in rodent with mutant Tyr-1138 dispensable for some neuroendocrine functions but irequired for POMC and AgRP expression and control of feeding behavior and energy expenditure. Stat3 signaling is important for adiposity-dependent regulation of glucose homeostasis but not for adiposity-independent regulation of glucose homeostasis by leptin.

LEPTIN RECEPTOR NEUROPHYSIOLOGY

The leptin receptor is expressed in various peripheral tissues and in various sites in the central nervous system *(93, 94)*. In the brain, the receptor is expressed in the hypothalamus but also in other sites including the brain stem and midbrain. The receptor is alternatively spliced giving rise to even more widespread distribution. Loss of either the leptin receptor or leptin leads to obesity. More specifically, it is the "long form" of the receptor, LRb, in the brain that mediates leptin's action on body weight *(95)*.

Within the hypothalamus, the LRb is expressed in the arcuate, dorsomedial, and ventromedial hypothalamus and activates these neurons *(14, 96)*. Within the arcuate, the receptor is found on two distinct populations of neurons: the POMC and the AgRP/NPY nuclei *(97, 98)*. Currently, the arcuate nucleus is considered a primary site of leptin action. It is proposed that leptin via the leptin receptor activates the POMC neurons while inhibiting the AgRP/NPY neurons. Indeed, several lines of evidence suggest this to be the case. First, fasting or leptin deficiency increase POMC expression while suppressing AgRP and NPY expression. Second, leptin increases c-fos expression only in POMC neurons, yet SOCS-3 is activated in both POMC and AgRP/NPY neurons indicating that leptin stimulates both sets of neurons but only activates the POMC neurons. Third, deletion of leptin receptor in the POMC neurons leads to a mild form of obesity with disturbances in glucose homeostasis *(99)*. Therefore, arcuate nuclei leptin receptors are important in regulation of energy balance and appear to be the first-order neurons in response to leptin signaling *(100)*.

The body weight effects of leptin are not limited to the arcuate hypothalamus *(14, 96)*. The long form of the leptin receptor is also found in the VMH and activates these nuclei as evidenced by SOCS3 expression and c-fos induction. VMH lesions in rodents lead to a massive obesity syndrome *(101)*. Development of the VMH is regulated by the transcription factor SF-1 (steroidogenic factor 1). Deletion of this transcription factor in mice results in a loss of VMH neurons and obesity *(102, 103)*. When mice were engineered with targeted deletion of the leptin receptor in the VMH, the mice were obese and highly sensitive to the high-fat and high-sucrose feeding *(104)*. These results strongly implicate the leptin receptor in the VMH regulation of energy balance.

Leptin receptor signaling in the brain is important for additional physiologic responses to leptin including reproductive functions and bone physiology *(105)*. Although these functions are central nervous system mediated, they do not appear to be regulated by the arcuate or ventromedial hypothalamic nuclei. Therefore, it is likely that other hypothalamic or extrahypothalamic nuclei are important for the regulation of these processes. Elucidation of this physiology awaits future research efforts.

INTEGRATION OF ADIPOSITY SIGNALS

Importantly, information about total body fat derived from insulin and leptin must be integrated with gut-derived satiety signals as well as other factors including learning, social situations, and stress for the control system to be maximally efficient. Although the nature of these interactions is not well understood, several generalizations can be made. First, negative-feedback circuits related to body fat and meal ingestion can be overridden by situational events. Second, because of these complex interactions, predictions about food intake within an individual meal based on recent energy expenditure or fat stores are futile, at least in the short-term. Rather, the influence of homeostatic signals becomes apparent only when intake is considered over longer intervals. That is, if homeostatic signals predominated, a relatively large intake in one meal should be compensated by reduced intake in the subsequent meal. However, detailed analyses have revealed that such compensation, if it occurs at all, is only apparent when intervals of one or more days are considered in humans *(106, 107)*. This phenomenon was initially demonstrated in a rigorous experiment using rabbits, where weekly intake correlated better with recent energy expenditure than did intake after 1 or 3 days *(108)*.

The homeostatic regulators of food intake are thought to act by changing the sensitivity to satiety signals. In this way, adiposity signals like insulin and leptin alter the effectiveness of signals like CCK. Hence, in the presence of excess weight and increased insulin and leptin, CCK is more efficacious to reduce meal size (*109–113*). This association continues until the individual or animal becomes obese and resistant to the adiposity signals leptin and insulin.

Consistent with the understanding that feeding circuits are integrated, satiety signals that influence meal size interact with vagal afferent fibers and continue into the hindbrain *(114, 115)* where meal size is likely determined *(116)*. In parallel, the hypothalamic arcuate nucleus receives input from adiposity signals (leptin and insulin) as well as information related to ongoing meals from the hindbrain. Through integration of these multiple signals, metabolism and ingestion are monitored (*11–14,117*).

Importantly, the two principal hormones may fill distinct niches in the endocrine system. Although leptin has been implicated in several systemic processes, such as angiogenesis, the primary role of leptin appears to be as a negative-feedback adiposity signal that acts in the brain to suppress food intake and net catabolic effector *(22, 118, 119)*. Consistent with this, animals that lack leptin or functional leptin receptors are grossly obese. In contrast with leptin, insulin has a primary action in the periphery to regulate blood glucose and stimulate glucose uptake by most tissues. Similar to leptin, however, deficits in insulin signaling are associated with hyperphagia in humans, and animals that lack normal insulin signaling in the brain are also obese (*22,118–121*).

The central redundancy between leptin and insulin has been highlighted by several recent studies demonstrating that they share both intracellular and neuronal signaling pathways. The central melanocortin system has long been known to mediate the central actions of leptin (see discussion on melanocortin below), though recent studies indicate insulin stimulated the expression of the melanocortin agonist precursor peptide POMC in fasted rats, and insulin-induced hypophagia is blocked by a nonspecific melanocortin receptor antagonist (*122–127*). Furthermore, phosphatidylinositol-3-OH kinase [PI-3K], a key mediator of intracellular insulin signaling *(128)*, also plays a crucial role in the leptin signal transduction pathway as well *(128)*. Finally, leptin functionally enhances some actions of insulin. The underlying molecular mechanisms for the insulin-sensitizing effects of leptin are unclear, and data are somewhat conflicting with regard to the effect of leptin on insulin-stimulated signal transduction. However, it is known that while the long form of the leptin receptor has the capacity to activate the JAK/Stat3 *(81, 129)* and mitogen-activated protein kinase (MAPK) pathways, leptin is also able to stimulate tyrosine phosphorylation of insulin receptor substrate (IRS-1) *(129, 130)*, and to increase transcription of fos, jun *(131)*.

CENTRAL SIGNALS RELATED TO ENERGY HOMEOSTASIS

Brain structures that regulate energy homeostasis can be subdivided into those that receive sensory information (afferent circuits), those that integrate the information, and those that control motor, autonomic, and endocrine responses (efferent circuits). Peptides and hormones such as insulin, leptin, and CCK represent afferent signals that influence food intake. Additional, more direct metabolic signals also arise within the brain itself and can influence food intake, and these are discussed below.

Importantly, nutrient substrates such as glucose and/or fatty acids are used in most cells in the body and can be captured or released as energy. As oxygen combines with these substrates in the mitochondria of the cell, water and carbon dioxide are produced, and the substrate's energy is transferred into molecules such as adenosine triphosphate (ATP) that can be used as needed to power cellular processes. Most cells in the body have complex means of maintaining adequate ATP generation because they are able to oxidize either glucose or fatty acids. Hence, if one or the other substrate becomes low, enzymatic changes occur to increase the ability of the cell rapidly to take up and oxidize the alternate fuel. Compromising the formation of ATP disables cells and, when it occurs in the brain, generates a signal that leads to increased eating (*32,132–134*).

It has been suggested that specific cells/neurons in the brain function as fuel sensors and thereby generate signals that interact with other neuronal systems to regulate energy homeostasis *(32, 134)*. The brain is sensitive to changes in glucose utilization because neurons primarily use glucose for energy. Additionally, glucose uptake and oxidation in neurons and glia occur in an insulin-independent manner. Importantly, it has been demonstrated that in addition to sensing changes in glucose levels, the brain also responds to and uses fatty acids as sensor to influence food intake.

In the presence of excess energy availability, most cells synthesize fatty acids from acetyl CoA (TCA cycle intermediate) and malonyl CoA by the cellular enzyme fatty acid synthase (FAS). Inhibition of FAS activity in the brain by the compound C75 causes animals to eat less food and, over the course of a few days, selectively lose body fat (*135–137*). One interpretation of these data is that some hypothalamic cells have the ability to sense the amount of available fatty acids, and these are a critical population of cells to energy homeostasis *(138)*. Interestingly, the anorexic activity of C75 appears to require brain carbohydrate metabolism *(139)*, further supporting a critical role of key hypothalamic cells in the regulation of energy homeostasis. Further, increases of either carbohydrate or long-chain fatty acid availability locally in the arcuate nucleus leads to reduced food intake and signals to the liver to reduce the secretion of energy-rich fuels into the blood *(140)*. Although much remains to be elucidated and understood, these findings collectively support the concept that some neurons can utilize either glucose or lipids for energy and hence function as overall energy sensors (e.g., see Refs. *31, 32, 141*).

Central glucose sensing cells have been characterized and appear to contain receptors and enzymes that are consistent with another type of cell that senses changes in glucose: the pancreatic β-cells. Like β-cells, certain populations of neurons and glia detect changes in glucose levels and generate signals that influence metabolism and behavior *(142, 143)*. Additional support of an integrated system comes from evidence that the same or proximal neurons contain receptors for both leptin and insulin. What can be hypothesized from the current research is that the brain is a critical "nutrient sensing" organ with populations of specialized neurons that collectively sample different classes of energy-rich molecules (i.e., glucose and fatty acids) as well as hormones that reflect adiposity throughout the body (i.e., insulin and leptin). These same neurons appear also to be sensitive to the myriad neuropeptides known to be important regulators of energy homeostasis *(32)*, which will be described more fully below.

CATABOLIC SYSTEMS

Systems that are activated during positive energy balance predispose to increased caloric expenditure and reduced food intake. Catabolic systems are defined here as those that are activated during positive energy balance and that act to reduce energy intake and/or to increase energy expenditure and thereby restore energy stores to its defended levels. These catabolic systems oppose those that are activated during negative energy balance. When animals and humans consume calories in excess of their requirements, they increase their fat stores. Importantly, if animals are experimentally forced to consume calories in excess of their needs, voluntary food intake drops to near zero and the animals gain body weight *(144, 145)*, and they will rapidly lose weight upon the termination of the experimental overfeeding. These data provide strong evidence that body weight is tightly regulated. That is, animals not only have potent regulatory responses to being in negative energy balance, but they also possess regulatory responses to being in positive energy balance.

CILIARY NEUROTROPHIC FACTOR AND AXOKINE

Ciliary neurotrophic factor (CNTF) is a neuronal survival factor shown to induce weight loss in rodents and humans *(146, 147)*. CNTF leads to a reduction in food intake and body weight apparently via activating pathways that mimic leptin, though unlike leptin CNTF is active in leptin resistant diet–induced obese mice *(148)*. Interestingly, CNTF-treated rodents and humans lose the weight and maintain the reduced body weight for a long period after cessation of treatment. The implication of these observations suggests that CNTF resets the body weight set point. But the reason was not understood, though recent data from the Flier Laboratory sheds light on a potential mechanism for the maintenance of the weight loss *(149)*. Flier and colleagues showed that CNTF induces neuronal cell proliferation in hypothalamic feeding centers. The new cells show functional leptin responsiveness. The data provide an explanation for the prolonged weight loss maintenance but do not explain how CNTF induces satiety and leads to weight loss. Initial data in rodents appeared to indicate that CNTF somehow suppresses the appetite-enhancing neuropeptide NPY *(150)*.

MELANOCORTINS

The action of leptin and possibly insulin on feeding behavior is transduced by the melanocortin signaling pathway in the hypothalamus *(151)*. The arcuate nuclei in the hypothalamus contain two distinct populations of neurons that highly express the leptin receptor. These neurons are the POMC and AgRP/NPY neurons, which project onto neurons in the paraventricular and lateral hypothalamic area known to express the melanocortin receptors. The POMC-containing neurons secrete the melanocortin agonist alpha melanocyte stimulating hormone (α-MSH), whereas the AgRP/NPY-containing neurons secrete the melanocortin antagonist AgRP. Leptin appears to reciprocally regulate these nuclei. Low leptin levels lead to increased expression of AgRP and reduced expression of POMC and α-MSH. In contrast, high leptin levels lead to increased expression of POMC and reduced expression of AgRP.

The importance of the melanocortin signaling pathway in feeding behavior and body weight was originally uncovered by mouse fanciers characterizing coat color phenotypes in the mouse *(152)*. One of these mutations, named agouti *lethal yellow,* had a yellow coat color and was obese. Over the past decade, the details of this unusual mutation were elucidated as well as its relevance to human obesity. The signaling system involves the melanocortin receptor and two functionally opposing ligands: an agonist derived from the POMC peptide and an antagonist, AgRP *(153, 154)*. Inactivating mutations in the receptor as well as the activating ligand, α-MSH, lead to hyperphagia and obesity in both rodents and humans (*155–157*). Likewise, overexpression of the antagonist, AgRP, also leads to obesity in rodents *(158)*.

There are five mammalian melanocortin receptor subtypes involved in diverse physiologic processes such as feeding behavior, energy balance, pigmentation, and stress response *(159, 160)*. The melanocortin-3 and -4 receptors (MC3R, MC4R) are expressed in the brain and implicated in body weight and feeding behavior regulation. The MC1R is expressed in the skin and implicated in skin and hair pigmentation. The MC2R is expressed in the adrenal gland and implicated in the stress response, part of the hypothalamic pituitary adrenal (HPA) axis. Finally, the MC5R is ubiquitously expressed in the periphery and implicated in sebaceous gland physiology.

The melanocortin receptors and particularly the MC4R have attracted significant pharmaceutical attention *(161)*. Indeed, pharmacologic validation for the role of the melanocortin receptors in feeding behavior derives based on the peptide nonspecific melanocortin agonist melanotan II (MTII) *(162, 163)*. Rodent and human studies with MTII indicate that melanocortin agonism leads to reduced food intake. The melanocortin receptors are involved in a variety of physiologic process, thus identifying a selective agonist has been quite complicated. Despite significant biotechnology and pharmaceutical interest, pharmacologic modulators of MC4R are not likely to appear in the clinic in the near future.

PLASTICITY IN THE SYSTEM

Numerous previous accounts have detailed important roles for energy balance and metabolic status in the plasticity of the central nervous system. Specifically, dysregulated energy balance including dietary-induced obesity and diabetes has been identified as a causative factor in the development of cognitive impairment and diseases of the CNS. For example, persons with insulin-insensitivity are predisposed to the development of Alzheimer disease (AD). Importantly, the severity of AD can be somewhat alleviated by experimental administration of very low doses of insulin. Additionally, mild glucose intolerance has been found to correlate with reduced memory performance even in young, healthy college students. Although numerous reports over the years have made similar observations, the data from animal studies are even more compelling. First, one long-recognized method to improve cognitive ability in experimental subjects is long-term caloric restriction. Consistent with human data, rats and mice exhibit greatly attenuated age-associated cognitive impairments when they are restricted to 65–80% of their ad libitum food intake. Second, animals that lack leptin, insulin, or their functional receptors all exhibit some form of dysregulated learning/memory performance and/or neural plasticity. Third, animals maintained on diets that promote obesity and diabetes exhibit impaired spatial cognition and reduced expression of neurotrophic factors in the hippocampus. Collectively, these data support the idea that diet and metabolism play significant roles in maintaining overall CNS function and point specifically to mechanisms involving neurotrophic factors like brain derived neurotrophic factor (BDNF).

Importantly, several recent reports have identified critical roles for mechanisms of plasticity in the control of food intake and body weight specifically in the hypothalamus. Two studies showed that exogenous administration of the hormone leptin results in increased axonal outgrowth in leptin-deficient ob/ob neonates *(164)*, to a similar extent seen in normal, wild-type mice. Additionally, leptin appears to regulate synaptic structure in hypothalamic tissue of adult rodents *(165)*. As mentioned above, previous work had already suggested a role for leptin in synaptic plasticity and neuronal outgrowth *(166, 167)*. Ob/ob mice exhibit impaired hippocampal long-term potentiation (LTP), and both ob/ob and leptin receptor–defective db/db mice are deficient in some memory tasks *(168, 169)*. However, the demonstrations of leptin action on plasticity in hypothalamic tissues suggests that the regulation of energy homeostasis systems may involve cellular mechanisms that have most often been relegated to CNS structures involved in learning. These data suggest that the energy balance regulatory system may be linked to structural plasticity systems.

In fact, synaptic changes may be important for melanocortin signaling as well *(165)*, and the hypothalamus expresses several key proteins that may mediate this process. Syndecan-3 and heparin-sulfate proteoglycan (HSPGs) are among those poised to regulate such plasticity around energy intake. An interesting observation that remains mechanistically unresolved is the prolonged activity of AgRP after a single 3rd ventricular (i3vt) injection of this peptide *(125)*. An initial hypothesis proposed that

AgRP simply has a very long-half life and exerts its prolonged effect on intake by continuing to act as an antagonist for melanocortin receptors. A more likely possibility is that the initial interaction of AgRP with melanocortin receptors produces a cascade of events perhaps involving genomic and protein synthesis or posttranslational modifications that result in an animal biased to consume more food over the next several days. Syndecan-3 or other proteoglycans may represent such a mechanism whereby AgRP influences structural or cellular plasticity, accounting for dramatic changes in food intake over many days. Consistent with this general hypothesis, families of proteoglycans are thought to provide exactly this function in regions of the CNS historically known for plasticity.

We have proposed that syndecan-3 facilitates AgRP and perhaps other neuropeptide action through regulation of synapse formation and function. Importantly, the syndecan-3 C-terminal 4 acids (EFYA) are a consensus-binding site for type II PDZ binding domain proteins. PDZ domain–containing proteins were named for the proteins PSD-95, discs large, and zonula occludens-1 proteins and are important in organizing and assembling protein complexes along the inner surface of plasma membranes at cell-cell contacts and synapses. In the face of altered energy balance (e.g., fasting vs. refeeding), these molecules can be cleaved from their cell anchors for rapid changes in cell-cell communication. This cleavage may 1) modify the structure of presynaptic terminals and 2) decrease the ability of ligands such as AgRP to reach their receptors (e.g., MC4R). Because cleavage is rapid, syndecan-3 (or other unidentified matrix molecules) may mediate immediate changes in the structure and number of excitatory and/or inhibitory synapses *(164, 165)*.

CONCLUSION

The ideas, work, and topics presented in this review are by no means the whole of CNS regulation of food intake and appetite. Indeed, there are rich areas of investigation of which we have only mentioned. The important conclusion is that the CNS control of this regulation is diverse and yet exquisitely integrated. From signals arising in the gastrointestinal tract, to hormones that convey adiposity information, to the multiple nuclei in the brain that receive and coordinate the behavioral response, each part of the system represents not an independent entity but rather an important piece of a complex whole.

REFERENCES

1. Stellar E. The physiology of motivation. Psychol Rev 1954;61:5–22.
2. Powley TL. The ventromedial hypothalamic syndrome, satiety, and a cephalic phase hypothesis. Psychol Rev 1977;84:89–126.
3. Sclafani A. The role of hyperinsulinema and the vagus nerve in hypothalamic hyperphagia reexamined. Diabetologia 1981;20(Suppl):402–410.
4. Bray GA, Sclafani A, Novin D. Obesity-inducing hypothalamic knife cuts: effects on lipolysis and blood insulin levels. Am J Physiol 1982;243:R445–R449.
5. Aravich PF, Sclafani A. Paraventricular hypothalamic lesions and medial hypothalamic knife cuts produce similar hyperphagia syndromes. Behav Neurosci 1983;97:970–983.
6. Grill HJ, Norgren R. Chronically decerebrate rats demonstrate satiation but not bait shyness. Science 1978;201:267–269.

7. Grill HJ, Norgren R. The taste reactivity test. II. Mimetic responses to gustatory stimuli in chronic thalamic and chronic decerebrate rats. Brain Res 1978;143: 281–297.
8. Grill HJ, Smith GP. Cholecystokinin decreases sucrose intake in chronic decerebrate rats. Am J Physiol 1988;254:R853–R856.
9. Flynn FW, Grill HJ. Intraoral intake and taste reactivity responses elicited by sucrose and sodium chloride in chronic decerebrate rats. Behav Neurosci 1988;102:934–941.
10. Kennedy GC. The role of depot fat in the hypothalamic control of food intake in the rat. Proc R Soc Lond (Biol) 1953;140:579–592.
11. Ahima RS, et al. Leptin regulation of neuroendocrine systems. Front Neuroendocrinol 2000;21: 263–307.
12. Cone RD, et al. The arcuate nucleus as a conduit for diverse signals relevant to energy homeostasis. Int J Obes Relat Metab Disord 2001;25(Suppl 5):S63–S67.
13. Elmquist JK, Elias CF, Saper CB. From lesions to leptin: hypothalamic control of food intake and body weight. Neuron 1999;22:221–232.
14. Schwartz MW, Woods SC, Porte D Jr, et al. Central nervous system control of food intake. Nature 2000;404:661–671.
15. Havel PJ, Kasim-Karakas S, Dubuc GR, et al. Gender differences in plasma leptin concentrations. Nat Med 1996;2:949–950.
16. Ahren B, Mansson S, Gingerich RL, et al. Regulation of plasma leptin in mice: Influence of age, high-fat diet and fasting. Am J Physiol 1997;273:R113–R120.
17. Havel PJ. Mechanisms regulating leptin production: Implications for control of energy balance. Am J Clin Nutr 1999;70:305–306.
18. Buchanan C, et al. Central nervous system effects of leptin. Trends Endocrinol Metab 1998; 9:146–150.
19. Bjorntorp P. Metabolic implications of body fat distribution. Diabetes Care 1991;14:1132–1143.
20. Bjorntorp P. Abdominal fat distribution and the metabolic syndrome. J Cardiovasc Pharmacol 1992;20(Suppl 8):S26–S28.
21. Bjorntorp P. Body fat distribution, insulin resistance, and metabolic diseases. Nutrition 1997;13: 795–803.
22. Woods SC, et al. Signals that regulate food intake and energy homeostasis. Science 1998;280: 1378–1383.
23. Schwartz MW, et al. Insulin in the brain: a hormonal regulator of energy balance. Endocri Rev 1992;13:387–414.
24. de Castro JM, Stroebele N. Food intake in the real world: implications for nutrition and aging. Clin Geriatr Med 2002;18:685–697.
25. de Castro JM. The control of eating behavior in free living humans. In: Stricker EM, Woods SC, eds. Handbook of neurobiology. Neurobiology of food and fluid intake, vol. 14, no. 2. New York: Kluwer Academic/Plenum Publishers; 2004:467–502.
26. de Graaf C, et al. Biomarkers of satiation and satiety. Am J Clin Nutr 2004;79:946–961.
27. Mayer J. Regulation of energy intake and the body weight: The glucostatic and lipostatic hypothesis. Ann N Y Acad Sci 1955;63:14–42.
28. Mayer J, Thomas DW. Regulation of food intake and obesity. Science 1967;156:328–337.
29. Friedman MI. Fuel partitioning and food intake. Am J Clin Nutr 1998;67(Suppl. 3):513S–518S.
30. Friedman MI. An energy sensor for control of energy intake. Proc Nutr Soc 1997;56:41–50.
31. Langhans W. Metabolic and glucostatic control of feeding. Proc Nutr Soc 1996;55:497–515.
32. Peters A, et al. The selfish brain: competition for energy resources. Neurosci Biobehav Rev 2004;28:143–180.
33. Strubbe JH, Woods SC. The timing of meals. Psychol Rev 2004;111:128–141.
34. Woods SC, Strubbe JH. The psychobiology of meals. Psychonom Bull Rev 1994;1:141–155.

35. Woods SC, et al. Food intake and the regulation of body weight. Annu Rev Psychol 2000;51:255–277.
36. Davis JD, Campbell CS. Peripheral control of meal size in the rat. Effect of sham feeding on meal size and drinking rate. J Comp Physiol Psychol 1973;83:379–387.
37. Davis JD, Smith GP. Learning to sham feed: behavioral adjustments to loss of physiological postingestional stimuli. Am J Physiol 1990;259:R1228–R1235.
38. Gibbs J, Young RC, Smith GP. Cholecystokinin elicits satiety in rats with open gastric fistulas. Nature 1973;245:323–325.
39. Gibbs J, Young RC, Smith GP. Cholecystokinin decreases food intake in rats. J Comp Physiol Psychol 1973;84:488–495.
40. Kissileff HR, et al. Cholecystokinin decreases food intake in man. Am J Clin Nutr 1981;34:154–160.
41. Muurahainenn N, et al. Effects of cholecystokinin-octapeptide (CCK-8) on food intake and gastric emptying in man. Physiol Behav 1988;44:644–649.
42. Moran TH, Schwartz GJ. Neurobiology of cholecystokinin. Crit Rev Neurobiol 1994;9:1–28.
43. Smith GP, Gibbs J. The development and proof of the cholecystokinin hypothesis of satiety. In: Dourish CT, et al., eds. Multiple cholecystokinin receptors in the CNS. Oxford: Oxford University Press; 1992:166–182.
44. Beglinger C, et al. Loxiglumide, a CCK-A receptor antagonist, stimulates calorie intake and hunger feelings in humans. Am J Physiol 2001;280:R1149–R1154.
45. Hewson G, et al. The cholecystokinin receptor antagonist L364,718 increases food intake in the rat by attenuation of endogenous cholecystokinin. Br J Pharmacol 1988;93:79–84.
46. Moran TH, et al. Blockade of type A, but not type B, CCK receptors postpones satiety in rhesus monkeys. Am J Physiol 1993;265:R620–R624.
47. Reidelberger RD, O'Rourke MF. Potent cholecystokinin antagonist L-364,718 stimulates food intake in rats. Am J Physiol 1989;257:R1512–R1518.
48. Kaplan JM, Moran TH. Gastrointestinal signaling in the control of food intake. In: Stricker EM, Woods SC, eds. Handbook of behavioral neurobiology. Neurobiology of food and fluid intake, vol. 4, no. 2. New York: Kluwer Academic/Plenum Publishing; 2004:273–303.
49. Smith GP, ed. Satiation: from gut to brain. New York: Oxford University Press; 1998.
50. Stein LJ, Woods SC. Gastrin releasing peptide reduces meal size in rats. Peptides 1982;3:833–835.
51. Ladenheim EE, Wirth KE, Moran TH. Receptor subtype mediation of feeding suppression by bombesin-like peptides. Pharmacol Biochem Behav 1996;54:705–711.
52. Okada S, et al. Enterostatin (Val-Pro-Asp-Pro-Arg), the activation peptide of procolipase, selectively reduces fat intake. Physiol Behav 1991;49:1185–1189.
53. Shargill NS, et al. Enterostatin suppresses food intake following injection into the third ventricle of rats. Brain Res 1991;544:137–140.
54. Lotter EC, et al. Somatostatin decreases food intake of rats and baboons. J Comp Physiol Psychol 1981;95:278–87.
55. Larsen PJ, et al. Systemic administration of the long-acting GLP-1 derivative NN2211 induces lasting and reversible weight loss in both normal and obese rats. Diabetes 2001;50:2530–2539.
56. Naslund E, et al. Energy intake and appetite are suppressed by glucagon-like peptide-1 (GLP-1) in obese men. Int J Obes Relat Metab Disord 1999;23:304–311.
57. Fujimoto K, et al. Effect of intravenous administration of apolipoprotein A-IV on patterns of feeding, drinking and ambulatory activity in rats. Brain Res 1993;608:233–237.
58. Batterham RL, et al. Gut hormone PYY(3-36) physiologically inhibits food intake. Nature 2002;418:650–654.
59. Chance WT, et al. Anorexia following the intrahypothalamic administration of amylin. Brain Res 1991;539:352–354.
60. Lutz TA, Del Prete E, Scharrer E. Reduction of food intake in rats by intraperitoneal injection of low doses of amylin. Physiol Behav 1994;55:891–895.

61. Geary N. Glucagon and the control of meal size. In: Smith GP, ed. Satiation. From Gut to Brain. New York: Oxford University Press: 1998:164–197.
62. Salter JM. Metabolic effects of glucagon in the Wistar rat. Am J Clin Nutr 1960;8:535–539.
63. Davison JS, Clarke GD. Mechanical properties and sensitivity to CCK of vagal gastric slowly adapting mechanoreceptors. Am J Physiol 1988;255:G55–G61.
64. Lorenz DN, Goldman SA. Vagal mediation of the cholecystokinin satiety effect in rats. Physiol Behav 1982;29:599–604.
65. Moran TH, et al. Vagal afferent and efferent contributions to the inhibition of food intake by cholecystokinin. Am J Physiol 1997;272:R1245–R1251.
66. Geary N, Le Sauter J, Noh U. Glucagon acts in the liver to control spontaneous meal size in rats. Am J Physiol 1993;264:R116–R122.
67. Langhans W. Role of the liver in the metabolic control of eating: what we know – and what we do not know. Neurosci Biobehav Rev 1996;20:145–153.
68. Lutz TA, Del Prete E, Scharrer E. Subdiaphragmatic vagotomy does not influence the anorectic effect of amylin. Peptides 1995;16:457–462.
69. Lutz TA, et al. Lesion of the area postrema/nucleus of the solitary tract (AP/NTS) attenuates the anorectic effects of amylin and calcitonin gene-related peptide (CGRP) in rats. Peptides 1998;19:309–317.
70. Edwards GL, Ladenheim EE, Ritter RC. Dorsomedial hindbrain participation in cholecystokinin-induced satiety. Am J Physiol 1986;251:R971–R977.
71. Moran TH, Ladenheim EE, Schwartz GJ. Within-meal gut feedback signaling. Int J Obes Relat Metab Disord 2001;25:S39–S41.
72. Moran TH, Kinzig KP. Gastrointestinal satiety signals II. Cholecystokinin. Am J Physiol Gastrointest Liver Physiol 2004;286:G183–G188.
73. Rinaman L, et al. Cholecystokinin activates catecholaminergic neurons in the caudal medulla that innervate the paraventricular nucleus of the hypothalamus in rats. J Comp Neurol 1995;360:246–256.
74. West DB, Fey D, Woods SC. Cholecystokinin persistently suppresses meal size but not food intake in free-feeding rats. Am J Physiol 1984;246:R776–R787.
75. West DB, et al. Lithium chloride, cholecystokinin and meal patterns: evidence the cholecystokinin suppresses meal size in rats without causing malaise. Appetite 1987;8:221–227.
76. Moran TH, et al. Disordered food intake and obesity in rats lacking cholecystokinin A receptors. Am J Physiol 1998;274: R618–R625.
77. Ahima RS. Central actions of adipocyte hormones. Trends Endocrinol Metab 2005;16:307–313.
78. Friedman JM, Halaas JL. Leptin and the regulation of body weight in mammals. Nature 1998;395: 763–770.
79. Munzberg H, Myers MG Jr. Molecular and anatomical determinants of central leptin resistance. Nat Neurosci 2005;8:566–570.
80. Bates SH, Myers MG Jr. The role of leptin receptor signaling in feeding and neuroendocrine function. Trends Endocrinol Metab 2003;14:447–452.
81. Tartaglia LA. The leptin receptor. J Biol Chem 1997;272:6093–6096.
82. White DW, et al. Leptin receptor (OB-R) signaling. Cytoplasmic domain mutational analysis and evidence for receptor homo-oligomerization. J Biol Chem 1997;272:4065–4071.
83. Zabeau L, et al. Leptin receptor activation depends on critical cysteine residues in its fibronectin type III subdomains. J Biol Chem 2005;280:22632–22640.
84. Banks AS, et al. Activation of downstream signals by the long form of the leptin receptor. J Biol Chem 2000;275:14563–14572.
85. Feng J, et al. Activation of Jak2 catalytic activity requires phosphorylation of Y1007 in the kinase activation loop. Mol Cell Biol 1997;17:2497–2501.

86. Li C, Friedman JM. Leptin receptor activation of SH2 domain containing protein tyrosine phosphatase 2 modulates Ob receptor signal transduction. Proc Natl Acad Sci USA 1999;96:9677–82.
87. Zhang EE, et al. Neuronal Shp2 tyrosine phosphatase controls energy balance and metabolism. Proc Natl Acad Sci USA 2004;101:16064–16069.
88. Bjorbaek C, et al. The role of SOCS-3 in leptin signaling and leptin resistance. J Biol Chem 1999;274:30059–30065.
89. Bjorbaek C, et al. Activation of SOCS-3 messenger ribonucleic acid in the hypothalamus by ciliary neurotrophic factor. Endocrinology 1999;140:2035–2043.
90. Bates SH, et al. STAT3 signaling is required for leptin regulation of energy balance but not reproduction. Nature 2003;421:856–859.
91. Bates SH, et al. LRb-STAT3 signaling is required for the neuroendocrine regulation of energy expenditure by leptin. Diabetes 2004;53:3067–3073.
92. Choudhury AI, et al. The role of insulin receptor substrate 2 in hypothalamic and beta cell function. J Clin Invest 2005;115:940–950.
93. Mercer JG, et al. Localization of leptin receptor mRNA and the long form splice variant (Ob-Rb) in mouse hypothalamus and adjacent brain regions by in situ hybridization. FEBS Lett 1996;387: 113–116.
94. Schwartz MW, et al. Identification of hypothalamic targets of leptin action. J Clin Invest 1996;98:1101–1106.
95. de Luca C, et al. Complete rescue of obesity, diabetes, and infertility in db/db mice by neuron-specific LEPR-B transgenes. J Clin Invest 2005;115:3484–3493.
96. Cheung CC, Clifton DK, Steiner RA. Proopiomelanocortin neurons are direct targets for leptin in the hypothalamus. Endocrinology 1997;138:4489–4492.
97. Marks DL, Cone RD. Central melanocortins and the regulation of weight during acute and chronic disease. Recent Prog Horm Res 2001;56:359–375.
98. Barsh GS, Schwartz MW. Genetic approaches to studying energy balance: perception and integration. Nat Rev Genet 2002;3:589–600.
99. Balthasar N, et al. Leptin receptor signaling in POMC neurons is required for normal body weight homeostasis. Neuron 2004;42:983–991.
100. Coppari R, et al. The hypothalamic arcuate nucleus: a key site for mediating leptin's effects on glucose homeostasis and locomotor activity. Cell Metab 2005;1:63–72.
101. Hetherington AW, Ranson SW. The spontaneous activity and food intake of rats with hypothalmic lesions. Am J Physiol 1942;136:609–617.
102. Dellovade TL, et al. Disruption of the gene encoding SF-1 alters the distribution of hypothalamic neuronal phenotypes. J Comp Neurol 2000;423:579–589.
103. Majdic G, et al. Knockout mice lacking steroidogenic factor 1 are a novel genetic model of hypothalamic obesity. Endocrinology 2002;143:607–614.
104. Dhillon H, et al. Leptin directly activates SF1 neurons in the VMH, and this action by leptin is required for normal body-weight homeostasis. Neuron 2006;49:191–203.
105. Elmquist JK, et al. Identifying hypothalamic pathways controlling food intake, body weight, and glucose homeostasis. J Comp Neurol 2005;493:63–71.
106. Birch LL, et al. The variability of young children's energy intake. N Engl J Med 1991;324:232–235.
107. de Castro JM. Prior day's intake has macronutrient-specific delayed negative feedback effects on the spontaneous food intake of free-living humans. J Nutr 1998;128:61–67.
108. Gasnier A, Mayer A. Recherche sur la régulation de la nutrition. II. Mécanismes régulateurs de la nutrition chez le lapin domestique. Ann Physiol Physicochem Biol 1939;15:157–185.
109. Barrachina MD, et al. Synergistic interaction between leptin and cholecystokinin to reduce short-term food intake in lean mice. Proc Natl Acad Sci USA 1997;94:10455–10460.

110. Figlewicz DP, et al. Intraventricular insulin enhances the meal-suppressive efficacy of intraventricular cholecystokinin octapeptide in the baboon. Behav Neurosci 1995;109:567–569.
111. Matson CA, et al. Synergy between leptin and cholecystokinin (CCK) to control daily caloric intake. Peptides 1997;18:1275–1278.
112. Matson CA, et al. Cholecystokinin and leptin act synergistically to reduce body weight. Am J Physiol 2000;278:R882–R890.
113. Riedy CA, et al. Central insulin enhances sensitivity to cholecystokinin. Physiol Behav 1995;58: 755–760.
114. Schwartz GJ, Moran TH. Sub-diaphragmatic vagal afferent integration of meal-related gastrointestinal signals. Neurosci Biobehav Rev 1996;20:47–56.
115. Schwartz GJ, et al. Relationships between gastric motility and gastric vagal afferent responses to CCK and GRP in rats differ. Am J Physiol 1997;272:R1726–33.
116. Grill HJ, Kaplan JM. The neuroanatomical axis for control of energy balance. Front Neuroendocrinol 2002;23:2–40.
117. Flier JS. Obesity wars: molecular progress confronts an expanding epidemic. Cell 2004;116:337–350.
118. Porte DJ, et al. Obesity, diabetes and the central nervous system. Diabetologia 1998;41:863–881.
119. Woods SC, et al. Insulin and the blood-brain barrier. Curr Pharm Design 2003;9:795–800.
120. Tartaglia LA, et al. Identification and expression cloning of a leptin receptor, OB-R. Cell 1995;83:1263–1271.
121. Bruning JC, et al. Role of brain insulin receptor in control of body weight and reproduction. Science 2000;289:2122–2125.
122. Seeley R, et al. Melanocortin receptors in leptin effects. Nature 1997;390:349.
123. Ollmann M, et al. Antagonism of central melanocortin receptors in vitro and in vivo by agouti-related protein. Science 1997;278:135–138.
124. Rossi M, et al. A C-terminal fragment of Agouti-related protein increases feeding and antagonizes the effect of alpha-melanocyte stimulating hormone in vivo. Endocrinology 1998;139:4428–4431.
125. Hagan MM, et al. Long-term orexigenic effects of AgRP-(83-132) involve mechanisms other than melanocortin receptor blockade. Am J Physiol 2000;279:R47–R52.
126. Fan W, et al. Role of melanocortinergic neurons in feeding and the agouti obesity syndrome. Nature 1997;385:165–168.
127. Hagan M, et al. Role of the CNS melanocortin system in the response to overfeeding. J Neurosci 1999;19:2362–2367.
128. Niswender KD, Schwartz MW. Insulin and leptin revisited: adiposity signals with overlapping physiological and intracellular signaling capabilities. Front Neuroendocrinol 2003;24:1–10.
129. Vaisse C, et al. Leptin activation of Stat3 in the hypothalamus of wild-type and ob/ob mice but not db/db mice. Nat Genet 1996;14:95–7.
130. Cohen B, Novick D, Rubinstein M. Modulation of insulin activities by leptin. Science 1996;274:1185–1188.
131. Van Dijk G, Thiele TE, Donahey JC, Campfield LA, Smith FJ, Burn P, Bernstein IL, Woods SC, Seeley RJ. Central infusions of leptin and GLP-1-(7-36) amide differentially stimulate c-FLI in the rat brain. Am J Physiol 1996;271:R1096–R1100.
132. Ainscow EK, et al. Dynamic imaging of free cytosolic ATP concentration during fuel sensing by rat hypothalamic neurones: evidence for ATP-independent control of ATP-sensitive K(+) channels. J Physiol 2002;544:429–445.
133. Even P, Nicolaidis S. Spontaneous and 2DG-induced metabolic changes and feeding: The ischymetric hypothesis. Brain Res Bull 1985;15:429–435.
134. Nicolaidis S, Even P. Mesure du métabolisme de fond en relation avec la prise alimentaire: hypothese iscymétrique. Comptes Rendus Academie de Sciences, Paris 1984;298:295–300.

135. Clegg, DJ, et al. Comparison of central and peripheral administration of C75 on food intake, body weight, and conditioned taste aversion. Diabetes 2002;51:3196–201.
136. Kumar MV, et al. Differential effects of a centrally acting fatty acid synthase inhibitor in lean and obese mice. Proc Natl Acad Sci USA 2002;99:1921–1925.
137. Loftus TM, et al. Reduced food intake and body weight in mice treated with fatty acid synthase inhibitors. Science 2000;288:2299–2300.
138. Obici S, et al. Inhibition of hypothalamic carnitine palmitoyltransferase-1 decreases food intake and glucose production. Nat Med 2003;9:756–761.
139. Wortman MD, et al. C75 inhibits food intake by increasing CNS glucose metabolism. Nat Med 2003;9:483–485.
140. Obici S, et al. Central administration of oleic acid inhibits glucose production and food intake. Diabetes 2002;51:271–275.
141. Nicolaidis S. Mecanisme nerveux de l'equilibre energetique. Journees Annuelles de Diabetologie de l'Hotel-Dieu 1978;1:152–156.
142. Levin BE, Dunn-Meynell AA, Routh VH. Brain glucose sensing and body energy homeostasis: role in obesity and diabetes. Am J Physiol 1999; 276:R1223–R1231.
143. Levin BE. Glucosensing neurons as integrators of metabolic signals. European Winter Conference on Brain Research (EWCBR) 2002;22:67.
144. Bernstein IL, Lotter EC, Kulkosky PJ. Effect of force-feeding upon basal insulin levels in rats. Proc Soc Exp Biol Med 1975;150:546–548.
145. Seeley RJ, et al. Behavioral, endocrine and hypothalamic responses to involuntary overfeeding. Am J Physiol 1996;271:R819–R823.
146. Ettinger MP, et al. Recombinant variant of ciliary neurotrophic factor for weight loss in obese adults: a randomized, dose-ranging study. JAMA 2003;289:1826–1832.
147. Anderson KD, et al. Activation of the hypothalamic arcuate nucleus predicts the anorectic actions of ciliary neurotrophic factor and leptin in intact and gold thioglucose-lesioned mice. J Neuroendocrinol 2003;15:649–660.
148. Kelly JF, et al. Ciliary neurotrophic factor and leptin induce distinct patterns of immediate early gene expression in the brain. Diabetes 2004;53:911–920.
149. Kokoeva MV, Yin H, Flier JS. Neurogenesis in the hypothalamus of adult mice: potential role in energy balance. Science 2005;310:679–683.
150. Pu S, et al. Neuropeptide Y counteracts the anorectic and weight reducing effects of ciliary neurotropic factor. J Neuroendocrinol 2000;12:827–832.
151. Cone RD. Anatomy and regulation of the central melanocortin system. Nat Neurosci 2005;8:571–578.
152. Yen T, et al. Obesity, diabetes, and neoplasia in yellow A(vy)/- mice: ectopic expression of the agouti gene. FASEB J 1994;8:479–488.
153. Zimanyi IA, Pelleymounter MA. The role of melanocortin peptides and receptors in regulation of energy balance. Curr Pharm Des 2003;9:627–41.
154. Stutz AM, Morrison CD, Argyropoulos G. The Agouti-related protein and its role in energy homeostasis. Peptides 2005;26:1771–1781.
155. Yaswen L, et al. Obesity in the mouse model of pro-opiomelanocortin deficiency responds to peripheral melanocortin. Nat Med 1999;5:1066–1070.
156. Krude H, et al. Severe early-onset obesity, adrenal insufficiency and red hair pigmentation caused by POMC mutations in humans. Nat Genet 1998;19:155–157.
157. Huszar D, et al. Targeted disruption of the melanocortin-4 receptor results in obesity in mice. Cell 1997;88:131–141.
158. Ollmann MM, et al. Antagonism of central melanocortin receptors in vitro and in vivo by agouti-related protein. Science 1997;278:135–138.

159. Cone RD, et al. The melanocortin receptors: agonists, antagonists, and the hormonal control of pigmentation. Recent Prog Hormone Res 1996; 51:287–320.
160. Seeley RJ, Drazen DL, Clegg DJ. The critical role of the melanocortin system in the control of energy balance. Annu Rev Nutr 2004;24:133–149.
161. Boyce RS, Duhl DM. Melanocortin-4 receptor agonists for the treatment of obesity. Curr Opin Invest Drugs 2004;5:1063–1071.
162. Bluher S, et al. Ciliary neurotrophic factorAx15 alters energy homeostasis, decreases body weight, and improves metabolic control in diet-induced obese and UCP1-DTA mice. Diabetes 2004;53:2787–2796.
163. Dorr RT, et al. Evaluation of melanotan-II, a superpotent cyclic melanotropic peptide in a pilot phase-I clinical study. Life Sci 1996;58:1777–1784.
164. Bouret SG, Draper SJ, Simerly RB. Trophic action of leptin on hypothalamic neurons that regulate feeding. Science 2004;304:108–110.
165. Pinto S, et al. Rapid rewiring of arcuate nucleus feeding circuits by leptin. Science 2004;304:110–115.
166. Shanley LJ, Irving AJ, Harvey J. Leptin enhances NMDA receptor function and modulates hippocampal synaptic plasticity. J Neurosci 2001;21:RC186.
167. Wayner MJ, et al. Orexin-A (hypocretin-1) and leptin enhance LTP in the dentate gyrus of rats in vivo. Peptides 2004;25:991–996.
168. Ohta R, et al. Conditioned taste aversion learning in leptin-receptor-deficient db/db mice. Neurobiol Learn Mem 2003;80:105–112.
169. Li XL, et al. Impairment of long-term potentiation and spatial memory in leptin receptor-deficient rodents. Neuroscience 2002;113:607–615.

3 Inactivating Melanocortin 4 Receptor Mutations and Human Obesity

Ya-Xiong Tao

CONTENTS

Abstract

Multiple lines of studies, including anatomic, pharmacologic, and mouse genetic, demonstrated the critical importance of the melanocortin 4 receptor (MC4R) as a regulator of energy homeostasis in rodents. Human genetic studies showed that mutations in the MC4R gene are the most common monogenic form of obesity. About 80 different mutations have been identified from cohorts from various ethnic origins. Functional analyses of the mutant receptors revealed multiple defects including cell surface expression, ligand binding, and signaling. Some variant receptors have the normal functions of the wild-type receptor. A classification scheme was proposed to catalogue the ever-increasing array of MC4R mutations. Based on studies from other G protein–coupled receptors, potential therapeutic approaches to correct the dysfunctional MC4Rs are highlighted.

Key Words: G protein–coupled receptor, melanocortin-4 receptor, mutation, obesity.

INTRODUCTION

Obesity and its associated disorders such as type 2 diabetes mellitus and cardiovascular disease are at epidemic levels, especially in developed countries such as the United States *(1)*, with tremendous economic and social costs. In the United States, two thirds of adults are either overweight or obese. The Centers for Disease Control and Prevention listed obesity as a major preventable cause of death just behind tobacco

From: *Contemporary Endocrinology: Energy Metabolism and Obesity: Research and Clinical Applications*
Edited by: P. A. Donohoue © Humana Press Inc., Totowa, NJ

use. Therefore, understanding the molecular mechanisms underlying the regulation of energy homeostasis and the defects of these regulations that result in obesity is of enormous interest to scientists in academia as well as in industry.

During the past decade, tremendous progress has been made in elucidating the neural pathways regulating energy homeostasis. Several neuropeptides were found to regulate energy balance (reviewed in Ref. 2). The leptin-regulated melanocortin circuit was found to be especially important. Leptin produced by the adipocytes binds to its receptors in two subsets of neurons in the arcuate nucleus of the hypothalamus. One subset of neurons expresses neuropeptide Y (NPY) and agouti-related protein (AgRP), another subset of neurons expresses pro-opiomelanocortin (POMC) and cocaine and amphetamine regulated transcript. AgRP is an antagonist for the brain melanocortin receptors (MCRs), the melanocortin 3 receptor (MC3R) and melanocortin 4 receptor (MC4R). POMC is processed posttranslationally to α-, β-, and γ-melanocyte stimulating hormone (MSH) and adrenocorticotropin (ACTH) (collectively called melanocortins) by prohormone convertases *(3)*. This processing is tissue-specific. In the hypothalamus, POMC is processed to MSHs, whereas in the pituitary gland, it is processed to ACTH. α-MSH and β-MSH activate both MC3R and MC4R, whereas all three MSH's activate MC3R.

Melanocortins regulate numerous physiologic functions, including pigmentation, adrenal steroidogenesis, energy homeostasis, sexual function, exocrine gland secretion, inflammation, cardiovascular function, and many others (reviewed in Ref. 4). MCRs mediate the diverse functions of melanocortins. There have been five subtypes of MCRs cloned and they are named MC1R to MC5R according to the sequence of their cloning *(4)*. These MCRs are members of the G protein–coupled receptor (GPCR) superfamily. They couple to the stimulatory heterotrimeric G protein Gs, therefore receptor activation results in increased intracellular cAMP production. Like other GPCRs, MCRs consist of seven transmembrane α-helices (TMs) connected by alternating intracellular and extracellular loops, with the N-terminus lying outside of the cell and the C-terminus lying on the inside of the cell.

MC4R AND RODENT ENERGY HOMEOSTASIS

Several lines of investigations, including anatomic, genetic, and pharmacologic studies, demonstrated convincingly the crucial importance of the MC4R in regulating food intake and energy homeostasis in rodents. The agonist α-MSH is expressed in neurons in the arcuate nucleus that coexpress leptin receptor and cocaine and amphetamine regulated transcript, whereas the antagonist AgRP is expressed in neurons in the arcuate nucleus that coexpress the leptin receptor and neuropeptide Y. These neurons project to the paraventricular nucleus, which abundantly expresses MC4R. AgRP expression is elevated in situations of negative energy balance and in the hypothalamus of *obese* and *diabetic* mice *(5–7)*, supporting a role for AgRP and MC4R in the regulation of feeding.

Pharmacologic studies also highlighted the importance of MC4R in regulating energy balance. Administration of the MC3/4R agonist melanotan II (a cyclic heptapeptide) into brain ventricles of rodents suppressed food intake and decreased body weight *(8, 9)*, and the MC3/4R antagonist SHU 9119 stimulated feeding and reversed the suppressive effects of melanotan II on food intake *(8)*. AgRP increases feeding and can antagonize the effect of α-MSH on food intake *(10)*. In addition to the arcuate and paraventricular nuclei as the possible sites of action for these melanocortin analogues, the brain stem, which has the highest expression of MC4R in the brain *(11)*, may also be involved in the control of feeding *(12)*.

Mouse genetic studies similarly showed the critical importance of the melanocortin circuit in regulating energy homeostasis. POMC knockout mice are obese; they also have defective adrenal gland development due to lack of MC2R signaling and altered pigmentation due to lack of MC1R signaling *(13)*. The agouti (A^y) mice, which overexpress agouti ectopically in the hypothalamus, are also obese, because agouti is a competitive antagonist of the MC4R *(14)*. Overexpression of AgRP also results in obesity *(6, 15)*. Finally, mice lacking MC4R had increased food intake and body weight, increased linear growth, and hyperinsulinemia *(16)*. Heterozygous mice have intermediate body weight, suggesting that one allele is not enough to maintain normal body weight.

NATURALLY OCCURRING MUTATIONS IN THE MC4R GENE AND HUMAN OBESITY

The melanocortin system is also critical in regulating energy balance in humans. This is clearly demonstrated by experiments of nature in which mutations in multiple molecules of the circuit, including leptin *(17, 18)*, leptin receptor *(19)*, POMC *(20)*, prohormone convertase 1 *(21)*, and MC4R, all result in severe early-onset obesity (reviewed in Ref. 22). Essentially, human genetic studies replicated the rodent genetic studies. For example, mutations in the POMC gene in humans result in the same phenotypes as in POMC knockout mice, including severe early-onset obesity, adrenal insufficiency, and red hair pigmentation.

In 1998, the first frameshift mutations in the MC4R gene were reported to be associated with severe early-onset obesity *(23, 24)*. Since then, about 80 mutations have been reported in numerous patient cohorts, including German, French, British, Swedish, Spanish, Caucasian American, African American, Japanese, and Chinese *(25–49)*. These mutations include frameshift, in-frame deletion, nonsense, and missense mutations, scattered throughout the MC4R (Fig. 3.1). Up to 6% of early-onset morbidly obese patients in some cohorts harbor MC4R mutations *(29)*, therefore mutations in the MC4R gene are likely to be the most common monogenic form of early-onset severe obesity. However, in some studies, very low frequency or no pathogenic mutations were identified *(34, 43, 50)*.

Although so many distinct mutations were reported following the two original reports, only an association rather than a causal relationship could be demonstrated in many of the earlier reports because functional analyses of the mutant receptors were not performed. Recently, detailed functional characterizations were performed on some of the mutant MC4Rs. These studies addressed two important questions: 1) Do these mutations result in loss-of-function therefore pathogenic for obesity? 2) What are the molecular defects in the loss-of-function mutants? These studies are briefly summarized here. A more detailed review has recently been published *(51)*.

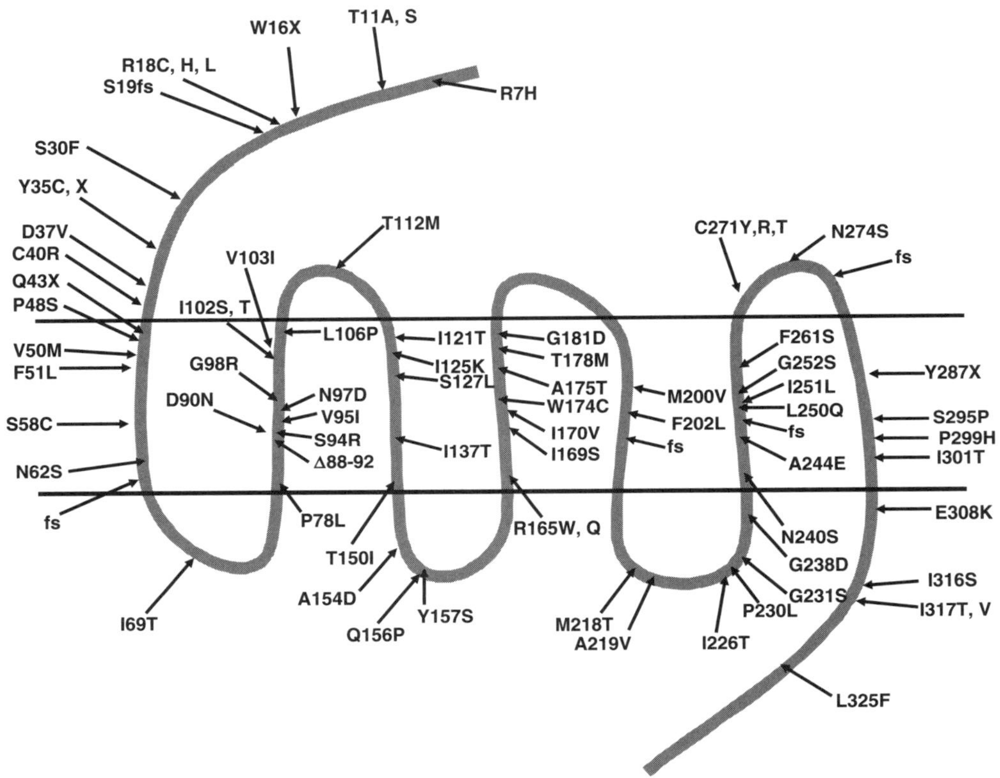

Fig. 3.1 The 80 naturally occurring MC4R mutations identified so far from various patient cohorts. Shown are their approximate locations in the snake plot. (Modified with permission from Tao YX. Molecular mechanisms of the neural melanocortin receptor dysfunction in severe early-onset obesity. Mol Cell Endocrinol 2005;239:1–14. Copyright © 2005, Elsevier.).

Functional Characterizations of the MC4R Mutations Identified from Obese Patients

MC4R is known to activate Gs after ligand binding, therefore resulting in increased intracellular cAMP levels. Measurement of intracellular cAMP directly or indirectly after agonist stimulation can ascertain whether a mutant is defective in signaling. If a mutant is defective in signaling, further studies are needed to identify the molecular defects. Defective protein synthesis, intracellular trafficking, ligand binding, and receptor activation all can cause defects in signaling. Even if the signaling is normal, it is still important to study the cell surface expression and ligand binding because of the existence of spare receptors in the transient expression system frequently used (see below).

In our studies, we used direct measurement of cAMP levels by radioimmunoassay to measure signaling properties of the mutant MC4Rs. In cells transfected with wild-type MC4R, the superpotent agonist [Nle^4,D-Phe^7]-α-MSH (NDP-MSH) increased intracellular cAMP levels in a dose-dependent manner *(52)*. Some mutant receptors have either decreased or absent signaling in response to NDP-MSH stimulation. Ligand binding studies showed that many of these mutants have either decreased or absent binding to iodinated NDP-MSH. To investigate whether these mutant receptors are expressed on the cell surface, confocal microscopy studies were performed on cells stably transfected with wild-type or mutant MC4Rs. In stably transfected cells, wild-type MC4R was expressed on the cell surface, although intracellular staining could also be observed. The mutant receptors that have decreased or absent binding were shown to have decreased or absent cell surface expression. In permeabilized cells, intracellular staining could be observed, suggesting that mutant receptors were expressed but retained intracellularly *(52)*.

Of the naturally occurring mutations in GPCRs that cause human diseases, intracellular retention is the most common defect for loss-of-function phenotype. This has been observed in numerous GPCRs, including rhodopsin, the V2 vasopressin receptor (V2R), the endothelin B receptor, the calcium-sensing receptor, the gonadotropin-releasing hormone receptor, the gonadotropin receptors, and the thyrotropin receptor (reviewed in Ref. 53). Any perturbations in the complex process of the folding of GPCRs will result in misfolded receptor detected by the cell's quality control system and prevented from exiting the endoplasmic reticulum *(54)*. Indeed, exiting the endoplasmic reticulum is the rate-limiting step in the receptor's maturation as demonstrated in δ-opioid receptor *(55)*. In rare cases, a mutation might specifically disrupt a motif important for cell surface targeting resulting in intracellular retention. For example, disruption of a dileucine motif at the proximal C-terminus was found to disrupt trafficking of the MC4R *(56)*.

Molecular Classification of Inactivating MC4R Mutations

Multiple defects in MC4R mutants were identified from the recent functional studies. We proposed the following scheme, modeled after the classification of mutations in low density lipoprotein (LDL) receptor and cystic fibrosis transmembrane conductance regulator *(57, 58)*, for classifying MC4R mutations *(52)* as schematically shown in Figure 3.2.

Class I: Null mutants. Due to defective protein synthesis and/or accelerated protein degradation, no receptor proteins are present in the cell. We speculate that nonsense mutants such as W16X, Y35X, Q43X, and L64X might belong to this class *(52)*. Expression studies are needed to confirm or refute this prediction experimentally.

Class II: Intracellularly retained mutants. The mutant receptors are produced but cannot be transported to the cell surface. This class comprises the largest set of MC4R mutations reported to date, including the frameshift mutations ΔCTCT at codon 211 and the TGAT insertion at codon 244 *(59)*, and Δ750-751GA *(38)*, S58C *(37, 52)*, N62S *(49, 52)*, P78L *(37, 52, 60)*, N97D *(49)*, G98R *(52)*, I102S *(37)*, L106P and I125K *(49)*, R165Q *(60)*, R165W *(37, 60)*, N240S *(60a)*, L250Q *(37)*, Y287X *(49)*, C271R *(46)*, C271Y *(49, 52)*, P299H *(37)*, I316S *(49)*, and I317T *(37, 56)*. Figure 3.3 shows examples of mutants (S58C, N62S, P78L, G98R, Y157S, and C271Y) that are expressed but are retained intracellularly.

Class III. Binding defective mutants. These mutant MC4Rs are expressed on the cell surface but are defective in ligand binding per se, with either decreased binding capacity and/or affinity, resulting in impairments in hormone-stimulated signaling. These mutants include N97D, L106P, I125K *(49)*, I137T *(31)*, I316S *(49)*, and Δ88-92 *(27)* (Fig. 3.4). We recently showed that I102S and I102T have partial defect in NDP-MSH binding *(60a)*. They are expressed on cell surface but have little or no binding.

Class IV. Signaling defective mutants. These mutant MC4Rs are expressed on the cell surface, bind ligand with normal affinity, but are defective in agonist-stimulated signaling

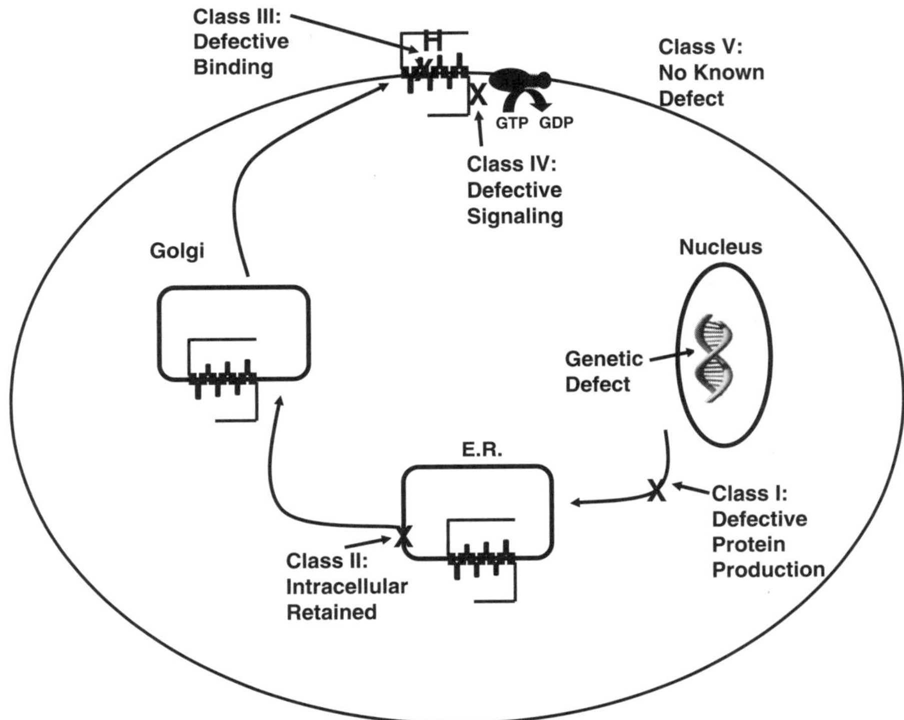

Fig. 3.2 Molecular classification of naturally occurring MC4R mutations in early-onset severe obesity. (Reprinted with permission from Tao YX. Molecular mechanisms of the neural melanocortin receptor dysfunction in severe early-onset obesity. Mol Cell Endocrinol 2005;239:1–14. Copyright © 2005, Elsevier.).

(decreased efficacy and/or potency). Mutants D90N *(25)*, I137T *(31)*, A175T and V253I *(49)* likely belong to this class.

Class V. Variants with apparently normal functions. These variants behave similarly as the wild-type MC4R in vitro in multiple functional assays. Some variants, such as T11A, Y35C, D37V, C40R, P48S, V50M, F51L, A154D, I170V, M200V, M218T, N274S, and S295P, exhibit normal cell surface expression, ligand binding, and agonist-stimulated cAMP production *(43, 60a, 52)*. Figure 3.3 shows examples of mutants (P48S, I170V, and N274S) that are expressed normally on the cell surface. Whether and how these variants cause energy imbalance and therefore obesity is unclear.

We recently identified three novel variants from obese Chinese subjects *(43)*. These variants are Y35C, C40R, and M218T. Although originally Y35C and M218T were identified from obese subjects, family studies showed that they do not cosegregate with the variants. The family of C40R could not be followed. More extensive screening in normal weight controls showed that Y35C occurs in similar frequency in normal weight and control subjects. Functional studies showed that all three variants have normal functions *(43)*. All these data showed that the novel variants are likely not the cause of obesity in the probands. It is important to recognize that environmental factors are also important for the pathogenesis of obesity. It is naïve to conclude that any variants identified from obese subjects are the cause of obesity.

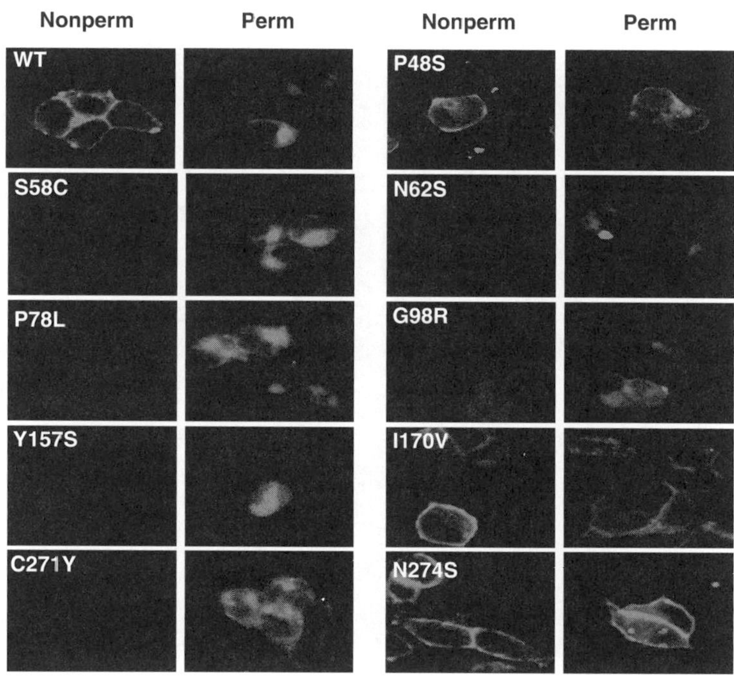

Fig. 3.3 Examples of mutants belonging to class II and class V. Mutants S58C, N62S, P78L, G98R, Y157S, and C271Y are class II mutants. They are retained intracellularly. Mutants P48S, I170V, and N274S are expressed on cell surface and function normally and belong to class V. (Reprinted with permission from Tao YX, Segaloff DL. Functional characterization of melanocortin-4 receptor mutations associated with childhood obesity. Endocrinology 2003;144:4544–4551. Copyright © 2003, The Endocrine Society.). (*see* Color Plate 1)

It is important to recognize that there are spare receptors in the transient expression systems currently used. For example, mutants such as S58C and I102T, with only 15–20% of wild-type binding capacity, have similar maximal response as wild-type MC4R *(60a, 52)*. In the arcuate nucleus, there are likely no spare receptors as suggested by the fact that heterozygous mutations of the MC4R cause obesity by haploinsufficiency. To avoid reaching an erroneous conclusion, it is important to measure cell surface expression, ligand binding, and signaling. Some mutants might be defective in cell surface expression and have decreased binding capacity but still have normal maximal response. If only the signaling is measured, these mutants will be erroneously considered as having normal functions.

Because most of the patients harboring MC4R mutations are heterozygous, an important question is whether obesity results from haploinsufficiency or dominant negative activity exerted by the mutant receptor. Co-transfection studies showed that most of the mutants do not have dominant negative activity *(30, 49, 59)*. The only mutation that has been shown to have dominant negative activity is the D90N mutation in which the most conserved Asp in TM2 was mutated to Asn *(25)*.

It is still unknown why most of the MC4R mutants that have been co-transfected with wild-type MC4R do not exert dominant negative activity. All the co-transfection studies were done in transient transfections, and the majority of the mutants are

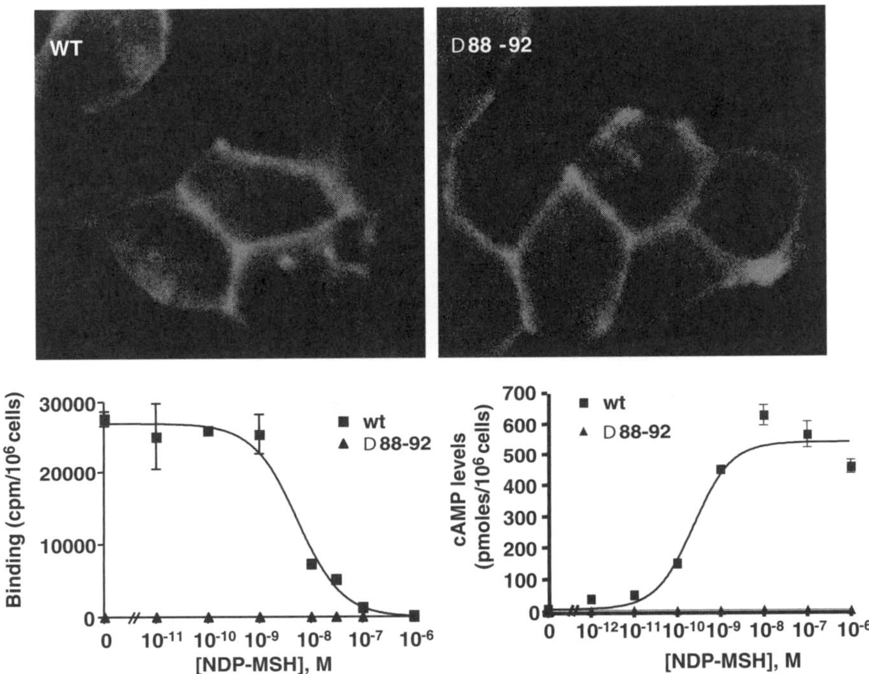

Fig. 3.4 Mutant Δ88-92 belongs to class III. Δ88-92 is expressed on cell surface but cannot bind to the ligand or signal. (Reprinted with permission from Donohoue PA, Tao YX, Collins M, Yeo GSH, O'Rahilly S, Segaloff DL. Deletion of codons 88–92 of the melanocortin-4 receptor gene: a novel deleterious mutation in an obese female. J Clin Endocrinol Metab 2003;88:5841–5845. Copyright © 2003, The Endocrine Society.). (*see* Color Plate 2)

intracellularly retained. Previous studies in other GPCRs have shown that in transient transfections, intracellularly retained mutant receptors decrease cell surface expression of co-transfected wild-type receptors *(61–64)*.

THERAPEUTIC IMPLICATIONS

Different approaches can be devised to treat obese patients with different classes of mutations. There are several nonsense and frameshift mutations in the MC4R that truncate the receptor prematurely. Previous studies showed that aminoglycoside antibiotics, by binding to the decoding site on the ribosome, could decrease the codon-anticodon proofreading efficiency resulting in read-through of the premature stop codon. A number of studies have explored the use of aminoglycosides as a therapeutic approach in treating diseases caused by premature terminations. For example, extensive studies in cystic fibrosis were performed, and very promising clinical results were obtained *(65)*. Similarly, studies in muscular dystrophy *(66)*, hemophilia *(67)*, ataxia-telangiectasia *(68)*, and spinal muscular atrophy *(69)* have all shown the feasibility of this approach.

In GPCRs, Schoneberg and colleagues investigated the potential of aminoglycoside antibiotics in treating nephrogenic diabetes insipidus caused by nonsense V2R mutations *(70, 71)*. It was shown that geneticin can rescue nonsense V2R mutations such as W200X, E242X, and R337X in vitro by increasing cell surface expression of full-length receptor and signaling capacity of the read-through receptor. In vivo, geneticin treatment in the transgenic mice expressing E242X increases urine osmolality in both normal and challenged conditions, suggesting that geneticin can partially rescue the nonsense mutation *(70)*. Whether aminoglycosides can induce read-through in MC4R nonsense mutations (such as W16X, Y35X, Q43X, and L64X) is worth investigating.

Because many of the loss-of-function mutations in the MC4R are retained intracellularly, obesity caused by these mutations can be considered as a trafficking disease. Studies in other protein trafficking diseases such as cystic fibrosis and nephrogenic diabetes insipidus have identified approaches of increasing cell surface expression of the mutant proteins in vitro. For example, treating the cells with chemical chaperones such as glycerol and DMSO increases the cell surface expression of the most common mutation (ΔF508) in the cystic fibrosis transmembrane conductance regulator gene that causes cystic fibrosis *(72, 73)*. In GPCRs, some of the mutations in V2R that cause nephrogenic diabetes insipidus also result in the mutant receptor trapped intracellularly *(74)*. Bouvier and colleagues were the first to identify small-molecule analogues that can cross the cell membrane and act as pharmacologic chaperones, increasing the cell surface expression of the mutant V2Rs *(75)*. Similar results were achieved subsequently in δ-opioid receptor *(76)*, μ-opioid receptor *(77)*, gonadotropin-releasing hormone receptor *(78)*, and the prototypical GPCR, rhodopsin *(79, 80)*. Indeed, it was shown that treatment of nephrogenic diabetes insipidus patients with the nonpeptide antagonist SR49059 decreased urine volume and water intake *(81)*.

AgRP, the endogenous antagonist of MC4R, has been shown to be an inverse agonist of the MC4R *(82, 83)*. Previous studies showed that inverse agonists could increase cell surface expression of constitutively active receptors (see Ref. 84 for an example). Because MC4R has constitutive activity, AgRP or its analogue might be able to enhance MC4R expression. Indeed, it was shown that the C-terminal fragment of AgRP could increase the cell surface expression of MC4R *(85)*. It will be of great interest to identify small-molecule agonists and antagonists that might act as pharmacological chaperones. The fact that some mutants, such as N62S, I102S, Y157S, and C271Y, can respond to NDP-MSH stimulation with increased cAMP production in spite of minimal binding capacity (less than 5% of wild type) *(51, 52)* suggests that these mutants are competent in G protein coupling and effector activation. Increasing their expression through pharmacological chaperones can be of therapeutic value.

Pharmacological chaperones cannot be used to treat mutants that are transported to the plasma membrane but are defective in ligand binding or G protein coupling/activation. If the mutant receptor is defective in ligand binding or signaling for the natural or superpotent agonists used in the functional studies or in clinics, it might be possible to design new agonists the can activate the mutant receptors. Therefore, it may prove fruitful to test those mutant receptors for binding to other ligands. A mutant receptor may be defective in binding to one ligand but not the others. For example, O'Rahilly and colleagues identified a MC4R mutation (I316S) that alters the relative affinities of the receptor for its endogenous agonist (α-MSH) and antagonist agouti-related protein *(49)*. A proof of principal of this strategy was shown in the lutropin (LH) receptor (LHR). A patient was found to have a mutation that results in deletion of exon 10 *(86)*. He presented with normal male development sustained by human chorionic gonadotropin (hCG) stimulation of fetal LHR during the fetal period. But as an adult, due to defective LH action, he was unable to initiate pubertal development and had hypogonadism (small testes and very low testosterone level) although he had high serum LH level. Functional analysis of the mutant receptor showed that it signals to hCG stimulation normally but failed to signal in response to LH stimulation *(87, 88)*. In the clinic, treatment with hCG was found to increase serum testosterone levels and testicular volumes and enhance spermatogenesis *(86)*. It remains to be seen whether we can identify analogues that can bind to and activate MC4R mutants defective in binding the natural ligands.

CONCLUSION

During the past few years, about 80 mutations in the MC4R gene have been identified with new mutations continuing to be identified. Functional studies of these mutants identified multiple defects, including cell surface expression, ligand binding, and signaling. Nonsense mutations might cause decreased expression of the mutant receptors. Some variants have normal functions therefore might not be pathogenic for obesity or other disorders such as binge eating disorder. Detailed functional studies are necessary to bridge the clinical studies identifying an association of the mutation with obesity or other disorders to a causative relationship. In addition, the identification of the exact defect is necessary for personalized treatment of mutation-harboring patients. We highlighted several potential therapeutic approaches, including aminoglycosides, pharmacological chaperones, and novel ligands, for personalized medicine.

REFERENCES

1. Cummings DE, Schwartz MW. Genetics and pathophysiology of human obesity. Annu Rev Med 2003;54:453–471.
2. Schwartz MW, Woods SC, Porte D Jr, Seeley RJ, Baskin DG. Central nervous system control of food intake. Nature 2000;404:661–671.
3. Smith AI, Funder JW. Proopiomelanocortin processing in the pituitary, central nervous system, and peripheral tissues. Endocr Rev 1988;9:159–179.
4. Gantz I, Fong TM. The melanocortin system. Am J Physiol 2003;284:E468–E474.
5. Mizuno TM, Mobbs CV. Hypothalamic agouti-related protein messenger ribonucleic acid is inhibited by leptin and stimulated by fasting. Endocrinology 1999;140:814–817.
6. Ollmann MM, Wilson BD, Yang YK, Kerns JA, Chen Y, Gantz I, Barsh GS. Antagonism of central melanocortin receptors in vitro and in vivo by agouti-related protein. Science 1997;278:135–138.
7. Shutter JR, Graham M, Kinsey AC, Scully S, Luthy R, Stark KL. Hypothalamic expression of ART, a novel gene related to agouti, is up-regulated in obese and diabetic mutant mice. Genes Dev 1997;11:593–602.
8. Fan W, Boston BA, Kesterson RA, Hruby VJ, Cone RD. Role of melanocortinergic neurons in feeding and the agouti obesity syndrome. Nature 1997;385:165–168.
9. Thiele TE, van Dijk G, Yagaloff KA, Fisher SL, Schwartz M, Burn P, Seeley RJ. Central infusion of melanocortin agonist MTII in rats: assessment of c-Fos expression and taste aversion. Am J Physiol 1998;274:R248–R254.
10. Rossi M, Kim MS, Morgan DG, et al. A C-terminal fragment of Agouti-related protein increases feeding and antagonizes the effect of alpha-melanocyte stimulating hormone *in vivo*. Endocrinology 1998;139:4428–4431.

11. Mountjoy KG, Mortrud MT, Low MJ, Simerly RB, Cone RD. Localization of the melanocortin-4 receptor (MC4-R) in neuroendocrine and autonomic control circuits in the brain. Mol Endocrinol 1994;8:1298–1308.
12. Grill HJ, Ginsberg AB, Seeley RJ, Kaplan JM. Brainstem application of melanocortin receptor ligands produces long-lasting effects on feeding and body weight. J Neurosci 1998;18:10128–10135.
13. Yaswen L, Diehl N, Brennan MB, Hochgeschwender U. Obesity in the mouse model of pro-opiomelanocortin deficiency responds to peripheral melanocortin. Nat Med 1999;5:1066–1070.
14. Lu D, Willard D, Patel IR, et al. Agouti protein is an antagonist of the melanocyte-stimulating-hormone receptor. Nature 1994;371:799–802.
15. Graham M, Shutter JR, Sarmiento U, Sarosi I, Stark KL. Overexpression of Agrt leads to obesity in transgenic mice. Nat Genet 1997;17:273–274.
16. Huszar D, Lynch CA, Fairchild-Huntress V, et al. Targeted disruption of the melanocortin-4 receptor results in obesity in mice. Cell 1997;88:131–141.
17. Montague CT, Farooqi IS, Whitehead JP, et al. Congenital leptin deficiency is associated with severe early-onset obesity in humans. Nature 1997;387:903–908.
18. Strobel A, Issad T, Camoin L, Ozata M, Strosberg AD. A leptin missense mutation associated with hypogonadism and morbid obesity. Nat Genet 1998;18:213–215.
19. Clement K, Vaisse C, Lahlou N, et al. A mutation in the human leptin receptor gene causes obesity and pituitary dysfunction. Nature 1998; 392:398–401.
20. Krude H, Biebermann H, Luck W, Horn R, Brabant G, Gruters A. Severe early-onset obesity, adrenal insufficiency and red hair pigmentation caused by POMC mutations in humans. Nat Genet 1998;19:155–157.
21. Jackson RS, Creemers JW, Ohagi S, et al. Obesity and impaired prohormone processing associated with mutations in the human prohormone convertase 1 gene. Nat Genet 1997;16:303–306.
22. O'Rahilly S, Farooqi IS, Yeo GS, Challis BG. Minireview: human obesity-lessons from monogenic disorders. Endocrinology 2003;144:3757–3764.
23. Vaisse C, Clement K, Guy-Grand B, Froguel P. A frameshift mutation in human MC4R is associated with a dominant form of obesity. Nat Genet 1998;20:113–114.
24. Yeo GS, Farooqi IS, Aminian S, Halsall DJ, Stanhope RG, O'Rahilly S. A frameshift mutation in MC4R associated with dominantly inherited human obesity. Nat Genet 1998;20:111–112.
25. Biebermann H, Krude H, Elsner A, Chubanov V, Gudermann T, Gruters A. Autosomal-dominant mode of inheritance of a melanocortin-4 receptor mutation in a patient with severe early-onset obesity is due to a dominant-negative effect caused by receptor dimerization. Diabetes 2003;52:2984–2988.
26. Buono P, Pasanisi F, Nardelli C, et al. Six novel mutations in the proopiomelanocortin and melanocortin receptor 4 genes in severely obese adults living in southern Italy. Clin Chem 2005;51:1358–1364.
27. Donohoue PA, Tao YX, Collins M, Yeo GSH, O'Rahilly S, Segaloff DL. Deletion of codons 88-92 of the melanocortin-4 receptor gene: a novel deleterious mutation in an obese female. J Clin Endocrinol Metab 2003;88:5841–5845.
28. Dubern B, Clement K, Pelloux V, Froguel P, Girardet JP, Guy-Grand B, Tounian P. Mutational analysis of melanocortin-4 receptor, agouti-related protein, and α-melanocyte-stimulating hormone genes in severely obese children. J Pediatr 2001;139:204–209.
29. Farooqi IS, Keogh JM, Yeo GS, Lank EJ, Cheetham T, O'Rahilly S. Clinical spectrum of obesity and mutations in the melanocortin 4 receptor gene. N Engl J Med 2003;348:1085–1095.
30. Farooqi IS, Yeo GS, Keogh JM, et al. Dominant and recessive inheritance of morbid obesity associated with melanocortin 4 receptor deficiency. J Clin Invest 2000;106:271–279.
31. Gu W, Tu Z, Kleyn PW, et al. Identification and functional analysis of novel human melanocortin-4 receptor variants. Diabetes 1999;48:635–639.

32. Hinney A, Hohmann S, Geller F, et al. Melanocortin-4 receptor gene: case-control study and transmission disequilibrium test confirm that functionally relevant mutations are compatible with a major gene effect for extreme obesity. J Clin Endocrinol Metab 2003;88:4258–4267.
33. Hinney A, Schmidt A, Nottebom K, et al. Several mutations in the melanocortin-4 receptor gene including a nonsense and a frameshift mutation associated with dominantly inherited obesity in humans. J Clin Endocrinol Metab 1999;84:1483–1486.
34. Jacobson P, Ukkola O, Rankinen T, et al. Melanocortin 4 receptor sequence variations are seldom a cause of human obesity: the Swedish Obese Subjects, the HERITAGE Family Study, and a Memphis cohort. J Clin Endocrinol Metab 2002;87:4442–4446.
35. Kobayashi H, Ogawa Y, Shintani M, et al. A novel homozygous missense mutation of melanocortin-4 receptor (MC4R) in a Japanese woman with severe obesity. Diabetes 2002;51:243–246.
36. Larsen LH, Echwald SM, Sorensen TI, Andersen T, Wulff BS, Pedersen O. Prevalence of mutations and functional analyses of melanocortin 4 receptor variants identified among 750 men with juvenile-onset obesity. J Clin Endocrinol Metab 2005;90:219–224.
37. Lubrano-Berthelier C, Durand E, Dubern B, et al. Intracellular retention is a common characteristic of childhood obesity-associated MC4R mutations. Hum Mol Genet 2003;12:145–153.
38. Lubrano-Berthelier C, Le Stunff C, Bougneres P, Vaisse C. A homozygous null mutation delineates the role of the melanocortin-4 receptor in humans. J Clin Endocrinol Metab 2004;89:2028–2032.
39. Ma L, Tataranni PA, Bogardus C, Baier LJ. Melanocortin 4 receptor gene variation is associated with severe obesity in Pima Indians. Diabetes 2004;53:2696–2699.
40. Marti A, Corbalan MS, Forga L, Martinez JA, Hinney A, Hebebrand J. A novel nonsense mutation in the melanocortin-4 receptor associated with obesity in a Spanish population. Int J Obes Relat Metab Disord 2003;27:385–388.
41. Mergen M, Mergen H, Ozata M, Oner R, Oner C. A novel melanocortin 4 receptor (MC4R) gene mutation associated with morbid obesity. J Clin Endocrinol Metab 2001:86:3448–3451.
42. Miraglia Del Giudice E, Cirillo G, Nigro V, et al. Low frequency of melanocortin-4 receptor (MC4R) mutations in a Mediterranean population with early-onset obesity. Int J Obes Relat Metab Disord 2002;26:647–651.
43. Rong R, Tao YX, Xu A, Cheung BMY, Cheung G, Lam KSL. Identification and characterization of three novel missense mutations of the human melanocortin-4 receptor gene in a Chinese obesity population. Clin Endocrinol (Oxf) 2006;65:198–205.
44. Santini F, Maffei M, Ceccarini G, et al. Genetic screening for melanocortin-4 receptor mutations in a cohort of Italian obese patients: description and functional characterization of a novel mutation. J Clin Endocrinol Metab 2004;89:904–908.
45. Shao XY, Jia WP, Cai SB, Fang QC, Zhang R, Lu JX, Xiang KS. Cloning and functional analysis of melanocortin 4 receptor mutation gene F261S. Zhonghua Yi Xue Za Zhi 2005;85:366–369.
46. Tarnow P, Schoneberg T, Krude H, Gruters A, Biebermann H. Mutationally induced disulfide bond formation within the third extracellular loop causes melanocortin 4 receptor inactivation in patients with obesity. J Biol Chem 2003;278:48666–48673.
47. Vaisse C, Clement K, Durand E, Hercberg S, Guy-Grand B, Froguel P. Melanocortin-4 receptor mutations are a frequent and heterogeneous cause of morbid obesity. J Clin Invest 2000;106:253–262.
48. Valli-Jaakola K, Lipsanen-Nyman M, Oksanen L, Hollenberg AN, Kontula K, Bjorbaek C, Schalin-Jantti C. Identification and characterization of melanocortin-4 receptor gene mutations in morbidly obese Finnish children and adults. J Clin Endocrinol Metab 2004;89:940–945.
49. Yeo GS, Lank EJ, Farooqi IS, Keogh J, Challis BG, O'Rahilly S. Mutations in the human melanocortin-4 receptor gene associated with severe familial obesity disrupts receptor function through multiple molecular mechanisms. Hum Mol Genet 2003;12:561–574.
50. Beckers S, Mertens I, Peeters A, Van Gaal L, Van Hul W. Screening for melanocortin-4 receptor mutations in a cohort of Belgian morbidly obese adults and children. Int J Obes (Lond) 2006;30:221–225.

51. Tao YX. Molecular mechanisms of the neural melanocortin receptor dysfunction in severe early-onset obesity. Mol Cell Endocrinol 2005;239:1–14.
52. Tao YX, Segaloff DL. Functional characterization of melanocortin-4 receptor mutations associated with childhood obesity. Endocrinology 2003;144:4544–4551.
53. Tao YX. Inactivating mutations of G protein-coupled receptors and diseases: structure-function insights and therapeutic implications. Pharmacol Ther 2006;111:949–973.
54. Ellgaard L, Helenius A. Quality control in the endoplasmic reticulum. Nat Rev Mol Cell Biol 2003;4:181–191.
55. Petaja-Repo UE, Hogue M, Laperriere A, Walker P, Bouvier M. Export from the endoplasmic reticulum represents the limiting step in the maturation and cell surface expression of the human delta opioid receptor. J Biol Chem 2000;275:13727–13736.
56. VanLeeuwen D, Steffey ME, Donahue C, Ho G, MacKenzie RG. Cell surface expression of the melanocortin-4 receptor is dependent on a C-terminal di-isoleucine sequence at codons 316/317. J Biol Chem 2003;278:15935–15940.
57. Hobbs HH, Russell DW, Brown MS, Goldstein JL. The LDL receptor locus in familial hypercholesterolemia: mutational analysis of a membrane protein. Annu Rev Genet 1990;24:133–170.
58. Welsh MJ, Smith AE. Molecular mechanisms of CFTR chloride channel dysfunction in cystic fibrosis. Cell 1993;73:1251–1254.
59. Ho G, MacKenzie RG. Functional characterization of mutations in melanocortin-4 receptor associated with human obesity. J Biol Chem 1999;274:35816–35822.
60. Nijenhuis WA, Garner KM, VanRozen RJ, Adan RA. Poor cell surface expression of human melanocortin-4 receptor mutations associated with obesity. J Biol Chem 2003;278:22939–22945.
60a. Tao YX, Segaloff DL. Functional analyses of melanocortin-4 receptor mutations identified from patients with binge eating disorder and nonobese or obese subjects. J Clin Endocrinol Metab 2005;90:5632–5638.
61. Benkirane M, Jin DY, Chun RF, Koup RA, Jeang KT. Mechanism of transdominant inhibition of CCR5-mediated HIV-1 infection by ccr5Δ32. J Biol Chem 1997;272:30603–30606.
62. Colley NJ, Cassill JA, Baker EK, Zuker CS. Defective intracellular transport is the molecular basis of rhodopsin-dependent dominant retinal degeneration. Proc Natl Acad Sci USA 1995;92:3070–3074.
63. Overton MC, Blumer KJ. G-protein-coupled receptors function as oligomers in vivo. Curr Biol 2000;10:341–344.
64. Tao YX, Johnson NB, Segaloff DL. Constitutive and agonist-dependent self-association of the cell surface human lutropin receptor. J Biol Chem 2004;279:5904–5914.
65. Wilschanski M, Yahav Y, Yaacov Y, et al. Gentamicin-induced correction of CFTR function in patients with cystic fibrosis and CFTR stop mutations. N Engl J Med 2003;349:1433–1441.
66. Barton-Davis ER, Cordier L, Shoturma DI, Leland SE, Sweeney HL. Aminoglycoside antibiotics restore dystrophin function to skeletal muscles of mdx mice. J Clin Invest 1999;104:375–381.
67. James PD, Raut S, Rivard GE, et al. Aminoglycoside suppression of nonsense mutations in severe hemophilia. Blood 2005;106:3043–3048.
68. Lai CH, Chun HH, Nahas SA, Mitui M, Gamo KM, Du L, Gatti RA. Correction of ATM gene function by aminoglycoside-induced read-through of premature termination codons. Proc Natl Acad Sci USA 2004;101:15676–15681.
69. Wolstencroft EC, Mattis V, Bajer AA, Young PJ, Lorson CL. A non-sequence-specific requirement for SMN protein activity: the role of aminoglycosides in inducing elevated SMN protein levels. Hum Mol Genet 2005;14:1199–1210.
70. Sangkuhl K, Schulz A, Rompler H, Yun J, Wess J, Schoneberg T. Aminoglycoside-mediated rescue of a disease-causing nonsense mutation in the V2 vasopressin receptor gene in vitro and in vivo. Hum Mol Genet 2004;13:893–903.

71. Schulz A, Sangkuhl K, Lennert T, et al. Aminoglycoside pretreatment partially restores the function of truncated V(2) vasopressin receptors found in patients with nephrogenic diabetes insipidus. J Clin Endocrinol Metab 2002;87:5247–5257.
72. Brown CR, Hong-Brown LQ, Biwersi J, Verkman AS, Welch WJ. Chemical chaperones correct the mutant phenotype of the delta F508 cystic fibrosis transmembrane conductance regulator protein. Cell Stress Chaperones 1996;1:117–125.
73. Sato S, Ward CL, Krouse ME, Wine JJ, Kopito RR. Glycerol reverses the misfolding phenotype of the most common cystic fibrosis mutation. J Biol Chem 1996;271:635–638.
74. Morello JP, Bichet DG. Nephrogenic diabetes insipidus. Annu Rev Physiol 2001:63: 607–630.
75. Morello JP, Salahpour A, Laperriere A, et al. Pharmacological chaperones rescue cell-surface expression and function of misfolded V2 vasopressin receptor mutants. J Clin Invest 2000;105: 887–895.
76. Petaja-Repo UE, Hogue M, Bhalla S, Laperriere A, Morello JP, Bouvier M. Ligands act as pharmacological chaperones and increase the efficiency of delta opioid receptor maturation. EMBO J 2002;21:1628–1637.
77. Chaipatikul V, Erickson-Herbrandson LJ, Loh HH, Law PY. Rescuing the traffic-deficient mutants of rat μ-opioid receptors with hydrophobic ligands. Mol Pharmacol 2003;64:32–41.
78. Janovick JA, Maya-Nunez G, Conn PM. Rescue of hypogonadotropic hypogonadism-causing and manufactured GnRH receptor mutants by a specific protein-folding template: misrouted proteins as a novel disease etiology and therapeutic target. J Clin Endocrinol Metab 2002;87:3255–3262.
79. Noorwez SM, Kuksa V, Imanishi Y, Zhu L, Filipek S, Palczewski K, Kaushal S. Pharmacological chaperone-mediated in vivo folding and stabilization of the P23H-opsin mutant associated with autosomal dominant retinitis pigmentosa. J Biol Chem 2003;278:14442–14450.
80. Noorwez SM, Malhotra R, McDowell JH, Smith KA, Krebs MP, Kaushal S. Retinoids assist the cellular folding of the autosomal dominant retinitis pigmentosa opsin mutant P23H. J Biol Chem 2004;279:16278–16284.
81. Bernier V, Morello JP, Zarruk A, et al. Pharmacologic chaperones as a potential treatment for X-linked nephrogenic diabetes insipidus. J Am Soc Nephrol 2006;17:232–243.
82. Haskell-Luevano C, Monck EK. Agouti-related protein functions as an inverse agonist at a constitutively active brain melanocortin-4 receptor. Regul Pept 2001;99:1–7.
83. Nijenhuis WA, Oosterom J, Adan RA. AgRP(83-132) acts as an inverse agonist on the human melanocortin-4 receptor. Mol Endocrinol 2001;15:164–171.
84. Lee TW, Cotecchia S, Milligan G. Up-regulation of the levels of expression and function of a constitutively active mutant of the hamster alpha1B-adrenoceptor by ligands that act as inverse agonists. Biochem J 1997;325:733–739.
85. Shinyama H, Masuzaki H, Fang H, Flier JS. Regulation of melanocortin-4 receptor signaling: agonist-mediated desensitization and internalization. Endocrinology 2003;144:1301–1314.
86. Gromoll J, Eiholzer U, Nieschlag E, Simoni M. Male hypogonadism caused by homozygous deletion of exon 10 of the luteinizing hormone (LH) receptor: differential action of human chorionic gonadotropin and LH. J Clin Endocrinol Metab 2000;85:2281–2286.
87. Muller T, Gromoll J, Simoni M. Absence of exon 10 of the human luteinizing hormone (LH) receptor impairs LH, but not human chorionic gonadotropin action. J Clin Endocrinol Metab 2003;88: 2242–2249.
88. Zhang FP, Kero J, Huhtaniemi I. The unique exon 10 of the human luteinizing hormone receptor is necessary for expression of the receptor protein at the plasma membrane in the human luteinizing hormone receptor, but deleterious when inserted into the human follicle-stimulating hormone receptor. Mol Cell Endocrinol 1998;142:165–174.

4 The Role of Central Melanocortins in Cachexia

Daniel L. Marks

CONTENTS

Abstract

Cachexia is a clinical syndrome of wasting that accompanies many chronic diseases including cancer, renal failure, and heart failure. This condition is marked by an increase in energy expenditure and preferential loss of lean body mass, creating a striking catabolic state. Cachexia contrasts with starvation, a state in which energy expenditure decreases and muscle mass is maintained while fat stores are consumed. In contrast, cachexia is accompanied by a paradoxical anorexia that occurs despite ongoing weight loss and negative calorie balance. This loss of appetite is a significant component of the decreased quality of life experienced by patients with cachexia. Few treatments have proved to be of significant benefit to patients suffering from cachexia. One new treatment that shows promise is pharmacologic blockade of the central melanocortin system. The importance of this system in maintaining normal body weight in humans is highlighted by the finding that disordered melanocortin signaling results in early-onset morbid obesity and dramatic increases in lean body mass in humans. Emerging evidence suggests that blocking this system via pharmacologic antagonists to the type 4 melanocortin receptor (MC4R) may restore appetite and lean body mass in subjects with cachexia caused by a variety of underlying disorders. This review will focus on current pathophysiologic mechanisms involved in cachexia and will outline the central melanocortin pathway as pertaining to these diseases and summarize early animal data using MC4R antagonists to treat cachexia.

Key Words: cachexia, cytokine, hypothalamus, inflammation, melanocortin.

From: *Contemporary Endocrinology: Energy Metabolism and Obesity: Research and Clinical Applications*
Edited by: P. A. Donohoue © Humana Press Inc., Totowa, NJ

INTRODUCTION

Cachexia is a clinical entity that has been described in the medical literature for centuries. Indeed, Hippocrates described all of the salient features of this metabolic disorder more than 2,400 years ago, and the term itself is derived from the ancient Greek terms *kakos* and *hexis*, which translate into the phrase "bad condition" *(1)*. The hallmark features of cachexia are relative anorexia, an increased basal metabolic rate, and a global wasting of lean body mass. Unfortunately, this condition is found in numerous chronic disease states and not only impairs quality of life but also strongly predicts mortality and limits therapeutic options (*2–5*). For example, in AIDS, wasting of 5–10% of body weight more than doubles mortality, making this the strongest predictor of mortality in this condition *(6)*. In chronic congestive heart failure, up to 15% of patients exhibit some degree of cachexia, whereas in renal failure this number approaches 40% *(7, 8)*. In both of these conditions, cachexia also strongly predicts poor outcome and mortality *(7, 9)*. Perhaps the most obvious and dramatic cachexia occurs in patients with cancer, and this not only predicts mortality but also often limits therapeutic options for treatment of the underlying disease *(10)*.

In spite of this long history and clinical impact, the physiologic mechanisms involved in the development of cachexia remain unclear. At this point, most investigations point toward the elaboration of proinflammatory cytokines into the circulation as being the most important initiating event *(11, 12)*. Several proinflammatory cytokines have been implicated in the initiation and maintenance of a cachectic state. In particular, evidence exists supporting the role of interleukin-1β (IL-1β), interleukin-6 (IL-6), tumor necrosis factor-α (TNF-α), and leukemia inhibitory factor (LIF) in this process (*13–15*). Indeed, there is sound clinical data linking elevations in various combinations of these cytokines to wasting and mortality in AIDS, cancer, heart failure, cystic fibrosis, rheumatoid arthritis, and renal failure (*9,10,16–21*).

It is now also widely accepted that although these cytokines may produce some of their effects by acting in the periphery, the central nervous system (CNS) is a critical site of action of cytokines in the development of cachexia (*22–24*). Indeed, numerous cytokine receptors are expressed in brain regions known to regulate appetite and metabolic rate, and central nervous system (CNS) injections of various proinflammatory cytokines can produce all of the features of cachexia, even at very small doses (*25–27*). As discussed below, we are now beginning to understand the specific neuronal systems involved in transducing the cytokine signal, and this knowledge is directing the search for new therapies. The need for new therapies is acute, as the currently available treatment modalities are of limited clinical utility. Initially, treatment strategies focused on increasing nutrient intake, by either enteral or parenteral means. However, these strategies proved to be unable to overcome the anorexia, increased metabolic rate, and altered fuel partitioning found in cachectic patients *(28)*. Glucocorticoids produce weight gain and improvement in quality of life scores, but they do not improve strength or lean body mass and are associated with numerous unwanted side effects typical of iatrogenic Cushing syndrome *(29)*. The most widely used agent in cachexia, megestrol acetate, produces similar results and may in fact exert many of its effects via binding to the glucocorticoid receptor *(30, 31)*. Other agents such as growth hormone and androgens have proved useful in selected situations, but the prohibitive cost and known side effects make their widespread use for this condition an untenable option. Thus, the need to search for new therapeutic options is obvious, and this search needs to be guided by the burgeoning new body of information regarding the regulation of body weight and body composition. This chapter will focus on a growing body of evidence that blockade of anorexigenic neural pathways may provide a novel and effective therapeutic option for cachexia.

CYTOKINE ACTION IN THE CENTRAL NERVOUS SYSTEM

The concept that inflammatory cytokines exert their effects, at least in part, by acting on feeding centers in the hypothalamus is derived from many sources. In fact, neurons and glia within the hypothalamus respond to proinflammatory stimuli by initiating the production of many of these cytokines, and this production is most notable in nuclei known to be directly involved in the regulation of food intake and metabolic rate (*32–35*). Furthermore, the receptors for these cytokines are found throughout the CNS, including in feeding centers in the hypothalamus and brain stem (*36–39*). Neurons in these same brain areas are also known to be activated during inflammation, as evidenced by the induction of markers of neuronal activation including c-Fos and nuclear factor kappa B (NF-κB) in these cells *(40,41)*. Finally, cytokines are known to have a much more potent effect on food intake and metabolic rate when injected centrally rather than peripherally and do not need to exceed normal pathophysiologic concentrations in the brain to achieve these effects *(26)*.

THE ARCUATE NUCLEUS

The arcuate nucleus (ARC) (also known as the infundibular nucleus in humans) has been known to be an important hypothalamic center for body weight regulation for decades, dating back to classic lesioning studies performed in the 1940s *(42,43)*. The importance of this nucleus in the tonic restraint on food intake and weight gain is also obvious in humans as damage to this area during tumor resection (e.g., during resection of a craniopharyngioma) often leads to severe hyperphagia and obesity *(44)*. Because the ARC occupies the highly vascular space between the floor of the third ventricle and the median eminence, it is thought to have an attenuated blood-brain barrier and therefore to have access to numerous circulating molecules *(45)*. It is well-known, for example, that neurons in this nucleus respond to a large variety of hormones including insulin, ghrelin, leptin, and other peptide hormones (*45–47*). The ARC also has extensive reciprocal connections with other hypothalamic nuclei, many of which are known to play a role in various physiologic responses to illness. It is also important to point out that this nucleus is known to express receptors for several proinflammatory cytokines (e.g., IL-1β, TNF-α, and LIF), raising the possibility that it provides an essential conduit for these molecules to produce various illness behaviors and metabolic changes typical of cachexia *(37,39,48,49)*.

THE ROLE OF THE CENTRAL MELANOCORTIN SYSTEM IN THE REGULATION OF FEEDING AND METABOLIC RATE

Pro-opiomelanocortin (POMC) is a propeptide precursor that is produced in neurons found in the ARC *(50)*. POMC neurons provide a critical tonic restraint on food intake and energy storage, primarily by cleaving POMC into α-melanocyte stimulating hormone (α-MSH) that in turn acts as a peptide neurotransmitter within the CNS. α-MSH binds to specific melanocortin receptors [including the type 4 melanocortin receptor (MC4R) and the type 3 melanocortin receptor (MC3R)] that are expressed in numerous hypothalamic nuclei and in other areas of the brain *(51,52)*. Whereas the role of MC3R in energy balance remains somewhat obscure, a great deal is now known about the role of MC4R. Experimental administration of MC4-R agonists inhibits food intake and stimulates metabolic rate, whereas administration of antagonists or genetic disruption of this receptor leads to overgrowth and obesity *(53,54)*. The importance of this receptor in body weight regulation in humans was first suggested by studies of two separate families with dominantly inherited obesity linked to a heterozygous frameshift mutation in the MC4R gene *(55,56)*. Subsequent studies have confirmed these findings and have gone on to demonstrate that mutations in this receptor account for nearly 5% of all childhood-onset obesity, making this the most common monogenic form of obesity described to date *(57)*. Collectively, the data in humans and in animals strongly support the idea that MC4R plays an important role in the regulation of food intake, basal metabolic rate, and the accumulation and maintenance of both lean body mass and fat mass. The fact that this receptor also plays a role in the central regulation of insulin release also suggests that it has important effects on nutrient partitioning *(58)*.

Agouti-Related Peptide

One unique feature of the central melanocortin system is the existence of a potent and highly regulated endogenous antagonist, agouti-related peptide (AgRP). AgRP fibers project to many of the same nuclei innervated by α-MSH, although there are also many MC4R expressing sites (particularly in the brain stem) that only receive α-MSH input *(59)*. Whereas the synthesis and release of α-MSH is thought to be relatively stable, its activity at the MC4R can be greatly modified by the action of AgRP, and the expression of AgRP is itself highly responsive to nutritional status *(60,61)*. As would be expected for an orexigenic peptide, AgRP expression is stimulated by fasting and inhibited by overfeeding and by leptin *(62)*. The ability of AgRP to produce sustained increases in food intake, growth, and accumulation of body energy stores was demonstrated when ectopic expression of AgRP in transgenic mice was found to cause an obesity syndrome analogous to that seen in the MC4R knockout (KO) animal *(61)*.

The idea that an MC4R antagonist would be a useful drug in the treatment of cachexia is therefore very appealing. However, it is important to point out in this context that although AgRP clearly functions as an MC4R antagonist, it is difficult to explain all of the effects of AgRP with this simple explanation of its action. For example, a single intracerebroventricular (ICV) injection of AgRP into a rat can induce hyperphagia for as long as a week, an observation that is difficult to ascribe to simple receptor antagonism *(63)*. Indeed, animals injected with AgRP remain normally sensitive to injections of α-MSH on days subsequent to the initial AgRP injection, indicating that the antagonist is no longer bound to the receptor and that the ongoing hyperphagia may be due to other properties of AgRP, including its ability to act as an inverse agonist at the MC4R *(64)*. Thus, any drugs that are effective AgRP mimetics should be able to produce sustained increases in food intake and would not be expected to have their efficacy limited by receptor tachyphylaxis.

THE ROLE OF THE CENTRAL MELANOCORTIN SYSTEM IN CACHEXIA

As pointed out above, acute inflammation is known to induce c-Fos expression in the arcuate nucleus *(40, 65)*. More recent data have confirmed these findings and gone on to demonstrate that this marker of neuronal activation is robustly expressed in POMC neurons within this nucleus *(66)*. Furthermore, POMC gene expression is increased during acute inflammation, and the anorexic response to lipopolysaccharide (LPS) is attenuated in animals with relatively low POMC expression (i.e., in fasting animals) (*67–69*). Thus, it is reasonable to suggest that inflammation-induced anorexia is mediated by POMC neurons, and the degree of this anorexia is dependent on overall melanocortin tone. There is a growing body of experimental evidence that supports this argument and further suggests that the strategy of interfering with melanocortin signaling will be of benefit in the setting of cachexia. The first studies used LPS or IL-1β to study the impact of melanocortin blockade in the setting of acute inflammation. Huang et al. investigated the impact of central administration of α-MSH or the MC3/MC4R antagonist SHU-9119 on LPS-induced anorexia and fever in rats *(70)*. In this study, the investigators found a significant potentiation of the suppressive effects of LPS on food intake with the coadministration of α-MSH and a reversal of LPS-induced anorexia with SHU-9119 administration. In another study, investigators found that MC4R KO mice resist the inhibition of locomotion normally brought about by IL-1β administration *(71)*. Pharmacologic blockade of central melanocortin signaling has also been shown to dramatically attenuate the anorexic but not the pyrogenic actions of IL-1β infusions in a rat model *(72)*. After these initial publications, a series of studies demonstrated that blockade of the central MC4R by genetic or pharmacologic methods attenuated all measurable features of cachexia brought about by either LPS or cancer in murine models *(73, 74)*. It is particularly important that these studies were able to utilize serial dual energy x-ray absorptiometry (DEXA) scans to demonstrate that MC4R KO animals are able to continue to accumulate both lean mass and fat mass in the face of tumor growth and that tumor growth itself was not affected in these animals. These data were confirmed and extended in a rat cancer model in which it was demonstrated that melanocortin antagonists were able to reverse cancer anorexia whereas other known orexigenic compounds (ghrelin and neuropeptide Y) were not *(75)*. Finally, recent studies have demonstrated that both genetic and pharmacologic blockade of melanocortin signaling were shown to reverse the hypophagia, growth failure, and elevated basal metabolic rate in a murine model of chronic renal failure *(76)*. Given that approximately 40% of patients with chronic renal failure develop some degree of cachexia, this study is particularly exciting from a clinical perspective *(8)*. An overall summary of the proposed role of melanocortin signaling in chronic disease is shown in Figure 4.1.

Small-Molecule Synthetic Melanocortin Antagonists

Obviously, the studies outlined above are limited by the necessity of using genetic manipulation or an intracerebroventricular route of injection of antagonists to achieve the experimental outcome. Fortunately, several companies have produced small-molecule melanocortin antagonists, and these compounds appear to be effective in experimental cachexia as well. Vos et al. published an initial study demonstrating

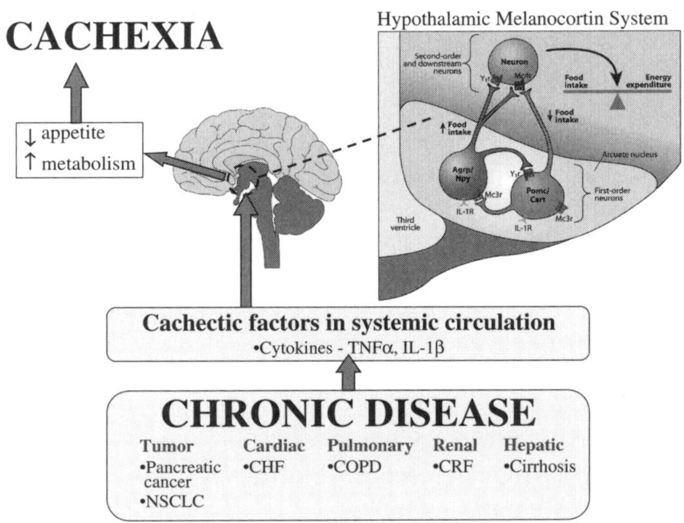

Fig. 4.1 Theoretical model for the role of the central melanocortin system in cachexia. AgRP, agouti-related peptide; CART, cocaine and amphetamine regulated transcript; CHF, congestive heart failure; COPD, chronic obstructive pulmonary disease; CRF, chronic renal failure; IL, interleukin; MC4R, melanocortin 4 receptor; NPY, neuropeptide Y; NSCLC, non–small cell lung cancer; POMC, pro-opiomelanocortin; Y1R, NPY receptor type 1. (Reproduced with permission from the Thompson Corporation and Foster AC, Chen C, Markison S, Marks DL. MC4 receptor antagonists: a potential treatment for cachexia. iDrugs 2005;8 *(4)*:314–319. Copyright © 2005, The Thompson Corporation.) (*see* Color Plate 3)

that subcutaneous administration of a small-molecule melanocortin antagonist could prevent weight loss due to cancer in a xenograft mouse model *(77)*. This study was limited in that there were no data regarding the effect on food intake, body composition, or metabolic rate, and there were no in vivo receptor specificity studies performed. In a subsequent publication, Markison et al. used peripheral (intraperitoneal) injections of a novel small-molecule melanocortin antagonist (NBI 12i; Neurocrine Biosciences, Inc., San Diego, CA, USA) to address all of these issues *(78)*. This compound was found to be a potent, selective, and bioavailable small-molecule MC4R antagonist both in vitro and in vivo. Furthermore, it was demonstrated that peripheral administration of this compound stimulated food intake in normal mice and dramatically attenuated cachexia in a murine cancer model. Thus, these studies demonstrate that the development of a melanocortin antagonist drug suitable for use in human trials is both technically feasible and based on sound experimental data.

CONCLUSION

Cachexia of chronic disease is composed of three primary cardinal features: 1) relative anorexia, even in an underweight state, 2) an elevated basal metabolic rate above that expected for the patient's existing lean body mass, 3) a rate of loss of lean body mass that greatly exceeds that found in simple starvation. This is a common condition and one that compromises quality of life (e.g,. strength, endurance, physical appearance) and strongly predicts morbidity and mortality in a variety of chronic diseases. This metabolic disorder has proved to be extraordinarily difficult to treat either by increasing nutrition or by pharmacologic means. The initiating event in cachexia is thought to be the elaboration and local production of proinflammatory cytokines that act on feeding centers in the brain to produce the observed behavioral and metabolic alterations. The central melanocortin system is a likely conduit for access of this inflammatory signal to higher brain centers and represents a logical target for therapeutic intervention. Studies to date strongly suggest that melanocortin antagonists are likely to be beneficial to patients suffering from cachexia.

REFERENCES

1. Katz, AM and Katz, PB, Diseases of the heart in the works of Hippokrates. Br Heart J, 1962. 24: p. 257–264.
2. Deans, C and Wigmore, SJ, Systemic inflammation, cachexia and prognosis in patients with cancer. Curr Opin Clin Nutr Metab Care, 2005. 8(3): p. 265–269.
3. Larkin, M, Thwarting the dwindling progression of cachexia. Lancet, 1998. 351: p. 1336.
4. Laviano, A, Meguid, MM, Inui, A, et al., Therapy insight: Cancer anorexia-cachexia syndrome–when all you can eat is yourself. Nat Clin Pract Oncol, 2005. 2(3): p. 158–165.
5. Maltoni, M, Caraceni, A, Brunelli, C, et al., Prognostic factors in advanced cancer patients: evidence-based clinical recommendations–a study by the Steering Committee of the European Association for Palliative Care. J Clin Oncol, 2005. 23(25): p. 6240–6248.
6. Guenter, P, Muurahainen, N, Simons, G, et al., Relationships among nutritional status, disease progression, and survival in HIV infection. J Acquir Immune Defic Syndr, 1993. 6(10): p. 1130–1138.
7. Anker, SD and Sharma, R, The syndrome of cardiac cachexia. Int J Cardiol, 2002. 85(1): p. 51–66.
8. Mehrotra, R and Kopple, JD, Nutritional management of maintenance dialysis patients: why aren't we doing better? Annu Rev Nutr, 2001. 21: p. 343–379.
9. Qureshi, AR, Alvestrand, A, Divino-Filho, JC, et al., Inflammation, malnutrition, and cardiac disease as predictors of mortality in hemodialysis patients. J Am Soc Nephrol, 2002. 13 Suppl 1: p. S28–36.
10. Tisdale, MJ, Cachexia in cancer patients. Nat Rev Cancer, 2002. 2(11): p. 862–871.
11. Gelin, J, Moldawer, LL, Lonnroth, C, et al., Role of endogenous tumor necrosis factor alpha and interleukin 1 for experimental tumor growth and the development of cancer cachexia. Cancer Res, 1991. 51(1): p. 415–421.
12. Plata-Salaman, CR, Immunomodulators and feeding regulation: A humoral link between the immune and nervous systems. Br Behav Immun, 1989. 3: p. 193–213.
13. Moldawer, LL, Andersson, C, Gelin, J, et al., Regulation of food intake and hepatic protein synthesis by recombinant-derived cytokines. Am J Physiol, 1988. 254(3 Pt 1): p. G450–456.
14. Plata-Salaman, CR, Immunomodulators and feeding regulation: a humoral link between the immune and nervous systems. Brain Behav Immun, 1989. 3(3): p. 193–213.
15. Scott, HR, McMillan, DC, Crilly, A, et al., The relationship between weight loss and interleukin 6 in non-small-cell lung cancer. Br J Cancer, 1996. 73(12): p. 1560–1562.
16. Abad, LW, Schmitz, HR, Parker, R, et al., Cytokine responses differ by compartment and wasting status in patients with HIV infection and healthy controls. Cytokine, 2002. 18(5): p. 286–293.
17. Bonfield, TL, Panuska, JR, Konstan, MW, et al., Inflammatory cytokines in cystic fibrosis lungs. Am J Respir Crit Care Med, 1995. 152(6 Pt 1): p. 2111–2118.
18. Levine, B, Kalman, J, Mayer, L, et al., Elevated circulating levels of tumor necrosis factor in severe chronic heart failure. N Engl J Med, 1990. 323(4): p. 236–241.
19. Roubenoff, R, Roubenoff, RA, Cannon, JG, et al., Rheumatoid cachexia: cytokine-driven hypermetabolism accompanying reduced body cell mass in chronic inflammation. J Clin Invest, 1994. 93(6): p. 2379–2386.

20. Torre-Amione, G, Kapadia, S, Benedict, C, et al., Proinflammatory cytokine levels in patients with depressed left ventricular ejection fraction: a report from the Studies of Left Ventricular Dysfunction (SOLVD). J Am Coll Cardiol, 1996. 27(5): p. 1201–1206.
21. Wigmore, SJ, Fearon, KC, Maingay, JP, et al., Down-regulation of the acute-phase response in patients with pancreatic cancer cachexia receiving oral eicosapentaenoic acid is mediated via suppression of interleukin-6. Clin Sci (Lond), 1997. 92(2): p. 215–221.
22. Inui, A, Cancer Anorexia-Cachexia Syndrome: Are Neuropeptides the Key? Cancer Res, 1999. 59: p. 4493–4501.
23. Plata-Salaman, CR, Brain mechanisms in cytokine-induced anorexia. Psychoneuroendocrinology, 1998. 24: p. 25–41.
24. Turrin, NP, Ilyin, SE, Gayle, DA, et al., Interleukin-1beta system in anorectic catabolic tumor-bearing rats. Curr Opin Clin Nutr Metab Care, 2004. 7(4): p. 419–426.
25. Plata-Salaman, CR and Borkoski, JP, Chemokines/intercrines and central regulation of feeding. Am J Physiol, 1994. 266: p. R1711–R1715.
26. Plata-Salaman, CR, Sonti, G, Borkoski, JP, et al., Anorexia induced by chronic central administration of cytokines at estimated pathophysiological concentrations. Phys Behav, 1996. 60: p. 867–875.
27. Szelenyi, J, Cytokines and the central nervous system. Brain Res Bull, 2001. 54(4): p. 329–338.
28. Barber, MD, Fearon, KC, Delmore, G, et al., Should cancer patients with incurable disease receive parenteral or enteral nutritional support? Eur J Cancer, 1998. 34(3): p. 279–285.
29. Della Cuna, GR, Pellegrini, A, and Piazzi, M, Effect of methylprednisolone sodium succinate on quality of life in preterminal cancer patients: a placebo-controlled, multicenter study. The Methylprednisolone Preterminal Cancer Study Group. Eur J Cancer Clin Oncol, 1989. 25(12): p. 1817–1821.
30. Loprinzi, CL, Schaid, DJ, Dose, AM, et al., Body-composition changes in patients who gain weight while receiving megestrol acetate. J Clin Oncol, 1993. 11(1): p. 152–154.
31. Mann, M, Koller, E, Murgo, A, et al., Glucocorticoidlike activity of megestrol. A summary of Food and Drug Administration experience and a review of the literature. Arch Intern Med, 1997. 157(15): p. 1651–1656.
32. Eriksson, C, Nobel, S, Winblad, B, et al., Expression of interleukin 1 alpha and beta, and interleukin 1 receptor antagonist mRNA in the rat central nervous system after peripheral administration of lipopolysaccharides. Cytokine, 2000. 12(5): p. 423-431.
33. Gayle, D, Ilyin, SE, Flynn, MC, et al., Lipopolysaccharide (LPS)- and muramyl dipeptide (MDP)-induced anorexia during refeeding following acute fasting: Characterization of brain cytokine and neuropeptide systems mRNAs. Brain Res, 1998. 795: p. 77–86.
34. Laye, S, Gheusi, G, Cremona, S, et al., Endogenous brain IL-1 mediates the response to peripheral LPS. Am J Phys Reg Integr Comp Physiol, 2000. 279(1): p. R93–R98.
35. Takao, T, Hashimoto, K, and De Souza, EB, Modulation of interleukin-1 receptors in the neuro-endocrine-immune axis. Int J Dev Neurosci, 1995. 13(3-4): p. 167–178.
36. Ericsson, A, C., L, Hart, RP, et al., Type 1 interleukin-1 receptor in the rat brain: distribution, regulation, and relationship to sites of IL-1-induced cellular activation. J Comp Neurol, 1995. 361(4): p. 681–698.
37. Nadeau, S and Rivest, S, Effects of circulating tumor necrosis factor on the neuronal activity and expression of the genes encoding the tumor necrosis factor receptors (p55 and p75) in the rat brain: a view from the blood-brain barrier. Neuroscience, 1999. 93(4): p. 1449–1464.
38. Utsuyama, M and Hirokawa, K, Differential expression of various cytokine receptors in the brain after stimulation with LPS in young and old mice. Exp Gerontol, 2002. 37(2-3): p. 411–420.
39. Yamakuni, H, Minami, M, and Satoh, M, Localization of mRNA for leukemia inhibitory factor receptor in the adult rat brain. J Neuroimmunol, 1996. 70(1): p. 45–53.
40. Elmquist, JK, Scammell, TE, Jacobsen, CD, et al., Distribution of Fos-like immunoreactivity in the rat brain following intravenous lipopolysaccharide administration. J Comp Neurol, 1996. 371(1): p. 85–103.

41. Laflamme, N and Rivest, S, Effects of systemic immunogenic insults and circulating proinflammatory cytokines on the transcription of the inhibitory factor kappaB alpha within specific cellular populations of the rat brain. J Neurochem, 1999. 73(1): p. 309–321.
42. Broback, JR, Tepperman, J, and Long, CNH, Experimental hypothalamic hyperphagia in the albino rat. Yale Journal of Biological Medicine, 1943. 15: p. 831–853.
43. Hotheriogtoa, AW and Ranson, SW, Hypothalamic lesions and adiposity in the rat. Anatomical Record, 1940. 78: p. 149–172.
44. Muller, HL, Bruhnken, G, Emser, A, et al., Longitudinal study on quality of life in 102 survivors of childhood craniopharyngioma. Childs Nerv Syst, 2005. 21(11): p. 975–980.
45. Cone, RD, Cowley, MA, Butler, AA, et al., The arcuate nucleus as a conduit for diverse signals relevant to energy homeostasis. Int J Obes Relat Metab Disord, 2001. 25 Suppl 5: p. S63–67.
46. Cowley, MA, Smith, RG, Diano, S, et al., The distribution and mechanism of action of ghrelin in the CNS demonstrates a novel hypothalamic circuit regulating energy homeostasis. Neuron, 2003. 37(4): p. 649–661.
47. Schwartz, MW, Seeley, RJ, Campfield, LA, et al., Identification of targets of leptin action in rat hypothalamus. J Clin Invest, 1996. 98(5): p. 1101–1106.
48. Rizk, NM, Joost, HG, and Eckel, J, Increased hypothalamic expression of the p75 tumor necrosis factor receptor in New Zealand obese mice. Horm Metab Res, 2001. 33(9): p. 520–524.
49. Yabuuchi, K, Minami, M, Katsumata, S, et al., Localization of type-1 interleukin-1 receptor mRNA in the rat brain. Brain Res Mol Brain Res, 1994. 27(1): p. 27–36.
50. Jacobowitz, DM and O'Donohue, TL, a-Melanocyte-stimulating hormone: immunohistochemical identification and mapping in neurons of rat brain. Proc Natl Acad Sci USA, 1978. 75: p. 6300–6304.
51. Benoit, S, Schwartz, M, Baskin, D, et al., CNS melanocortin system involvement in the regulation of food intake. Horm Behav, 2000. 37(4): p. 299–305.
52. Cone, RD, Anatomy and regulation of the central melanocortin system. Nat Neurosci, 2005. 8(5): p. 571–578.
53. Fan, W, Boston, BA, Kesterson, RA, et al., Role of melanocortinergic neurons in feeding and the agouti obesity syndrome. Nature, 1997. 385: p. 165–168.
54. Huszar, D, Lynch, CA, Fairchild-Huntress, V, et al., Targeted disruption of the melanocortin-4 receptor results in obesity in mice. Cell, 1997. 88: p. 131–141.
55. Vaisse, C, Clement, K, Guy-Grand, B, et al., A frameshift mutation in human MC4R is associated with a dominant form of obesity. Nature Genetics, 1998. 20: p. 113–114.
56. Yeo, GS, Farooqi, IS, Aminian, S, et al., A frameshift mutation in MC4R associated with dominantly inherited human obesity. Nat Genet, 1998. 20(2): p. 111–112.
57. Farooqi, IS, Keogh, JM, Yeo, GS, et al., Clinical spectrum of obesity and mutations in the melanocortin 4 receptor gene. N Engl J Med, 2003. 348(12): p. 1085–1095.
58. Fan, W, Dinulescu, DM, Butler, AA, et al., The central melanocortin system can directly regulate serum insulin levels. Endocrinology, 2000. 141(9): p. 3072–3079.
59. Haskell-Luevano, C, Chen, P, Li, C, et al., Characterization of the neuroanatomical distribution of agouti-related protein immunoreactivity in the rhesus monkey and the rat. Endocrinology, 1999. 140(3): p. 1408–1415.
60. Fong, TM, Mao, C, MacNeil, C, et al., ART (protein product of agouti-related transcript) as an antagonist of MC-3 and MC-4 receptors. Biochem Biophys Res Commun, 1997. 237: p. 629–631.
61. Ollmann, MM, Wilson, BD, Yang, YK, et al., Antagonism of central melanocortin receptors in vitro and in vivo by agouti-related protein. Science, 1997. 278(5335): p. 135–138.
62. Mizuno, TM and Mobbs, CV, Hypothalamic agouti-related protein messenger ribonucleic acid is inhibited by leptin and stimulated by fasting. Endocrinology, 1999. 140(2): p. 814–817.
63. Hagan, MM, Rushing, PA, Pritchard, LM, et al., Long-term orexigenic effects of AgRP-(83-132) involve mechanisms other than melanocortin receptor blockade. Am J Physiol Regul Integr Comp Physiol, 2000. 279(1): p. R47–R52.

64. Nijenhuis, WA, Oosterom, J, and Adan, RA, AGRP (83-132) acts as an inverse agonist on the human melanocortin-4 receptor. Mol Endocrinol, 2001. 15(1): p. 164–171.
65. Rivest, S and Laflamme, N, Neuronal activity and neuropeptide gene transcription in the brains of immune-challenged rats. J Neuroendocrinol, 1995. 7(7): p. 501–525.
66. Scarlett, JM, Joppa, MA, Markison, S, et al., Direct activation of the hypothalamic melanocortin system by interleukin-1. Abs Endocr Soc (2004):OR6-3, 2005.
67. Lennie, TA, Relationship of body energy status to inflammation-induced anorexia and weight loss. Physiol Behav, 1998. 64(4): p. 475–481.
68. Lennie, TA, Wortman, MD, and Seeley, RJ, Activity of body energy regulatory pathways in inflammation-induced anorexia. Physiol Behav, 2001. 73(4): p. 517–523.
69. Sergeyev, V, Broberger, C, and Hokfelt, T, Effect of LPS administration on the expression of POMC, NPY, galanin, CART and MCH mRNAs in the rat hypothalamus. Brain Res Mol Brain Res, 2001. 90(2): p. 93–100.
70. Huang, QH, Hruby, VJ, and Tatro, JB, Role of central melanocortins in endotoxin-induced anorexia. Am J Physiol, 1999. 276(3 pt 2): p. R864–R871.
71. Tatro, JB, Huszar, D, Fairchild-Huntress, V, et al., Role of the melanocortin-4 receptor in thermoregulatory responses to central IL-1. Society for Neuroscience Abstracts, 1999. 25(624.4): p. 1558.
72. Lawrence, CB and Rothwell, NJ, Anorexic but not pyrogenic actions of interleukin-1 are modulated by central melanocortin-3/4 receptors in the rat. J Neuroendocrinol, 2001. 13(6): p. 490–495.
73. Marks, DL, Butler, AA, Turner, R, et al., Differential role of melanocortin receptor subtypes in cachexia. Endocrinology, 2003. 144(4): p. 1513–1523.
74. Marks, DL, Ling, N, and Cone, RD, Role of the Central Melanocortin System in Cachexia. Cancer Res, 2001. 61(4): p. 1432–1438.
75. Wisse, BE, Frayo, RS, Schwartz, MW, et al., Reversal of cancer anorexia by blockade of central melanocortin receptors in rats. Endocrinology, 2001. 142(8): p. 3292–3301.
76. Cheung, W, Yu, PX, Little, BM, et al., Role of leptin and melanocortin signaling in uremia-associated cachexia. J Clin Invest, 2005. 115(6): p. 1659–1665.
77. Vos, TJ, Caracoti, A, Che, JL, et al., Identification of 2-[2-[2-(5-bromo-2- methoxyphenyl)-ethyl]-3-fluorophenyl]-4,5-dihydro-1H-imidazole (ML00253764), a small molecule melanocortin 4 receptor antagonist that effectively reduces tumor-induced weight loss in a mouse model. J Med Chem, 2004. 47(7): p. 1602–1604.
78. Markison, S, Foster, AC, Chen, C, et al., The regulation of feeding and metabolic rate and the prevention of murine cancer cachexia with a small-molecule melanocortin-4 receptor antagonist. Endocrinology, 2005. 146(6): p. 2766–2773.

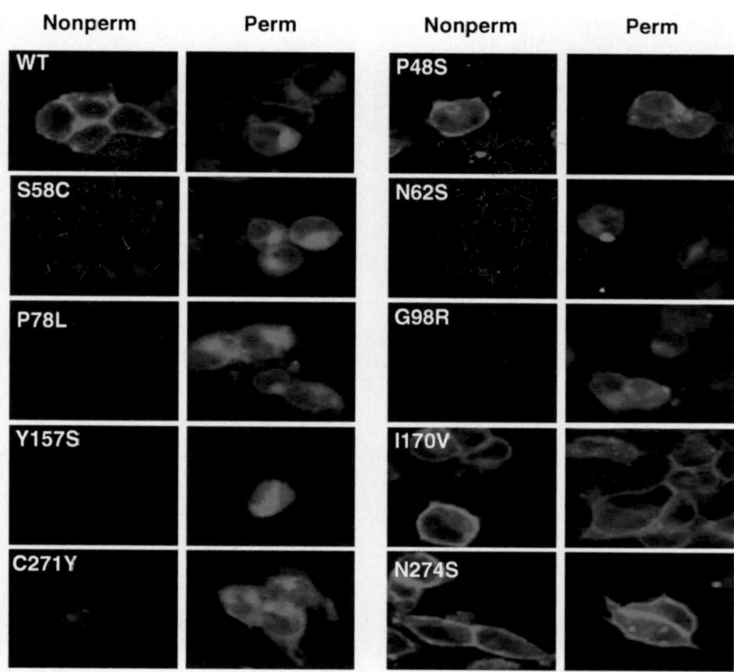

Plate 1. Examples of mutants belonging to class II and class V. Mutants S58C, N62S, P78L, G98R, Y157S, and C271Y are class II mutants. They are retained intracellularly. Mutants P48S, I170V, and N274S are expressed on cell surface and function normally and belong to class V. (Reprinted with permission from Tao YX, Segaloff DL. Functional characterization of melanocortin-4 receptor mutations associated with childhood obesity. Endocrinology 2003;144:4544–4551. Copyright © 2003, The Endocrine Society.). (see Figure 3.3)

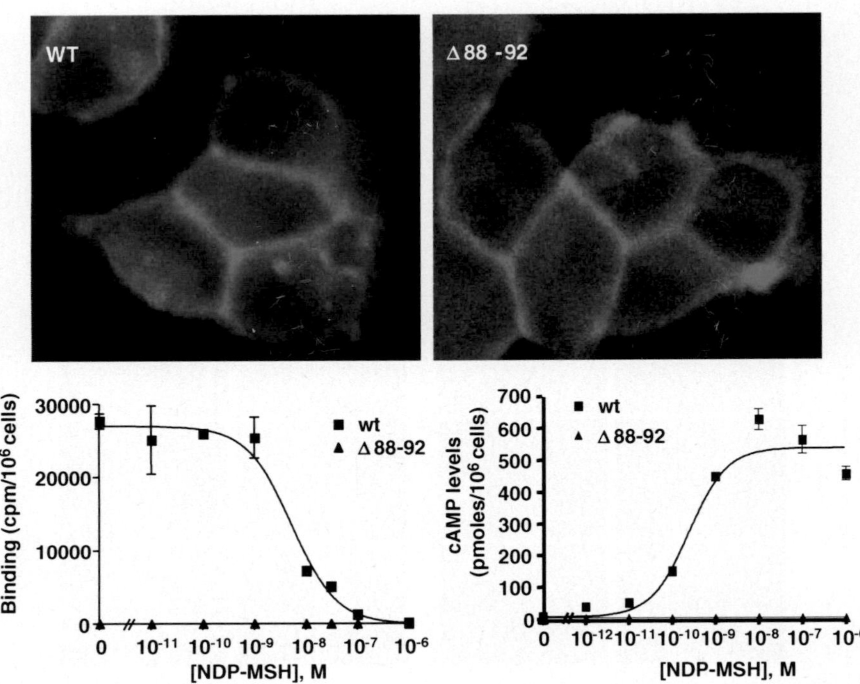

Plate 2. Mutant Δ88-92 belongs to class III. Δ88-92 is expressed on cell surface but cannot bind to the ligand or signal. (Reprinted with permission from Donohoue PA, Tao YX, Collins M, Yeo GSH, O'Rahilly S, Segaloff DL. Deletion of codons 88–92 of the melanocortin-4 receptor gene: a novel deleterious mutation in an obese female. J Clin Endocrinol Metab 2003;88:5841–5845. Copyright © 2003, The Endocrine Society.). (see Figure 3.4)

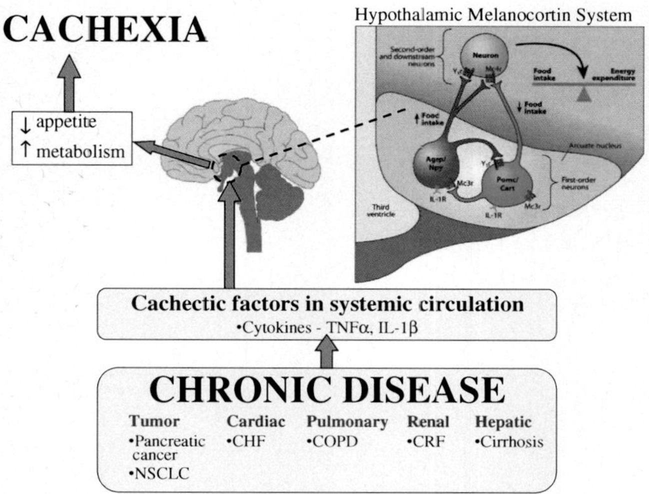

Plate 3. Theoretical model for the role of the central melanocortin system in cachexia. AgRP, agouti-related peptide; CART, cocaine and amphetamine regulated transcript; CHF, congestive heart failure; COPD, chronic obstructive pulmonary disease; CRF, chronic renal failure; IL, interleukin; MC4R, melanocortin 4 receptor; NPY, neuropeptide Y; NSCLC, non–small cell lung cancer; POMC, pro-opiomelanocortin; Y1R, NPY receptor type 1. (Reproduced with permission from the Thompson Corporation and Foster AC, Chen C, Markison S, Marks DL. MC4 receptor antagonists: a potential treatment for cachexia. iDrugs 2005;8 *(4)*:314–319. Copyright © 2005, The Thompson Corporation.) (see Figure 4.1)

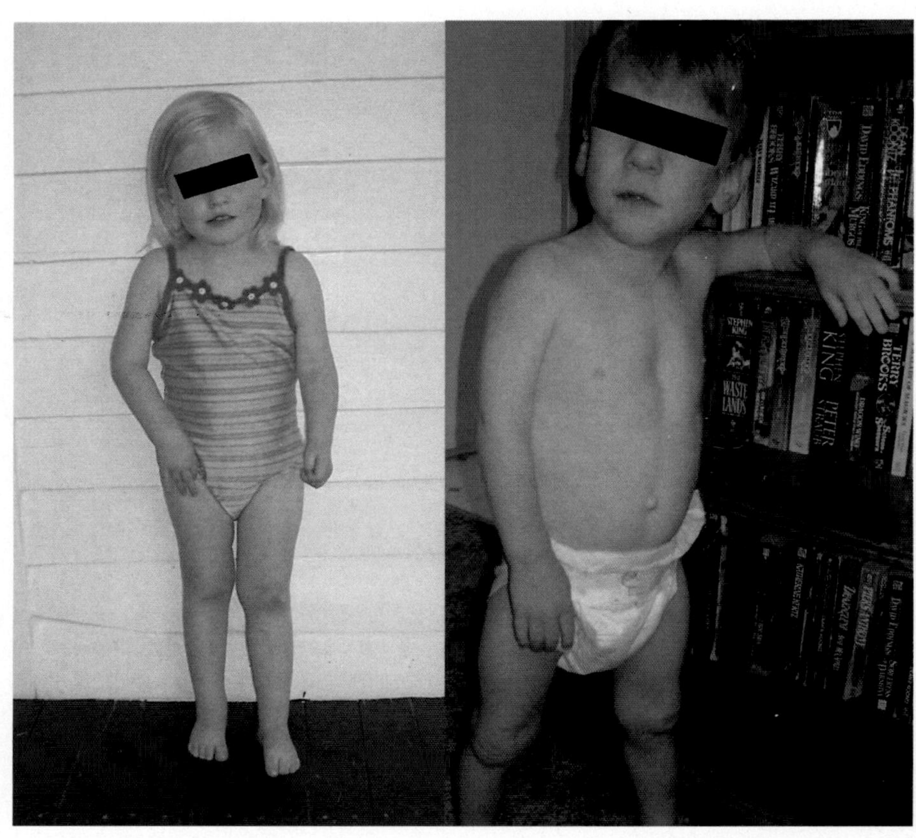

Plate 4. Typical physical features of PWS appearing in a $2\frac{1}{2}$-year-old girl and a 2-year-old boy with PWS. (see Figure 11.1)

5 The Efferent Arm of the Energy Balance Regulatory Pathway: Neuroendocrinology and Pathology

Robert H. Lustig

Contents

Abstract

The regulation of energy balance is unique among neuroendocrine homeostatic systems, as it does not involve the pituitary gland. It is accomplished through afferent neural and hormonal signals reaching the hypothalamus, with resultant efferent projections of the autonomic nervous system innervating the muscles, viscera, and adipose tissue. The efferent system is of particular interest, as it has its own pathologies, which can be modulated to achieve weight loss. The sympathetic nervous system promotes energy expenditure by increasing movement and thermogenesis and inhibiting insulin secretion. The vagus nerve promotes energy storage by increasing alimentary tract digestion and absorption, adipose tissue insulin sensitivity, and insulin secretion. These two pathways are clearly demonstrated in the starvation response, in which sympathetic activity decreases to conserve energy, and vagal activity increases to store energy. Hypothalamic obesity, an example of "organic" leptin resistance, manifests similarly. Finally, anorexia nervosa is an example of dissociation between weight loss, but with increased sympathetic modulation. Understanding the relationship between these two efferent arms is essential to treatment of energy balance disorders.

Key Words: anorexia nervosa, hypothalamic obesity, insulin, parasympathetic, starvation, sympathetic, thermogenesis, vagus.

From: *Contemporary Endocrinology: Energy Metabolism and Obesity: Research and Clinical Applications*
Edited by: P. A. Donohoue

INTRODUCTION

The prevalence of obesity continues to rise both in adults and children *(1, 2)*, as do the comorbidities related to obesity, including type 2 diabetes and the metabolic syndrome. In evaluating obesity, the first law of thermodynamics prevails: energy is neither created nor destroyed but can be transformed into matter, and vice versa. In human terms, caloric intake = energy expenditure + weight gain. This had led to the lay concept that in order to promote weight loss, diet and exercise are all that are necessary to treat the majority of obese persons. But obesity is not that simple; it does not have one etiology, one pathogenesis, and certainly not one treatment. Obesity is in fact a phenotype of different pathologies, which involve dysfunction of the negative feedback regulatory pathway of energy balance (Fig. 5.1). This complex pathway consists of an afferent arm (represented primarily by hormonal signals from the adipocyte and gastrointestinal tract to the hypothalamus and a central processing unit within the hypothalamus that integrates this information) and an efferent arm consisting of signals that travel via the autonomic nervous system to the gastrointestinal (GI) tract, β-cell, and adipocyte. Dysregulation may occur at any point, which can promote or prevent weight loss or gain. Many investigators have focused on defects in the afferent arm of this regulatory pathway. Although these will be referenced for completeness, in this chapter, the focus will be on the efferent arm of this pathway and in particular on its contribution to the pathogenesis of obesity.

THE AFFERENT ARM OF THE ENERGY BALANCE PATHWAY

Neuroendocrinology

The peripheral afferent hormones leptin, ghrelin, peptide YY_{3-36} (PYY), and insulin all have receptors located on neurons within the ventromedial hypothalamus (VMH). These hormonal signals are transduced by the VMH as indications of hunger (ghrelin), satiety (PYY), metabolism short-term energy accrual (insulin), and long-term energy accrual (leptin). Normally, in the fed state, both insulin and leptin levels are increased, which increase the synthesis and processing of hypothalamic pro-opiomelanocortin (POMC) to its component peptides, including α-melanocyte stimulating hormone (α-MSH), which along with its colocalized neuromodulator, cocaine amphetamine regulated transcript (CART), act at the lateral hypothalamic area (LHA) and paraventricular nucleus (PVN) to alter melanocortin receptor 4 (MC4R) occupancy, which decreases appetite and food intake (*3–6*). Insulin and leptin also directly inhibit the release of neuropeptide Y (NPY) and agouti-related protein (AgRP), further limiting feeding and providing for unantagonized MC4R occupancy *(7)*. Furthermore, PYY_{3-36} levels are elevated, and this hormone binds to the Y_2 receptor in the VMH, activating γ-aminobutyric acid (GABA), which inhibits the orexigenic signal transduction of NPY *(8)*. Conversely, in the fasting state, gastric secretion of ghrelin is increased *(9, 10)*, while leptin, insulin, and PYY_{3-36} levels are low, which leads to stimulation of hypothalamic NPY/AgRP and antagonism of α-MSH/CART. The resultant lack of anorexogenic pressure on the MC4R results in increased feeding behavior and energy efficiency (with reduced fat oxidation), in order to store energy substrate as fat. This is accomplished through signal transduction within the efferent pathway, consisting of the sympathetic and parasympathetic nervous systems (see below).

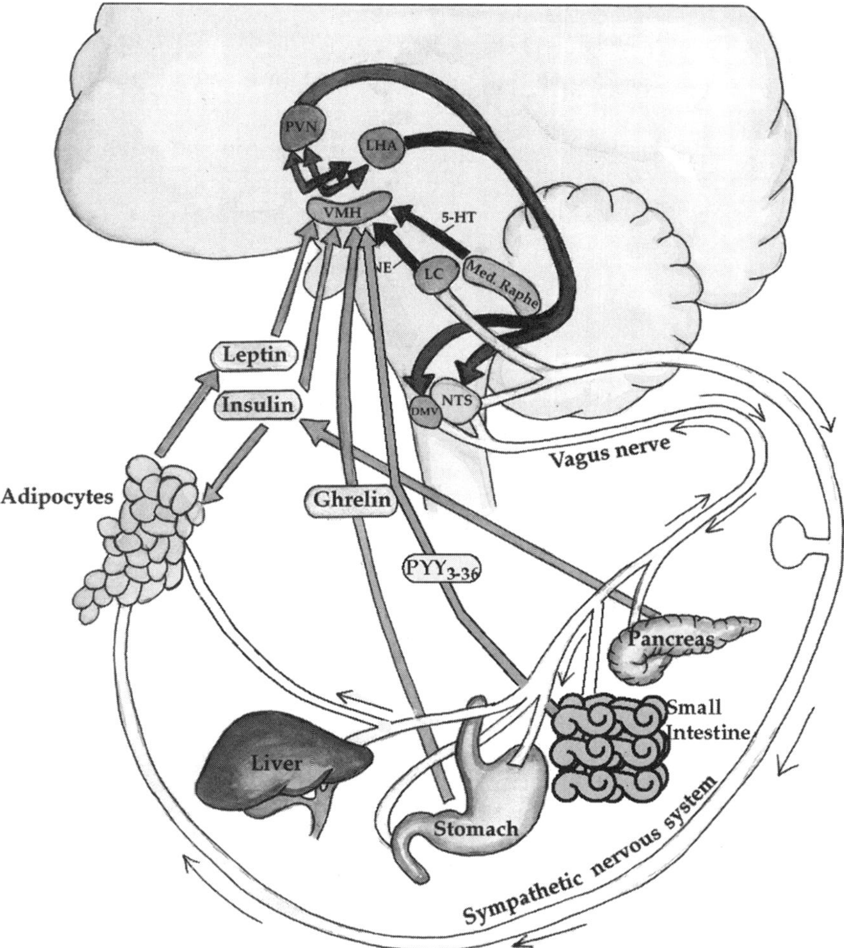

Fig. 5.1 Neuroendocrine regulation of energy balance. The afferent system: Neural (e.g., vagal) and hormonal (ghrelin, insulin, leptin) signals are generated from the liver, gut, pancreas, and adipose. In addition, norepinephrine from the locus coeruleus (LC) and serotonin (5-HT) from the median raphe are elaborated. These signals of satiety versus hunger and thinness versus fatness are interpreted by the nucleus tractus solitarius (NTS) and the ventromedial hypothalamus (VMH). These signals are integrated in the paraventricular nucleus (PVN) and lateral hypothalamus (LHA). The efferent system: Efferent signals from these areas in turn stimulate the sympathetic nervous system (SNS) to expend energy by activating β_3-adrenergic receptors and uncoupling proteins in the adipocyte, to release energy in the form of lipolysis, heat, or physical activity. Conversely, the parasympathetic nervous system (efferent vagal) increases insulin secretion, with resultant adipogenesis and energy storage and also increases insulin sensitivity through direct effects on the adipose tissue. (Reproduced from Lustig RH. The neuroendocrinology of childhood obesity. Pediatr Clin North Am 2001;48:909–930, with permission of Elsevier.).

Pathology

Numerous obesity syndromes with organic bases have been described over the past 10 years *(11)*. These include rare disorders such as congenital leptin deficiency *(12, 13)*, leptin receptor deficiency *(14)*, POMC splicing mutation *(15)*, and prohormone convertase-1 deficiency *(16)*, melanocortin 3 receptor (MC3R) mutations *(17)*, and more common disorders such as MC4R mutations *(18)*, which appear to account for up to 5% of morbid obesity. Through the identification of these disorders of the afferent arm of the regulatory pathway, it is now hypothesized that obesity is neither a behavior nor a disease but rather a general phenotype of numerous pathologic biochemical processes impinging on this complex negative feedback pathway for the control of energy balance. Indeed, the efferent pathway also contains disorders that lead to either weight loss or gain.

THE EFFERENT ARM OF THE ENERGY BALANCE PATHWAY

Neuroendocrinology

From the VMH, PVN, and LHA, efferent projections synapse in the locus coeruleus (LC), which controls the sympathetic nervous system (SNS), and in the dorsal motor nucleus of the vagus nerve (DMV), which controls the vagus nerve, the chief output of the parasympathetic nervous system. The SNS increases energy expenditure primarily through skeletal muscle energy utilization and lipolysis; and the vagus increases energy storage, primarily through its effects on insulin secretion and adipocyte insulin sensitivity. In this way, the afferent hormonal systems are entrained with the efferent neural systems to accomplish the fine-tuning required to coordinate energy intake, storage, and expenditure.

The SNS

The SNS and Energy Expenditure

The afferent hormones leptin and insulin activate the central processing unit indirectly through effects on the MC4R. The resultant pressure on the anorexigenic arm of the central processing pathway leads to decreased food intake and increased energy expenditure, in part, through activation of the SNS *(19)*. For instance, leptin administration to *ob/ob* mice promotes increased brown adipose tissue lipolysis, thermogenesis, renovascular activity, and increased movement, all associated with increased energy expenditure, which assists in weight loss *(20)*; however, this effect is not seen in the Zucker fatty rat, which has a mutation in the leptin receptor *(21)*. Similarly, insulin administration increases SNS activity in normal rats and in humans *(22, 23)*.

The SNS and Modulation of Thermogenesis and Lipolysis

Activation of the SNS by leptin and insulin acts to increase energy expenditure at the level of the skeletal muscle. At the muscle, SNS activation stimulates glycogenolysis, myocardial energy expenditure, increases glucose and fatty acid oxidation, and increases protein synthesis *(24)*. This is accomplished through activation of β_2-adrenergic receptors *(25)*, which in turn increase the expression of numerous genes in skeletal muscle *(26)*, especially those involved in carbohydrate metabolism.

In rodents, SNS activation of brown adipose tissue stimulates the β_3-adrenergic receptor to promote lipolysis. Mice with targeted disruption of the β_3-adrenergic receptor exhibit consistently increased weight gain and adipose tissue size *(27)*. Catecholamine binding to the β_3-adrenergic receptor increases cAMP, which activates protein kinase A (PKA). PKA acts in two separate molecular pathways to increase energy expenditure. First, PKA phosphorylates cyclic AMP response element binding protein (CREB), which induces expression of peroxisome proliferation activated receptor (PPAR) gamma coactivator (PGC)-1. PGC-1 binds to enhancer elements on the uncoupling protein (UCP)1 gene, which increases in the expression and activity of UCP 1 and 2 *(28, 29)*. UCP1 is an inner membrane mitochondrial protein that uncouples proton entry from ATP synthesis *(30)*; therefore, UCP1 expression dissipates energy as heat, thus reducing the energy efficiency of the adipose tissue. Second, PKA activation activates the enzyme hormone specific lipase (HSL), which is responsible for lipolysis of intracellular triglyceride to its component free fatty acids (FFAs). The FFAs also induce UCP1, further increasing energy expenditure. The FFAs released from the adipocyte also travel to the liver where they are utilized for energy by metabolizing into two-carbon fragments. This reduces leptin expression; thus a negative feedback loop is achieved through leptin signal transduction. Thus, leptin promotes increasing energy expenditure through its effects on the SNS, which are mediated peripherally (Fig. 5.2).

The SNS and Modulation of β-cell Function

Thoracic and upper lumbar preganglionic fibers of the SNS stimulate the paravertebral sympathetic chain, with postganglionic norepinephrine efferents to the β-cell. Furthermore, adrenal epinephrine circulates in response to SNS activation, such as in exercise. Both catecholamines activate α_{2a}- and α_{2c}-adrenoreceptors on the β-cell, which stimulate G_i and inhibit adenyl cyclase, lower cAMP (Fig. 5.3), and maintain potassium channels in an open configuration with a negative resting membrane potential *(31)*. This reduces the insulin response to glucose. Lastly, catecholamines stimulate glucagon secretion, which inhibits insulin secretion indirectly through paracrine effects on the

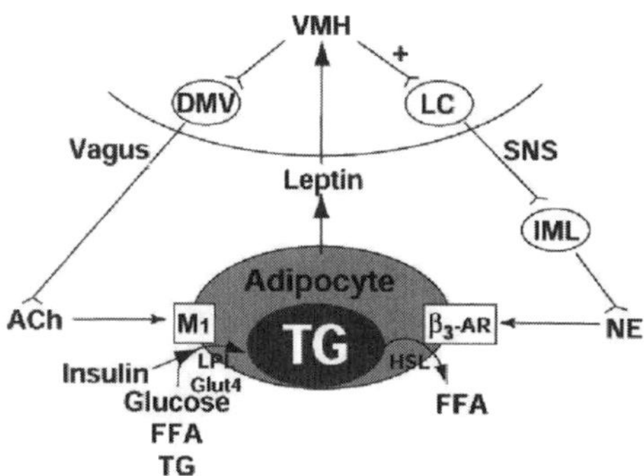

Fig. 5.2 Autonomic innervation of the adipocyte. The VMH transduces the peripheral leptin signal as one of sufficiency or deficiency. In the state of leptin sufficiency, efferents from the VMH synapse in the locus coeruleus (LC), which stimulates the sympathetic nervous system (SNS). SNS preganglionic motor neurons synapse in the intermediolateral cell column (IML) of the spinal cord. From there, postganglionic fibers emanate outward to white adipose tissue. Here, norepinephrine (NE) binds to the β_3-adrenergic receptor and stimulates hormone-sensitive lipase (HSL), which promotes lipolysis of stored triglyceride (TG) into free fatty acids (FFA), which are released. In the state of leptin deficiency, efferents from the VMH synapse in the dorsal motor nucleus of the vagus (DMV). From there, the vagus nerve emanates outward to white adipose tissue. Here, acetylcholine (ACh) binds to the M_1 muscarinic receptor. Activation of this receptor increases adipose tissue insulin sensitivity, promotes glucose uptake through activation of the glucose transporter Glut4, promotes uptake of FFA for lipogenesis, and promotes triglyceride uptake from circulating lipoproteins through activation of lipoprotein lipase (LPL).

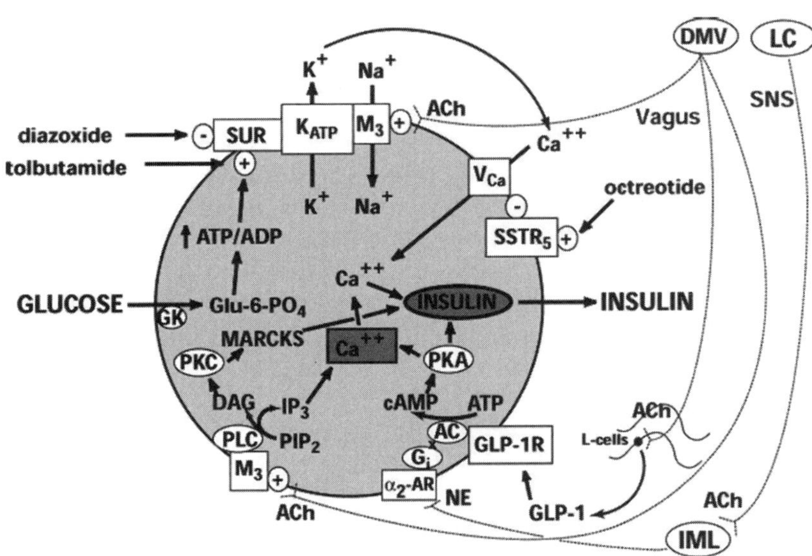

Fig. 5.3 Autonomic innervation of the β-cell. Glucose entering the cell is converted to glucose-6-phosphate, generating ATP. ATP accumulation closes an ATP-dependent potassium channel, resulting in cellular depolarization. A voltage-gated calcium channel (V_{Ca}) opens, allowing for intracellular calcium influx, which activates neurosecretory mechanisms necessary for insulin vesicular exocytosis. The vagus nerve stimulates insulin secretion through three overlapping mechanisms *(47)*: 1) acetylcholine (ACh) binds to a M_3 muscarinic receptor, opening a sodium channel. This augments the ATP-dependent cell depolarization, increasing the calcium influx, and insulin exocytosis. 2) ACh increases phospholipase activity (PLA, PLC, PLD), which hydrolyzes intracellular phosphatidylinositol (PIP_2) to diacylglycerol (DAG) and inositol triphosphate (IP_3). DAG stimulates protein kinase C (PKC), which phosphorylates myristoylated alanine-rich protein kinase C substrate (MARCKS), which binds actin and calcium-calmodulin and induces insulin exocytosis. IP_3 promotes calcium release from intracellular stores, which also promotes insulin secretion. 3) The vagus nerve innervates the L-cells of the small intestine, which secrete glucagon-like peptide-1 (GLP-1) into the circulation. GLP-1 binds to its receptor on the β-cell, which induces calcium-calmodulin–sensitive adenyl cyclase (AC), with conversion of intracellular ATP to cAMP, which then activates protein kinase A (PKA). PKA causes both the release of intracellular calcium stores and the phosphorylation of vesicular proteins, each contributing to an increase in insulin exocytosis. Octreotide binds to a somatostatin receptor ($SSTR_5$) on the β-cell, which is coupled to the voltage-gated calcium channel, thus limiting calcium influx and the amount of insulin released in response to glucose. The SNS inhibits insulin secretion, as norepinephrine (NE) binds to β_2-adrenoceptors (β_2-AR) on the β-cell membrane to stimulate G_i and decrease adenyl cyclase and its product cAMP, which reduces PKA and insulin release. (Reproduced from Lustig RH. Autonomic dysfunction of the β-cell and the pathogenesis of obesity. Rev Endocr Metab Dis 2003;4:23–32, with permission of Springer-Verlag.).

β-cell *(32)*. The net result of SNS activation is a decrease in insulin secretion and increase in the degree of glycemia, for use in β-oxidation by skeletal muscle.

The Vagus

The Vagus and Energy Storage

The vagus nerve serves essentially the opposite role of the SNS in the regulation of energy balance, in that it promotes energy deposition into adipose tissue. By slowing the heart rate, myocardial oxygen consumption is reduced, and through its effects on the alimentary tract, the vagus nerve promotes peristalsis and energy substrate absorption. Through direct effects on the adipocyte, the vagus nerve promotes insulin sensitivity to increase the clearance of energy substrate into adipose tissue, and finally, through effects on the β-cell, increased vagal tone results in a postprandial insulin hypersecretion, which promotes further energy deposition into fat (*33–35*).

The Vagus and Modulation of Adipogenesis

Although the effects of the SNS on lipolysis are well-known, it is not widely appreciated that vagal innervation of the adipocyte is crucial to lipogenesis. Retrograde tracing of white adipose tissue reveals a wealth of efferents originating at the DMV *(36)*. These efferents synapse on the M_1 muscarinic receptor on the adipocyte, which increases insulin sensitivity of the adipocyte. Denervation of white adipose tissue results in reduction of glucose and FFA uptake in response to a euglycemic hyperinsulinemic clamp and also results in the induction of HSL, which promotes lipolysis; both of which reduce the efficiency of insulin-induced energy storage. Thus, vagal modulation of the adipocyte augments storage of both glucose and FFAs by improving adipose insulin sensitivity *(37)* (Fig. 5.2).

The Vagus and Modulation of β-cell Function

In the efferent pathway, insulin is responsible for shunting blood-borne nutrients into adipose for storage (see above). Indeed, the primary hormonal signal for adipogenesis is insulin *(38)*. The amplitude and duration of pancreatic insulin secretion, and the activity of the insulin molecule at the adipose insulin receptor, play integral roles in the genesis of lipogenesis and weight gain. Within the adipocyte, insulin increases a) glucose transporter (Glut) 4 expression; b) acetyl-CoA carboxylase; c) fatty acid synthase; and d) lipoprotein lipase *(39)*. Thus, the net effect of insulin on the adipocyte is the rapid clearance and storage of circulating glucose and lipid. Thus, increasing insulin promotes increased energy storage.

In response to declining levels of leptin and/or under persistent orexigenic pressure, the LHA and PVN send efferent projections residing in the medial longitudinal fasciculus to the dorsal motor nucleus of the vagus nerve (DMV) *(40)*. The DMV in turn sends efferent projections throughout the alimentary system, including the β-cells of the pancreas *(41)*. This pathway is responsible for the "cephalic" or preabsorptive phase of insulin secretion, which is glucose-independent and can be blocked by atropine *(42)*. VMH lesions damage this pathway, leading to an increase in vagal firing rate *(43)*. For example, rats with VMH lesions exhibit both increased insulin levels and food intake; however, this can be prevented by pancreatic vagotomy (*44–46*). Overactive vagal neurotransmission increases insulin secretion from β-cells through three distinct but overlapping mechanisms *(47)* (Fig. 5.3):

1. Vagal firing increases acetylcholine availability and binding to the M_3 muscarinic receptor on the β-cell, which is coupled to a sodium channel within the pancreatic β-cell membrane *(48)*. Under resting conditions, the ATP-dependent potassium channel within the β-cell membrane remains open and leads to a negative β-cell resting membrane potential of approximately −70 mV, with essentially no insulin release. In this state, activation of the sodium channel by acetylcholine only minimally increases β-cell

resting membrane potential to −65 mV and has relatively minimal effects on insulin secretion and peripheral insulin levels. This is the "cephalic" phase of insulin secretion, described above *(42)*. As glucose enters the β-cell after ingestion of a meal, the enzyme glucokinase phosphorylates glucose to form glucose-6-phosphate. This increases the generation of intracellular ATP, which induces closure of the β-cell's ATP-dependent potassium channel. Upon channel closure, the β-cell experiences an ATP concentration-dependent β-cell depolarization *(49, 50)* and the opening of a separate voltage-gated calcium channel within the membrane. Intracellular calcium influx increases acutely, which results in rapid insulin vesicular exocytosis. Concomitant opening of the sodium channel by acetylcholine augments the β-cell depolarization, which in turn augments the intracellular calcium influx and results in insulin hypersecretion *(44, 51, 52)*. Conversely, knock-out of the β-cell M_3 receptor in mice reduces vagal-mediated insulin secretion and results in a hypophagic and lean phenotype *(53)*.

2. Vagally mediated acetylcholine increases phospholipases A_2, C, and D within the β-cell, which hydrolyze intracellular phosphatidylinositol to diacylglycerol (DAG) and inositol triphosphate (IP_3) *(47)*. DAG is a potent stimulator of protein kinase C (PKC) *(54)*, which phosphorylates myristoylated alanine-rich protein kinase C substrate (MARCKS), which then binds actin and calcium-calmodulin and induces insulin vesicular exocytosis *(55)*. IP_3 potentiates release of calcium within β-cells from intracellular stores, which also promotes insulin secretion *(56)*.
3. The vagus also stimulates the release of glucagon-like peptide-1 (GLP-1) from intestinal L-cells, which circulates and binds to a GLP-1 receptor within the β-cell membrane. Activation of this receptor induces a calcium-calmodulin–sensitive adenyl cyclase, with conversion of intracellular ATP to cAMP, which then activates protein kinase A (PKA). PKA causes both the release of intracellular calcium stores and the phosphorylation of vesicular proteins, each contributing to an increase in insulin exocytosis *(57, 58)*.

Measurement of Autonomic Function in Humans

Routine measurement of autonomic function has become possible in the past 10 years, as the phenomenon of heart rate variability (HRV) has been defined. Electrocardiographic (ECG) tracings demonstrate beat-to-beat variability of the R-R interval, which can be quantified by a computer, and a power spectral analysis system using a mathematical function called fast Fourier transform can separate the R-R interval variations of the ECG into characteristic frequencies of the underlying rhythm. Spectral analysis quantifies the proportional amount of variation at each component frequency. The power or amplitude of a frequency period demonstrates its relative contribution to overall HRV. Two discrete components in the frequency domain are determined: power in the low-frequency (LF) band (0.04–0.15 Hz), which estimates primarily sympathetic along with some parasympathetic and baroreceptor modulation; and power in the high-frequency (HF) band (0.15–0.40 Hz), which represents almost exclusively parasympathetic modulation. A report sheet indicating low- and high-frequency power values in units of natural log milliseconds squared [$\ln(ms^2)$] is obtained and used to determine the low-frequency:high-frequency ratio (LHR). The LHR is an index of the balance between sympathetic and parasympathetic modulation. As both LF and HF exhibit components of parasympathetic modulation, the LHR cancels these out, and it has been suggested as a more accurate indicator of sympathetic modulation. HRV has been previously used to quantify cardiovascular autonomic function in normal *(33)* and obese (*59–61*) subjects.

Alternatively, autonomic function can be measured directly by infusing the muscarinic antagonist atropine and the sympatholytic agent esmolol in tandem *(62)*. The change in beat-to-beat heart rate variability in response to each of these maneuvers is a direct index of the degree of sympathetic and vagal modulation. Studies in obesity generally demonstrate increased sympathetic tone in the obese, which would tend to mediate against further energy storage; indeed, this phenomenon is thought by some to be a protective mechanism to prevent further energy accumulation *(62)*.

A final method for assessing SNS reserve is by measuring catecholaminergic responses to insulin-induced hypoglycemia. As both norepinephrine and epinephrine reduce insulin release, and as epinephrine is a counterregulatory hormone, their rise in response to hypoglycemia is a direct indication of the function of the SNS in a pathologic situation, as is seen in diabetic-associated hypoglycemia *(63)*.

Pathology

The Starvation Response and the Autonomic Nervous System

In response to caloric restriction, leptin levels decline even before weight loss is manifest *(64)*. This leptin decline is interpreted by the hypothalamus as starvation; α-MSH and CART are decreased, whereas NPY and AgRP are increased. This leads to decreased MC4R occupancy. In response, the efferent pathway of energy balance coordinates efforts at improving energy efficiency and increasing energy storage. Total and resting energy expenditure decline in at attempt to conserve energy *(65)*. Specifically, UCP1 levels within adipose tissue decline *(66)*, as a result of decreased SNS activity in response to starvation, which can be seen during esmolol infusion *(59)*. Yet, in spite of decreased SNS tone at the adipocyte, there is clearly an obligate lipolysis (due to insulin suppression and upregulation of HSL), which is necessary to maintain energy delivery to the musculature and brain in the form of liver-derived ketone bodies. Conversely, in the starved state, vagal tone is increased in order to slow the heart rate and myocardial oxygen consumption, increase insulin secretion in response to glucose, and increase adipose insulin sensitivity; all directed to increase energy storage *(59)*. These revert back to baseline once caloric sufficiency is reestablished, and leptin levels rise.

Anorexia nervosa is unique among starvation paradigms. SNS activity, as measured by norepinephrine response to numerous stimuli, is markedly diminished *(67)*. However, using in vivo microdialysis techniques, it appears that SNS activity at the level of the adipocyte is actually increased versus controls *(68)*. This regiospecificity of SNS activity at the adipocyte (in comparison with starvation) leads to increased lipolysis in the face of caloric restriction and contributes rapidly to the emaciation seen in this syndrome.

Hypothalamic Obesity, Autonomic Dysfunction, and Energy Storage

It is well-known that bilateral electrolytic lesions or deafferentation of the VMH in rats leads to intractable weight gain *(44,52,69–71)*, even upon food restriction *(72)*. Originally, the obesity was felt to be due to damage to a "satiety" center, which promoted hyperphagia and increased energy storage *(73)*. In humans, hypothalamic damage, either due to CNS tumor, surgery, radiation, or trauma, can alter both the afferent and efferent pathway of energy balance and lead to severe and intractable weight gain *(74, 75)*. In this syndrome of "hypothalamic obesity," hypothalamic insult prevents integration of these peripheral energy and adiposity signals; thus, the VMH cannot transduce these signals into a sense of energy sufficiency and a subjective state of satiety *(70, 76)*. However, we now recognize that the weight gain in this syndrome is akin to the starvation response as stated above, in that it is actually secondary to 1) overactivation of the vagus, which promotes an obligate insulin hypersecretion and energy storage; and 2) defective activation of the SNS, which retards lipolysis and energy expenditure *(77)*.

1. Vagally mediated insulin hypersecretion and increased energy storage: Children with hypothalamic obesity exhibit weight gain, even in response to forced caloric restriction *(78)*. This seems paradoxical, as one would expect that if hyperphagia were the reason for the obesity, then caloric restriction would be effective. The reason for this paradox is that similar to the *db/db* mouse, these subjects exhibit "organic leptin resistance"; that is, the inability to respond to their own leptin due to the CNS damage that takes place, thus, their VMH cannot transduce the leptin signal. This elicits the starvation response, which increases vagal tone and augments insulin secretion via through the mechanisms described above. Indeed, children with hypothalamic obesity on oral glucose tolerance testing demonstrate insulin hypersecretion [as measured by an increased corrected insulin response, or CIR *(79)*] and increased insulin sensitivity [as measured by an increased composite insulin sensitivity index, or CISI *(80)*] compared with body mass index (BMI)-matched otherwise healthy obese children *(81)*. The hypothesis that vagally mediated insulin hypersecretion is the etiology of their obesity is further evidenced by the fact that insulin suppression with the somatostatin analogue octreotide reduces weight and increases spontaneous physical activity in many of these children *(82)*.
2. Defective activation of the SNS, physical activity, and energy expenditure: The adipocyte also responds to sympathetic nervous system activation to promote lipolysis and thermogenesis *(29)*. One of the most prominent and concerning complaints in patients with hypothalamic obesity is the persistent fatigue, lack of energy, and lack of physical activity. This generalized malaise is not due to hypopituitarism, as it persists even after full hormonal replacement. Recently, voluntary energy expenditure of patients with craniopharyngioma, as measured by accelerometry, was shown to be significantly decreased compared with BMI-matched, otherwise healthy, obese controls *(83)*. This decrease in energy expenditure may be mediated through defects in the regulation of the SNS. Two recent reports demonstrate an impaired ability of such patients to mount an epinephrine response to insulin-induced hypoglycemia *(84, 85)* and document decreased 24-hour epinephrine excretion *(85)*, although norepinephrine excretion was similar to controls. It is thought that this malaise and decrease in sympathetic tone may account for decreased rates of lipolysis through the adipocyte β_3-adrenergic receptor *(86)*, which result in decreased resting and voluntary energy expenditure. Thus, the mechanisms of adipogenesis in the syndrome of hypothalamic obesity are due to autonomic endocrinopathy, similar to that seen in the starvation response; a combination of parasympathetic hyperactivity and sympathetic hypoactivity secondary to VMH damage.

Adult Obesity, Autonomic Modulation, and Insulin Dynamics

Obesity is usually associated with fasting hyperinsulinemia, insulin resistance, and often manifests with glucose intolerance and type 2 diabetes and increased risk for developing the metabolic syndrome and its cardiovascular complications (*87–91*). Obesity is also routinely associated with increased SNS activity, which may be a function of the hyperleptinemia in affected patients, and which may be important in the development of the cardiovascular sequelae seen in most obese subjects *(33, 92, 93)*. Yet not all obese subjects exhibit metabolic decompensation; indeed, the bottom quintile of waist:hip ratio, indicating a preponderance of subcutaneous rather than visceral fat, has the same odds ratio for cardiovascular mortality as does the general population *(94)*.

Conversely, increased vagal tone has been postulated to result in postprandial insulin hypersecretion, which has been shown to precede weight gain in both children *(95)* and adults *(96)*, even without cranial insult. We identified a subcohort of obese subjects, who exhibit increased vagal modulation rather than sympathetic modulation. We recruited 44 severely obese (mean weight 123 kg, mean BMI 44.4 kg/m^2) but otherwise healthy adults into an open-label study using octreotide-LAR, 40 mg intramuscularly every for 28 days to suppress the early phase of insulin secretion, but without changes in lifestyle, diet, or exercise *(97)*. Of the 44 subjects, 8 exhibited steady and consistent weight loss over 6 months (Δweight -12.6 kg or 10% of initial body weight, ΔBMI -4.4), whereas the other 36 exhibited little or no weight loss. The eight responders exhibited significantly lower waist:hip ratio than the nonresponders, suggesting more subcutaneous and less visceral fat. In addition, the responders exhibited different baseline insulin dynamics, with a rapid insulin rise peaking by 60 min, and an equally rapid fall, indicating insulin hypersecretion with insulin sensitivity. Conversely, the other 36 subjects exhibited a slower insulin rise, which plateaued from 60 to 150 min, and a slow decline, indicating insulin resistance and poor insulin clearance. Octreotide treatment suppressed the early insulin rise only in the eight responders. The degree of insulin suppression correlated with BMI change, and the degree of pretreatment β-cell activity was an a priori predictor of response to octreotide; the higher the pretreatment β-cell activity, the more weight was lost. Total daily caloric intake was reduced equally by 500 kcal/day in responders and nonresponders. However, the number and percentage of calories consumed as carbohydrate in the responders was reduced from 900 to 350 kcal/day, and from 47% to 35%, respectively *(97)*. These data support the notion that the insulin hypersecretion in this subgroup was the proximate cause of their obesity, and that their food intake was secondary to their insulin dynamic abnormality.

We also assessed the utility of HRV as a surrogate marker of autonomic innervation of the β-cell in this cohort. At baseline, HF (vagal modulation) was *positively* correlated with β-cell activity, as measured by the corrected insulin response *(79)* (Fig. 5.4a), and *negatively* correlated with fasting insulin, a measure of insulin resistance (Fig. 5.4b). Conversely, LHR was *positively* correlated with fasting insulin (Fig. 5.4d) *(35)*. Thus, in this cohort, increased SNS tone correlated with insulin resistance, and increased vagal tone correlated with insulin hypersecretion and insulin sensitivity, reminiscent of the starvation response noted above.

The wide range of vagal and SNS modulation and the wide range of insulin hypersecretion versus resistance within a cohort of otherwise healthy, obese individuals suggests diversity among autonomic parameters and possibly neural regulation of the β-cell. Increased vagal modulation was correlated with increased β-cell activity and insulin sensitivity. Conversely, increased SNS modulation was correlated with insulin resistance. It should be pointed out that in each of these correlations, cause and

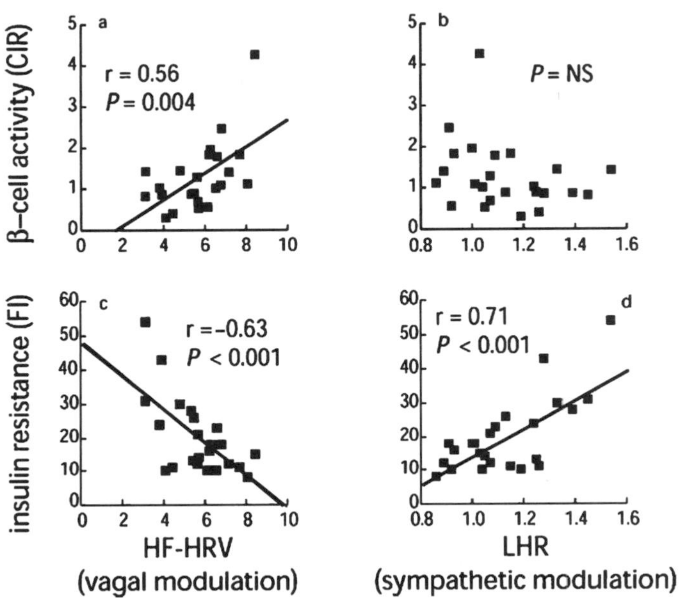

Fig. 5.4 Correlations between high-frequency heart rate variability (HF-HRV; an index of vagal modulation) and the low:high ratio (LHR; an index of SNS modulation), with (**a, b**) β-cell activity, as measured by the corrected insulin response (CIR) *(79)*; and (**c, d**) insulin resistance, as measured by fasting insulin (FI), in obese adults. (Reproduced from Lustig RH. Autonomic dysfunction of the β-cell and the pathogenesis of obesity. Rev Endocr Metab Dis 2003;4:23–32, with permission of Springer-Verlag.).

effect remain unknown. However, the wide disparity among these two HRV domains within the obese population argue that the autonomic nervous system is not merely a bystander in the genesis of obesity. The concomitant correlations of vagal modulation with insulin secretion and sensitivity and SNS modulation with insulin resistance are very compelling, particularly within the framework of hypothalamic control of energy balance and the constellation of insulin resistance, cardiovascular disease, and hypertension. The association of vagal activation with starvation, and weight loss response to insulin suppression only in those with vagally mediated insulin hypersecretion suggests within the global phenotype of obesity, there is a cadre of obese individuals in whom their weight gain is a manifestation of the starvation response mediating vagal hyperactivity, which also prevents them from manifesting adverse cardiovascular sequelae.

CONCLUSION

In this review, the role of the autonomic nervous system as the efferent arm of the energy balance pathway is substantiated. The SNS controls energy expenditure, whereas the vagus is primarily involved in energy storage. Normally, signal transduction of leptin at the level of the VMH results in activation of the SNS. These two efferent systems can be functionally yoked together through the starvation response, in which defective leptin signal transduction (as seen in the *ob/ob* or *db/db* mice, and in humans with hypothalamic obesity) increases vagal tone and decreases SNS tone to reduce energy expenditure and increase energy storage. However, these two systems can dissociate, as is seen in anorexia nervosa in which SNS modulation is high despite low leptin levels. Conversely, defects in obesity can present with either increased SNS modulation with insulin resistance or increased vagal modulation with insulin hypersecretion and insulin sensitivity. The author postulates that none of the well-known afferent syndromes of energy balance would be manifest without a corresponding dysfunction of the efferent arm. Furthermore, defects in the efferent arm of energy balance are modulable with drugs that are currently available. Therefore, the efferent arm of the energy balance regulatory pathway represents a crucial, diagnosable, and modifiable approach to the treatment of both obesity and cachexia.

ACKNOWLEDGMENTS

The author would like to thank Dr. Pedro Velasquez and Dr. Ann Cashion of the University of Tennessee, Dr. Pam Hinds, Dr. Melissa Hudson, and colleagues at St. Jude Children's Research Hospital, and Dr. Michele Mietus-Snyder, Dr. Andrea Garber, Dr. Cam-Tu Tran, Dr. Kristine Madsen, and Dr. Renee de la Torre of UCSF for all of their hard work and assistance in the enactment of these studies.

REFERENCES

1. Mokdad AH, Bowman BA, Ford ES, Vinicor F, Marks JS, Koplan JP. The continuing epidemics of obesity and diabetes in the United States. JAMA 2001;286:1195–200.
2. Styne DM. Childhood and adolescent obesity: prevalence and significance. Pediatr Clin North Am 2001;48:823–854.
3. Kalra SP, Dube MG, Pu S, Xu B, Horvath TL, Kalra PS. Interacting appetite-regulating pathways in the hypothalamic regulation of body weight. Endocr Rev 1999;20:68–100.
4. Schwartz MW, Woods SC, Porte D, Seeley RJ, Baskin DG. Central nervous system control of food intake. Nature 2000;404:661–671.
5. Elmquist JK, Elias CF, Saper CB. From lesions to leptin: hypothalamic control of food intake and body weight. Neuron 1999;22:221–232.
6. Lustig RH. The neuroendocrinology of childhood obesity. Pediatr Clin North Am 2001;48:909–930.
7. Elmquist JK, Ahima RS, Elias CF, Flier JS, Saper CB. Leptin activates distinct projections from the dorsomedial and ventromedial hypothalamic nuclei. Proc Natl Acad Sci USA 1998;95:741–746.
8. Small CJ, Bloom SR. Gut hormones and the control of appetite. Trends Endocrinol Metab 2004;15:259–263.
9. Tschöp M, Smiley DL, Heiman ML. Ghrelin induces adiposity in rodents. Nature 2000;407:908–913.
10. Kamegai J, Tamura H, Shimizu T, Ishii S, Sugihara H, Wakabayashi I. Central effect of ghrelin, an endogenous growth hormone secretagogue, on hypothalamic peptide gene expression. Endocrinology 2000;141:4797–4800.
11. Farooqi IS, O'Rahilly S. Monogenic human obesity syndromes. Recent Prog Horm Res 2004;59:409–424.
12. Farooqi IS, Jebb SA, Langmack G, et al. Effects of recombinant leptin therapy in a child with congenital leptin deficiency. N Engl J Med 1999;341:913–915.
13. Montague CT, Farooqi IS, Whitehead JP, et al. Congenital leptin deficiency is associated with severe early-onset obesity in humans. Nature 1997;387:903–908.
14. Clement K, Vaisse C, Lahlou N, et al. A mutation in the human leptin receptor gene causes obesity and pituitary dysfunction. Nature 1998;392:398–401.

15. Krude H, Biebermann H, Luck W, Horn R, Brabant G, Grüters A. Severe early-onset obesity, adrenal insufficiency, and red hair pigmentation caused by POMC mutations in humans. Nat Genet 1998;19:155–157.
16. Jackson RS, Creemers JW, Ohagi S, et al. Obesity and impaired prohormone processing associated with mutations in the prohormone convertase 1 gene. Nat Genet 1997;16:303–306.
17. Lee YS, Poh LKS, Loke KY. A novel melanocortin-3 receptor gene (MC3R) mutation associated with severe obesity. J Clin Endocrinol Metab 2002;87:1423–1426.
18. Vaisse C, Clement K, Durand E, Hercberg S, Guy-Grand B, Frougel P. Melanocortin-4 receptor mutations are a frequent and heterogeneous cause of morbid obesity. J Clin Invest 2000;106:253–262.
19. Rahmouni K, Haynes WG, Morgan DA, Mark AL. Role of melanocortin-4 receptors in mediating renal sympathoactivation to leptin and insulin. J Neurosci 2003;23(14):5998–6004.
20. Collins S, Kuhn CM, Petro AE, Swick AG, Chrunyk BA, Surwit RS. Role of leptin in fat regulation. Nature 1996;380:677.
21. Haynes WG, Morgan DA, Walsh SA, Mark AL, Sivitz WI. Receptor-mediated regional sympathetic nerve activation by leptin. J Clin Invest 1997;100:270–278.
22. Muntzel M, Morgan DA, Mark AL, Johnson AK. Intracerebroventricular insulin produces non-uniform regional increases in sympathetic nerve activity. Am J Physiol 1994;267:R1350–R1355.
23. Vollenweider L, Tappy L, Owlya R, Jequier E, Nicod P, Scherrer U. Insulin-induced sympathetic activation and vasodilation in skeletal muscle. Effects of insulin resistance in lean subjects. Diabetes 1995;44:641–645.
24. Navegantes LC, Migliorini RH, do Carmo Kettelhut I. Adrenergic control of protein metabolism in skeletal muscle. Curr Opin Clin Nutr Metab Care 2002;5:281–286.
25. Blaak EE, Saris WH, van Baak MA. Adrenoceptor subtypes mediating catecholamine-induced thermogenesis in man. Int J Obesity 1993;17:S78–S81.
26. Viguerie N, Clement K, Barbe P, et al. In vivo epinephrine-mediated regulation of gene express in human skeletal muscle. J Clin Endocrinol Metab 2004;89:2000–2014.
27. Susulic VS, Frederich RC, Lawitts J, et al. Targeted disruption of the beta 3-adrenergic receptor gene. J Biol Chem 1995;270:29483–29492.
28. Boss O, Bachman E, Vidal-Puig A, Zhang CY, Peroni O, Lowell BB. Role of the β_3-adrenergic receptor and/or a putative β_3-adrenergic receptor on the expression of uncoupling proteins and peroxisome proliferator-activated receptor-$_g$ coactivator-1. Biochem Biophys Res Commun 1999;261: 870–876.
29. Lowell BB, Spiegelman BM. Towards a molecular understanding of adaptive thermogenesis. Nature 2000;404:652–660.
30. Klingenberg M, Huang SG. Structure and function of the uncoupling protein from brown adipose tissue. Biochem Biophys Acta 1999;1415:271–296.
31. Sharp GW. Mechanisms of inhibition of insulin release. Am J Physiol 1996;271:C1781–C1799.
32. Kurose T, Seino Y, Nishi S, et al. Mechanism of sympathetic neural regulation of insulin, somatostatin, and glucagon secretion. Am J Physiol 1990;258:E220–E227.
33. Peles E, Goldstein DS, Akselrod S, et al. Interrelationships among measures of autonomic activity and cardiovascular risk factors during orthostasis and the oral glucose tolerance test. Clin Autonom Res 1995;5:271–278.
34. Rohner-Jeanrenaud F, Jeanrenaud B. Involvement of the cholinergic system in insulin and glucagon oversecretion of genetic preobesity. Endocrinology 1985;116:830–834.
35. Lustig RH. Autonomic dysfunction of the β-cell and the pathogenesis of obesity. Rev Endocr Metab Dis 2003;4:23–32.
36. Kreier F, Fliers E, Voshol PJ, et al. Selective parasympathetic innervation of subcutaneous and intra-abdominal fat-functional implications. J Clin Invest 2002;110:1243–1250.
37. Boden G, Hoeldtke RD. Nerves, fat, and insulin resistance. N Engl J Med 2003;349:1966–1967.

38. Marin P, Russeffé-Scrive A, Smith J, Bjorntorp P. Glucose uptake in human adipose tissue. Metabolism 1988;36:1154–1164.
39. Ramsay TG. Fat cells. Endocrinol Metab Clin North Am 1996;25:847–870.
40. Powley TL, Laughton W. Neural pathways involved in the hypothalamic integration of autonomic responses. Diabetologia 1981;20:378–387.
41. D'Alessio DA, Kieffer TJ, Taborsky GJ, Havel PJ. Activation of the parasympathetic nervous system is necessary for normal meal induced-insulin secretion in rhesus macaques. J Clin Endocrinol Metab 2001;86:1253–1259.
42. Ahren B, Holst JJ. The cephalic insulin response to meal ingestion in humans is dependent on both cholinergic and noncholingergic mechanisms and is important for postprandial glycemia. Diabetes 2001;50:1030–1038.
43. Lee HC, Curry DL, Stern JS. Direct effect of CNS on insulin hypersecretion in obese Zucker rats: involvement of vagus nerve. Am J Physiol 1989;256:E439–E444.
44. Berthoud HR, Jeanrenaud B. Acute hyperinsulinemia and its reversal by vagotomy following lesions of the ventromedial hypothalamus in anesthetized rats. Endocrinology 1979;105:146–151.
45. Tokunaga K, Fukushima M, Kemnitz JW, Bray GA. Effect of vagotomy on serum insulin in rats with paraventricular or ventromedial hypothalamic lesions. Endocrinology 1986;119:1708–1711.
46. Inoue S, Bray GA. The effect of subdiaphragmatic vagotomy in rats with ventromedial hypothalamic lesions. Endocrinology 1977;100:108–114.
47. Gilon P, Henquin JC. Mechanisms and physiological significance of the cholinergic control of pancreatic β-cell function. Endocr Rev 2001;22:565–604.
48. Miura Y, Gilon P, Henquin JC. Muscarinic stimulation increases Na^+ entry in pancreatic β-cells by a mechanism other than the emptying of intracellular Ca^{2-} pools. Biochem Biophys Res Commun 1996;224:67–73.
49. Zawalich WS, Zawalich KC, Rasmussen H. Cholinergic agonists prime the β-cell to glucose stimulation. Endocrinology 1989;125:2400–2406.
50. Nishi S, Seino Y, Ishida H, et al. Vagal regulation of insulin, glucagon, and somatostatin secretion *in vitro* in the rat. J Clin Invest 1987;79:1191–1196.
51. Komeda K, Yokote M, Oki Y. Diabetic syndrome in the Chinese hamster induced with monosodium glutamate. Experientia 1980;36:232–234.
52. Rohner-Jeanrenaud F, Jeanrenaud B. Consequences of ventromedial hypothalamic lesions upon insulin and glucagon secretion by subsequently isolated perfused pancreases in the rat. J Clin Invest 1980;65:902–910.
53. Yamada M, Miyakawa T, Duttaroy A, et al. Mice lacking the M3 muscarinic acetylcholine receptor are hypophagic and lean. Nature 2001;410:207–212.
54. Tian YM, Urquidi V, Ashcroft SJH. Protein kinase C in β-cells: expression of multiple isoforms and involvement in cholinergic stimulation of insulin secretion. Mol Cell Endocrinol 1996;119:185–193.
55. Arbuzova A, Murray D, McLaughlin S. MARCKS, membranes, and calmodulin: kinetics of their interaction. Biochim Biophys Acta 1998;1376:369–379.
56. Blondel O, Bell GI, Moody M, Miller RJ, Gibbons SJ. Creation of an inositol 1,4,5-triphosphate-sensitive Ca^{2+} store in secretory granules of insulin-producing cells. J Biol Chem 1994;269: 27167–27170.
57. Rocca AS, Brubaker PL. Role of the vagus nerve in mediating proximal nutrient-induced glucagon-like peptide-1 secretion. Endocrinology 1999;140:1687–1694.
58. Kiefer TJ, Habener JF. The glucagon-like peptides. Endocri Rev 1999;20:876–913.
59. Aronne LJ, Mackintosh R, Rosenbaum M, Leibel RL, Hirsch J. Autonomic nervous system activity in weight gain and weight loss. Am J Physiol 1995;269:R222–R225.
60. Hirsch J, Leibel RL, Mackintosh R, Aguirre A. Heart rate variability as a measure of autonomic function during weight change in humans. Am J Physiol 1991;261:R1418–R1423.

61. Karason K, Molgaard H, Wikstrand J, Sjostrom L. Heart rate variability in obesity and the effect of weight loss. Am J Cardiol 1999;83:1242–1247.
62. Aronne LJ, Mackintosh R, Rosenbaum M, Leibel RL, Hirsch J. Cardiac autonomic nervous system activity in obese and never-obese young men. Obes Res 1997;5:354–359.
63. Cryer PE. Diverse causes of hypoglycemia-associated autonomic failure in diabetes. N Engl J Med 2004;350(22):2272–2279.
64. Keim NL, Stern JS, Havel PJ. Relation between circulating leptin concentrations and appetite during a prolonged, moderate energy deficit in women. Am J Clin Nutr 1998;68:794–801.
65. Leibel RL, Rosenbaum M, Hirsch J. Changes in energy expenditure resulting from alered body weight. N Engl J Med 1995;332:621–628.
66. Champigny O, Ricquier D. Effects of fasting and refeeding on the level of uncoupling protein mRNA in rat brown adipose tissue: evidence for diet-induced and cold-induced responses. J Nutr 1990;120:1730–1736.
67. Pirke KM. Central and peripheral noradrenalin regulation in eating disorders. Psychiatr Res 1996;62:43–49.
68. Bartak V, Vybiral S, Pepezova H, Dostalova I, Pacak K, Nedvidkova J. Basal and exercise-induced sympathetic nervous activity and lipolysis in adipose tissue of patients with anorexia nervosa. Eur J Clin Invest 2004;34(5):371–377.
69. Jeanrenaud B. An hypothesis on the aetiology of obesity: dysfunction of the central nervous system as a primary cause. Diabetologia 1985;28:502–513.
70. Satoh N, Ogawa Y, Katsura G, et al. Pathophysiological significance of the *obese* gene product, leptin in ventromedial hypothalamus (VMH)-lesioned rats: evidence for loss of its satiety effect in VMH-lesioned rats. Endocrinology 1997;138:947–954.
71. Bray GA, Inoue S, Nishizawa Y. Hypothalamic obesity. Diabetologia 1981;20:366–377.
72. Bray GA, Nishizawa Y. Ventromedial hypothalamus modulates fat mobilization during fasting. Nature 1978;274:900–902.
73. Sklar CA. Craniopharyngioma: endocrine sequalae of treatment. Pediatr Neurosurg 1994;21: 120–123.
74. Bray GA. Syndromes of hypothalamic obesity in man. Pediatr Ann 1984;13:525–536.
75. Daousi C, Dunn AJ, Foy PM, MacFarlane IA, Pinkney JH. Endocrine and neuroanatomic predictors of weight gain and obesity in adult patients with hypothalamic damage. Am J Med 2005;118:45–50.
76. Thornton JE, Cheung CC, Clifton DK, Steiner RA. Regulation of hypothalamic proopiomelanocortin mRNA by leptin in *ob/ob* mice. Endocrinology 1997;138:5063–5066.
77. Lustig RH. Hypothalamic obesity: the sixth cranial endocrinopathy. Endocrinologist 2002;12:210–217.
78. Bray GA, Gallagher TF. Manifestations of hypothalamic obesity in man: a comprehensive investigation of eight patients and a review of the literature. Medicine 1975;54:301–33.
79. Sluiter WJ, Erkelens DW, Terpstra P, Reitsma WD, Doorendos H. Glucose intolerance and insulin release, a mathematical approach. 1. Assay of the beta cell response after glucose loading. Diabetes 1976;25:241–244.
80. Matsuda M, DeFronzo RA. Insulin sensitivity indices obtained from oral glucose tolerance testing: comparison with the euglycemic insulin clamp. Diabetes Care 1999;22:1462–1470.
81. Preeyasombat C, Bacchetti P, Lazar AA, Lustig RH. Racial and etiopathologic dichotomies in insulin secretion and resistance in obese children. J Pediatr 2005;146:474–481.
82. Lustig RH, Hinds PS, Ringwald-Smith K, et al. Octreotide therapy of pediatric hypothalamic obesity: a double-blind, placebo-controlled trial. J Clin Endocrinol Metab 2003;88:2586–2592.
83. Harz KJ, Muller HL, Waldeck E, Pudel V, Roth C. Obesity in patients with craniopharyngioma: assessment of food intake and movement counts indicating physical activity. J Clin Endocrinol Metab 2003;88(11):5227–5231.

84. Schofl C, Schleth A, Berger D, Terkamp C, Von Zur Muhlen A, Brabant G. Sympathoadrenal counterregulation in patients with hypothalamic craniopharyngioma. J Clin Endocrinol Metab 2002;87(2):624–669.
85. Coutant R, Maurey H, Rouleau S, et al. Defect in epinephrine production in children with craniopharyngioma: functional or organic origin? J Clin Endocrinol Metab 2003;88(12):5969–5975.
86. al-Adsani H, Hoffer LJ, Silva JE. Resting energy expenditure is sensitive to small dose changes in patients on chronic thyroid hormone replacement. J Clin Endocrinol Metab 1997;82:1118–1125.
87. Bonadonna RC, Groop L, Kraemer N. Obesity and insulin resistance in humans: a dose response study. Metabolism 1990;39:452–459.
88. Muscelli E, Camastra S, Gastaldelli A, et al. Influence of duration of obesity on the insulin resistance of obese non-diabetic patients. Int J Obes 1998;22:262–267.
89. Bodkin NL, Hannah JS, Ortmeyer HK, Hansen BC. Central obesity in rhesus monkeys: association with hyperinsulinemia, insulin resistance, and hypertriglyceridemia? Int J Obes 1993;17:53–61.
90. Haffner S, Stern M, Mitchell B, Hazuda H, Patterson J. Incidence of Type II diabetes in Mexican Americans predicted by fasting insulin and glucose levels, obesity, and body fat distribution. Diabetes 1990;39:283–287.
91. Reaven GM. Pathophysiology of insulin resistance in human disease. Physiol Rev 1995;75(3): 473–486.
92. Landsberg L. Diet, obesity, and hypertension: an hypothesis involving insulin, the sympathetic nervous system, and adaptive thermogenesis. Q J Med 1986;61:1081–1090.
93. Richter WO, Geiß HC, Aleksic S, Schwandt P. Cardiac autonomic nerve function and insulin sensitivity in obese subjects. International J Obes 1996;20:966–969.
94. Chan JM, Rimm EB, Colditz GA, Stampfer MJ, Willett WC. Obesity, fat distribution, and weight gain as risk factors for clinical diabetes in men. Diabetes Care 1994;17:961–969.
95. LeStunff C, Bougneres P. Early changes in postprandial insulin secretion, not in insulin sensitivity, characterize juvenile obesity. Diabetes 1994;43:696–702.
96. Sigal RJ, El-Hashimy M, Martin BC, Soeldner JS, Krolewski AS, Warram JH. Acute post-challenge hyperinsulinemia predicts weight gain. Diabetes 1997;46:1025–1029.
97. Velasquez-Mieyer PA, Cowan PA, Buffington CK, et al. Suppression of insulin secretion promotes weight loss and alters macronutrient preference in a subset of obese adults. Int J Obes 2003;27: 219–226.

6 Adiponectin: A Multifunctional Adipokine

Kristen J. Clarke and Robert L. Judd

CONTENTS

INTRODUCTION

Adipose tissue was once known primarily as a storage organ for excess energy in the form of triglycerides *(1, 2)*. However, during the past decade, adipose tissue has been recognized as an active endocrine organ, playing an important role in the regulation of whole body energy homeostasis, insulin sensitivity, and lipid/carbohydrate metabolism through the secretion of several hormones (*1–4*). These adipose-derived hormones (also known as adipocytokines, or adipokines) are secreted into the plasma where they circulate and have direct actions on peripheral tissues. The list of adipose tissue–derived secretory products includes leptin, tumor necrosis factor-α (TNF-α), interlukin-6 (IL-6), plasminogen activator inhibitor-1 (PAI-1), angiotensinogen, adipsin, and insulin-like growth factor 1 (IGF-1), among others. One adipocyte-derived factor

From: *Contemporary Endocrinology: Energy Metabolism and Obesity: Research and Clinical Applications*
Edited by: P. A. Donohoue © Humana Press Inc., Totowa, NJ

receiving widespread attention due to its insulin-sensitizing properties is adiponectin. Recent studies have demonstrated that adiponectin has antiatherogenic and anti-inflammatory properties in addition to its insulin-sensitizing properties (*5–9*). Similar to another adipocytokine, adipsin, adiponectin secretion from fat is regulated by insulin, suggesting a possible role for nutrition in the regulation of adiponectin expression and secretion *(10, 11)*. Adiponectin is one of the most abundant plasma proteins accounting for approximately 0.01–0.05% of total plasma proteins, and decreases in circulating adiponectin levels have been observed in obese humans and mice (*12–14*). Decreased adiponectin levels have been correlated with decreased insulin sensitivity *(13, 15, 16)*. It has been suggested that hormones such as TNF-α may play a role in the regulation of adiponectin secretion from adipocytes thereby mediating their effects on insulin metabolism and sensitivity *(17, 18)*. Adiponectin levels increase after treatment with thiazolidinediones (TZDs), a class of diabetic drugs that enhance insulin sensitivity (*19–22*). Therefore, adiponectin may provide a link between obesity and insulin resistance as well as provide clues to the mechanism of action of the insulin-sensitizing properties of TZDs. The purpose of this review is to summarize our current knowledge of adiponectin, with particular focus on the effects of adiponectin on whole body energy metabolism.

DISCOVERY OF ADIPONECTIN

Adiponectin [also known as complement-related protein 30 (Acrp30), adipose most dominant gene transcript 1 (apml), and AdipoQ], was discovered at the same time as leptin (1995–1996), but the importance of this discovery was not recognized for a number of years due to clinical correlation issues and difficulty in analytical measurements *(23)*. Adiponectin was discovered independently by four different laboratories using four different techniques. In 1995, Scherer et al. identified adiponectin using subtractive cDNA screening to identify mRNAs induced during differentiation of 3T3-L1 adipocytes *(10)*. Northern blot analysis of one specific clone showed a 100-fold increase in induction during differentiation; the resulting full-length cDNA was isolated and sequenced, and the protein encoded by this cDNA was discovered to be novel. It was subsequently described as having sequence and structural homology to complement factor C1q, and therefore was named adipocyte-derived complement-related protein of 30 kDa, or Acrp30 *(10)*.

In 1996, Hu et al. used mRNA differential display to isolate a novel adipose cDNA they named AdipoQ *(12)*. The expression of AdipoQ was specific to adipose tissue in both mouse and rat and encoded a protein consisting of 247 amino acids with significant homology to complement factor C1q. The encoded protein contained a collagenous structure in its N-terminus as well as a globular domain in its C-terminus. AdipoQ was found to be highly regulated during the differentiation of adipocytes, and Hu et al. were the first to describe a significant downregulation of AdipoQ mRNA in fat tissues collected from obese humans and mice *(12)*.

Maeda et al. isolated a novel adipose-specific gene, adipose most abundant gene transcript (apM1), from human adipose tissue *(24)*. The transcript of apM1 is the most abundant of all mRNA from adipose tissue. Northern blotting of RNAs from several different human tissues including skeletal muscle, small intestine, placenta, uterus, ovary, kidney, liver, lung, brain, heart, and bladder revealed that apM1 was specifically expressed in adipose tissue. Further studies revealed that apM1 encodes the adiponectin protein.

In 1996, Nakano et al. used gel chromatography to identify a novel protein from human plasma they named gelatin binding protein of 28 kDa, or GBP28 *(25)*. GBP28 was identified by its affinity to gelatin-Cellulofine. The protein purified from the column was described as having a molecular mass of 28 kDa under reducing conditions and 68 kDa under nonreducing conditions. Further analysis revealed that the cDNA clone apM1 previously discovered by Maeda et al. encoded a protein containing all the sequences of GBP28 and it was concluded that apM1 encoded GBP28 *(25)*. The amino acid sequence for GBP28 showed 82.7% homology to Acrp30, which is thought to be the murine equivalent of GBP28 *(25)*.

ADIPONECTIN PROTEIN STRUCTURE

Adiponectin is a 30-kDa monomeric protein. Human adiponectin consists of 244 amino acid residues *(10)* and is composed of an N-terminal signal sequence, a nonhomologous region, an amino-terminal collagenous domain, and a domain containing 22 Gly-X-Pro or GLY-X-X repeats (Fig. 6.1). This suggests that adiponectin has a straight collagen stalk as opposed to the kinked collagen domain present in the protein C1q *(10)*. There is a globular domain in the carboxy-terminus of the protein that bears structural homology to a number of other proteins including the globular domains of type VIII and type X collagens, the subunits of complement factor C1q, and TNF-α *(10, 24)*. The three-dimensional structure of adiponectin is very similar to that of TNF-α *(12)*.

Adiponectin is secreted from adipocytes and posttranslationally modified into different multimers *(26)*. Two-dimensional gel electrophoresis of recombinant adiponectin produced by *Escherichia coli* revealed only one multimer of adiponectin, suggesting that multiple isoforms of adiponectin are the result of posttranslational processing in mammalian adipocytes *(26)*. Several isoforms of adiponectin purified from 3T3-L1 adipocytes are hydroxylated and subsequently glycosylated, which may contribute to the heterogeneity of the protein. Wang et al. revealed that the glycosylation was neither N-linked nor O-linked; however the glycosylation occurred on four lysine residues in the collagen domain of the protein *(26)*. Replacement of the

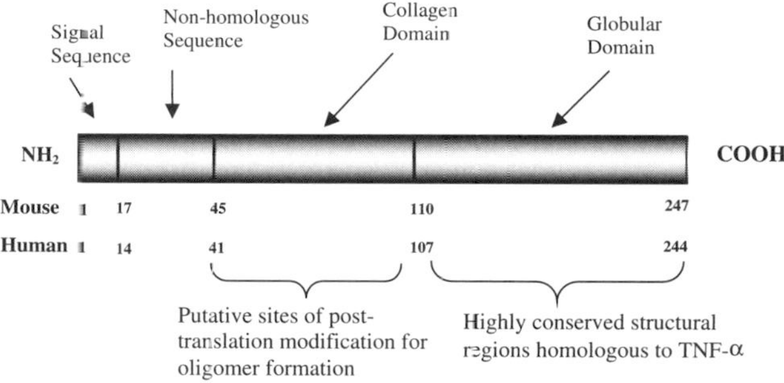

Fig. 6.1 Schematic representation of murine and human adiponectin. (Adapted from Ukkola O, Santaniemi M. J Adiponectin: a link between excessive adiposity and associated comorbidities Mol Med 2002;80:696–702; and from Berg AH, Combs TP, Scherer PE. ACRP30/adiponectin: an adipokine regulating glucose and lipid metabolism. Trends Endocrinol Metab 2002;13:84–89.).

lysine residues with arginine residues resulted in decreased action of insulin to suppress hepatic glucose production indicating that the glycosylated lysine residues are required for the biological activity of adiponectin *(26)*. In later studies, Wang et al. purified adiponectin from fetal bovine serum and demonstrated that four proline residues in the collagenous domain are hydroxylated (Pro39, 42, 48 and 86), and a total of five lysine residues in the collagenous domain are hydroxylated and subsequently glycosylated (Lys28, 60, 63, 72 and 96) *(27)*.

Adiponectin circulates in the plasma in remarkably high concentrations (10 μg/ml), accounting for approximately 0.01–05% of the total serum protein. It circulates in protein complexes or multimers. Figure 6.2 describes the formation of these complexes. Monomers are single 30-kDa proteins that can form trimers through associations in their globular domains *(28)*. Trimers associate with other trimers through disulfide bonds in their collagen domains to form higher-molecular-weight structures *(28)*. Adiponectin has been identified in human serum in two higher-order structures: a dimer of trimers [known as the low-molecular-weight (LMW) complex, approximately 180 kDa] or higher-order structures that are larger complexes of 12–18 subunits (4–6 trimers, approximately 360–540 kDa) *(29)*. These higher-order complexes are known as high-molecular-weight (HMW) complexes and are the predominant form found in human serum. Multimer (LMW, HMW) formation depends on disulfide bond formation mediated by Cys-39 *(29)*. The LMW and HMW complexes form inside the adipocyte and are secreted into the circulation where they may undergo further proteolytic cleavage. For example, the globular domain of adiponectin has been identified in

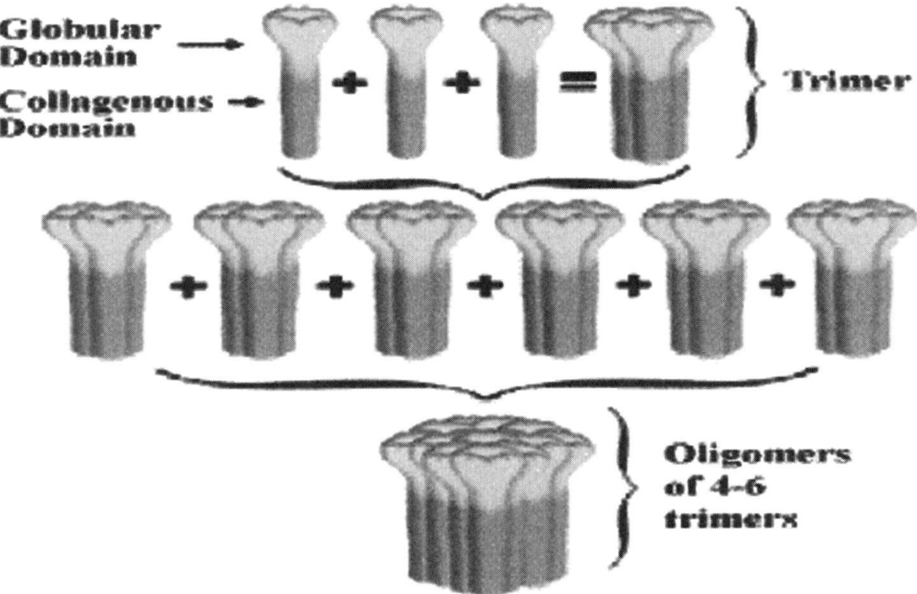

Fig. 6.2 Model for assembly of adiponectin complexes. Three monomers form a trimer through associations between their globular domains. Four to six trimers associate noncovalently through their collagenous domains to form high-molecular-weight oligomers, which circulate in the plasma. (Adapted from Chandran M, Phillips SA, Ciaraldi T, Henry RR. Adiponectin: more than just another fat cell hormone? Diabetes Care 2003;26:2442–2450.).

human plasma at physiologically significant levels and has been identified as having biological activity *(30, 31)*. Waki et al. recently identified the enzyme leukocyte elastase as an enzyme capable of cleaving adiponectin in its collagenous domain resulting in a globular fragment of 18–25 kDa *(32)*.

Adiponectin circulates in serum as a hexamer of relatively LMW and large multimer structure of HMW. There has been controversy regarding the biological activity of the individual complexes. Numerous studies have correlated inflammation, obesity, diabetes, and atherosclerosis with total adiponectin concentrations. However, in cases where changes in insulin sensitivity cannot be explained on the basis of differences in absolute serum adiponectin concentrations alone, Pajvani et al. have proposed an index S_A *(33)*. S_A is calculated as the ratio of HMW/HMW + LMW, and has implications as a strong indicator of hepatic insulin sensitivity, suggesting that the liver and not muscle is the primary target site of action for the full-length protein *(33)*. Pajvani et al. also suggested that the HMW multimer is the active form of adiponectin *(33)*.

ADIPONECTIN GENE EXPRESSION

Northern blot analysis demonstrated that adiponectin is encoded for by the human adipose most abundant gene transcript 1 (apM1) *(24)*. The adiponectin gene spans 17 kb on human chromosome 3q27, which has been identified as a susceptibility locus for diabetes *(34)*. apM1 consists of three exons and two introns and has been detected in human adipose tissue but not skeletal muscle, small intestine, placenta, uterus, kidney, liver, lung, brain, or heart. Therefore, it is believed that apM1 is expressed exclusively in adipose tissue *(24)*. The specificity of apM1 holds true for other species as well, including the rat and mouse *(12)*. Expression of apM1 is highly restricted to mature fat cells, and initial expression of the gene does not appear until approximately day 4 after induction of differentiation of preadipocytes into adipocytes *(12, 24)*. apM1 is not expressed in 3T3-L1 fibroblasts, however it is induced more than 100-fold after differentiation of 3T3-L1 fibroblasts into 3T3-L1 adipocytes *(10)*.

Specific mutations in apM1 have been observed to result in lower plasma levels of adiponectin. A G/T polymorphism has been reported in exon 2 and a missense mutation (R112C) in exon 3 *(35)*. Although the plasma levels of adiponectin in patients with the G/T polymorphism were low, they were not significantly different from plasma levels of adiponectin in normal patients *(35)*. The one subject with the missense mutation (R112C) showed very low plasma levels of adiponectin suggesting the missense mutation was responsible for the low levels of the protein. Kondo et al. characterized three more missense mutations of the adiponectin gene in locations encoding the globular domain of the protein *(36)*. These mutations include I164T, R221S, and H241P. The frequency of the I164T mutation was significantly higher in type 2 diabetic patients than in age-matched and body mass index (BMI)-matched control subjects *(36)*. Plasma levels of adiponectin in individuals carrying this mutation were also significantly lower than adiponectin levels in individuals without the mutation, and all patients identified with this mutation had at least one feature of the metabolic syndrome such as hypertension, hyperlipidemia, diabetes, or atherosclerosis *(36)*. These results give further evidence to support the role of adiponectin in the development of type 2 diabetes or other components of the metabolic syndrome.

More recent studies have investigated the association between adiponectin encoding gene variants, insulin resistance, and cardiovascular disease *(37,38)*. An association of the T-G polymorphism in apM1 (exon 2) was associated with obesity and diabetes in a family cohort *(39)*. Additional studies demonstrated that adiponectin variants predispose individuals to the development of severe childhood and adult obesity, but further investigations are required to determine the physiologic mechanisms responsible for this process *(40)*.

ADIPONECTIN RECEPTORS

Yamauchi et al. were the first to describe functional receptors for adiponectin in 2003 *(41)*. They identified two receptor subtypes by a series of expression cloning experiments and named them AdipoR1 and AdipoR2 *(41)*. Although these receptors are expressed ubiquitously, AdipoR1 is more highly expressed in skeletal muscle, and AdipoR2 is more highly expressed in the liver. AdipoR1 is a high-affinity receptor for globular adiponectin and a low-affinity receptor for full-length adiponectin, whereas AdipoR2 is an intermediate receptor for both globular and full-length adiponectin *(41)*. The globular domain of the protein by itself has been demonstrated to have more potent effects on fatty acid oxidation in skeletal muscle than the full-length protein *(42)*. However, the full-length form of the protein is believed to be the predominant circulating form of adiponectin.

Both receptor subtypes are predicted to contain seven-transmembrane domains, however they are functionally and structurally distinct from G protein–coupled receptors *(41)*. The N-terminus of the adiponectin receptor lies on the internal surface of the cell membrane, whereas the C-terminus is on the external surface of the cell membrane, opposite the structural topology of typical G protein–coupled receptors *(41)*. Although the full signal transduction pathway upon adiponectin binding to its receptor is currently unknown, it has been reported that binding of globular and full-length adiponectin to AdipoR1 or AdipoR2 increases peroxisome proliferator-activated receptor-alpha (PPAR-α) ligand activity and increases the phosphorylation of adenosine monophosphate protein kinase (AMPK), acetyl coenzyme A carboxylase (ACC), and p38 mitogen-activated protein kinase. These events result in increased glucose uptake and fatty acid oxidation in skeletal muscle (AdipoR1) and decreased glucose output by the liver (AdipoR2) *(41)*.

Recent *in vivo* and *in vitro* studies investigated whether AdipoR1 and AdipoR2 expression levels are altered in pathophysiologic states. Civitarese et al. suggested that AdipoR1and AdipoR2 expression levels in muscle are lower in subjects with a family history of type 2 diabetes than in those without *(43)*. Importantly, the expression of both receptors correlated positively with insulin sensitivity. In contrast with these results, Debard et al. did not demonstrate any significant differences in expression of AdipoR1 or AdipoR2 in skeletal muscle of type 2 diabetic patients *(44)*. Staiger et al. also investigated the expression levels of AdipoR1 and AdipoR2 from human myotubes and found that neither AdipoR1 nor AdipoR2 correlated with insulin sensitivity *(45)*. It is clear that further investigation of the expression of AdipoR1 and AdipoR2 will be necessary to elucidate whether there is indeed a correlation between adiponectin receptor levels and insulin sensitivity.

There is recent evidence that AdipoR1 and AdipoR2 expression levels are under nutritional control in mice *(46)*. Fasting upregulated AdipoR1 and AdipoR2 expression increased in both liver and skeletal muscle of mice compared with mice fed ad libitum *(46)*. Refeeding subsequently downregulated AdipoR1 and AdipoR2 expression in both liver and skeletal muscle. However, Beylot et al. were unable to demonstrate the same nutritional regulation of AdipoR1 or AdipoR2 in rats *(47)*. Neither high fat feeding nor fasting modified AdipoR1 in normal Wistar rats *(47)*. A slight decrease in AdipoR2 was observed in livers of high-fat-fed Wistar rats *(47)*. Using obese Zucker rats as a model of insulin resistance, Beylot et al. found no difference in the expression of AdipoR1 or AdipoR2 in muscle *(47)*. However, a slight decrease in expression of AdipoR1 and AdipoR2 in adipose tissue and a slight increase in AdipoR1 and AdipoR2 in liver was observed *(47)*. It is unclear whether these conflicting results are species specific. However, it is clear that further investigation of the potential role for nutritional regulation of adiponectin receptors is necessary.

Adiponectin receptor expression may also be under hormonal influence. Tsuchida et al. demonstrated that adiponectin receptors are negatively regulated by insulin *(46)*. Insulin regulation of AdipoR1 and AdipoR2 was suppressed by the PI3-kinase inhibitor LY294002 suggesting that insulin regulation of AdipoR1 and AdipoR2 occurs through the PI3-kinase pathway *(46)*.

AdipoR1 and AdipoR2 expression has also been investigated in skeletal muscle and liver from two different models of diabetic mice. Expression of AdipoR1 and AdipoR2 was upregulated in skeletal muscle of streptozotocin (STZ) diabetic mice *(46)*. Treatment of STZ mice with insulin reduced expression levels of AdipoR1 and AdipoR2. Expression of AdipoR1 and AdipoR2 was not significantly different in the livers of STZ diabetic mice compared with non–STZ mice, however insulin significantly decreased expression of both receptors in the livers of STZ-treated mice *(46)*. AdipoR1 and AdipoR2 expression levels were reduced in muscle and adipose tissue but not in liver of *ob/ob* mice, a model commonly used to study type 2 diabetes. The authors suggest that downregulation of adiponectin receptors in *ob/ob* mice is correlated with decreased adiponectin sensitivity *(46)*.

In 2004, Hug et al. reported that the T-cadherin receptor was capable of binding adiponectin in C2C12 myoblasts but not in the liver *(48)*. T-cadherin is a member of the cadherin family of receptors involved in calcium mediated cell-cell interactions and is structurally distinct from AdipoR1 and AdipoR2 *(48)*. T-cadherin receptors are expressed on smooth muscle cells as well as endothelial cells and bind eukaryotically produced high-molecular-weight as well as hexameric forms of adiponectin but not the trimeric or globular forms of adiponectin *(48)*. They do not bind bacterially produced adiponectin suggesting that posttranslational modifications are necessary for the binding of adiponectin to the T-cadherin receptors *(48)*.

PHYSIOLOGIC FUNCTIONS OF ADIPONECTIN

A wide array of physiologic functions in a variety of tissues including skeletal muscle, liver, and the vasculature occur after adiponectin binding to its receptors. Adiponectin has been demonstrated to have anti-inflammatory and antiatherogenic properties. Studies showed that adiponectin suppressed activation of the transcription factor, NF-κB, in the vascular endothelium *(49)*. TNF-α regulates the activation of NF-κB, which results in the accumulation of cAMP. This activation is blocked by adenyl cyclase and protein kinase A (PKA) inhibitors suggesting that adiponectin mediates this inflammatory response through the cAMP-PKA and NF-κB pathways *(49)*. Recent studies suggest some of adiponectin's anti-inflammatory action may be due to neutralization of lipopolysaccharide (LPS)-mediated inflammatory events *(50, 51)*. Adiponectin was also shown to adhere to injured vascular walls, preventing the adhesion of macrophages as well as plaque formation *(52)*. Interestingly, diabetic patients with coronary artery disease (CAD) had lower levels of adiponectin than did diabetic patients without CAD suggesting that adiponectin deficiency may play a role in the development of CAD *(53, 54)*.

Adiponectin may also be an important link between obesity, insulin resistance, and the development of type 2 diabetes. Adiponectin levels are reduced in obese adults as well as in adults with type 2 diabetes *(53, 55)*. Studies suggest that serum adiponectin concentrations are determined predominately by visceral fat content *(56)*. In vivo and in vitro studies demonstrate that adiponectin secretion is higher from visceral adipose tissue compared with subcutaneous adipose tissue (*57–59*). In contrast, leptin is secreted primarily from subcutaneous adipose tissue *(56, 57)*. Recent studies suggest that low adiponectin levels are more strongly correlated with insulin resistance and hyperinsulinemia than degree of adiposity and glucose tolerance *(60, 61)*. Low basal levels of adiponectin in a population of Pima Indians were found to predict decreased insulin sensitivity in this population regardless of adiposity *(62)*. In addition, adiponectin levels are positively correlated with high-density lipoprotein (HDL) levels; low levels of adiponectin are associated with high levels of low-density lipoprotein (LPL) as well as other metabolic parameters involved in the development of the metabolic syndrome *(63)*. These studies point to a role of adiponectin in increasing insulin sensitivity and suggest decreased plasma concentrations of this hormone are associated with increased insulin resistance.

There is an abundant amount of experimental evidence supporting the role of adiponectin as an insulin-sensitizing hormone. Interestingly, Pajvani et al. demonstrated that the HMW complex of adiponectin dose-dependently decreases serum glucose levels *(33)*. Intraperitoneal injection of adiponectin lowered serum glucose levels and free fatty acids without changes in insulin levels in mice *(15, 16)*. Chronic injections of full-length adiponectin resulted in decreased body weight in high-fat-fed mice *(15)* and improved insulin sensitivity in insulin-resistant mice *(64)*. Surprisingly, injections of the isolated C-terminal globular domain had the same, if not more potent, metabolic effects than the full-length protein *(15, 16, 64)*.

Skeletal muscle is a major target for adiponectin's physiologic functions. Improved insulin sensitivity may be the result of increased fatty acid oxidation and decreased triglyceride content in muscle *(15, 64)*. Yamauchi et al. demonstrated that globular and full-length adiponectin phosphorylated and activated AMPK in skeletal muscle *(42)*. Activation of AMPK resulted in phosphorylation of acetyl coenzyme A carboxylase (ACC), fatty acid oxidation, glucose uptake, and lactate production in C2C12 myocytes *(42)*.

Liver is another primary target organ of adiponectin's insulin-sensitizing properties. Adiponectin enhances insulin action in primary hepatocytes by decreasing gluconeogenesis and hepatic glucose output *(16)*. However, exposure to the isolated globular C-terminus did not have the same metabolic effects in isolated hepatocytes, indicating that the full-length protein is necessary for adiponectin's insulin-sensitizing effects in the liver *(16)*. Adiponectin mediates these insulin-sensitizing effects by increasing fatty acid oxidation through activation of AMPK and PPAR-α *(42)*. Activation of AMPK in the liver is followed by increased phosphorylation of ACC, decreased malonyl-CoA, and increased fatty acid oxidation *(42)*. Activation of PPAR-α also results in increased gene expression of enzymes involved in fatty acid oxidation *(65)*. The expression levels of enzymes such as phosphoenolpyruvate carboxykinase (PEPCK) and glucose-6-phosphatase (G6Pase) involved in gluconeogenesis were decreased in mice infused with Acrp30 *(66)*. These results suggest that adiponectin lowers circulating glucose levels by decreasing hepatic glucose output *(66)*.

Recent studies also suggest adiponectin is present and has effects in the brain *(67)*. Qi et al. demonstrated that adiponectin is transported from the serum to the cerebrospinal fluid (CSF) *(67)*. Intracerebroventricular (ICV) injections of adiponectin in normal mice reduced the body weight of these mice without affecting food intake. Increased oxygen consumption as well as increased expression of uncoupling protein-1 (UCP-1) in brown adipose tissue were also observed in these mice. These results suggest that ICV injections of adiponectin increased thermogenesis in these animals. Importantly, ICV injections of adiponectin in Agouti mice did not affect body weight or thermogenesis, suggesting that adiponectin's effects are mediated at least in part through the melanocortin pathway *(67)*. However, two recent studies suggest that adiponectin is not detectable in human CSF *(68)* due to the fact that it does not cross the blood-brain barrier *(69)*. However, it has been demonstrated that adiponectin can modify cytokine expression of brain endothelial cells *(68)*. Figure 6.3 represents a hypothetical model for the actions of adiponectin in its target tissues including liver, skeletal muscle, brain, and the endothelium *(70)*.

Further characterization of adiponectin as an insulin-sensitizing hormone has been undertaken using genetically modified or knockout mice. However, these studies have produced conflicting data. Maeda et al. reported that mice lacking a functional adiponectin gene and fed a normal diet did not show any differences in growth rate, food intake, body weight, or other metabolic parameters measured at 12 and 16 weeks of age compared with wild-type mice *(71)*. However, these knockout mice did show delayed clearance of free fatty acids in plasma, low levels of fatty acid transport protein-1 (FATP-1) mRNA in muscle, as well as high levels of TNF-α mRNA in adipose tissue and high circulating levels of TNF-α *(71)*. Additionally, knockout mice fed a high-fat/high-sucrose diet for 2 weeks had significantly higher plasma glucose levels and insulin concentrations compared with wild-type mice. Six weeks on the high-fat/high-sucrose diet did not result in increased body weight or adiposity compared with wild-type mice. However, it did result in the development of severe insulin resistance *(71)*. Adenovirus-mediated increased adiponectin expression in the knockout mice reversed the reduction of FATP-1 as well as the increase in TNF-α and the diet-induced insulin resistance. In a subset of these studies, mice were also generated heterozygote for adiponectin expression. No significant differences in any of the metabolic parameters measured as well as insulin sensitivity were recorded between these mice on either the normal diet or the high-fat/high-sucrose diet compared with wild-type mice *(71)*.

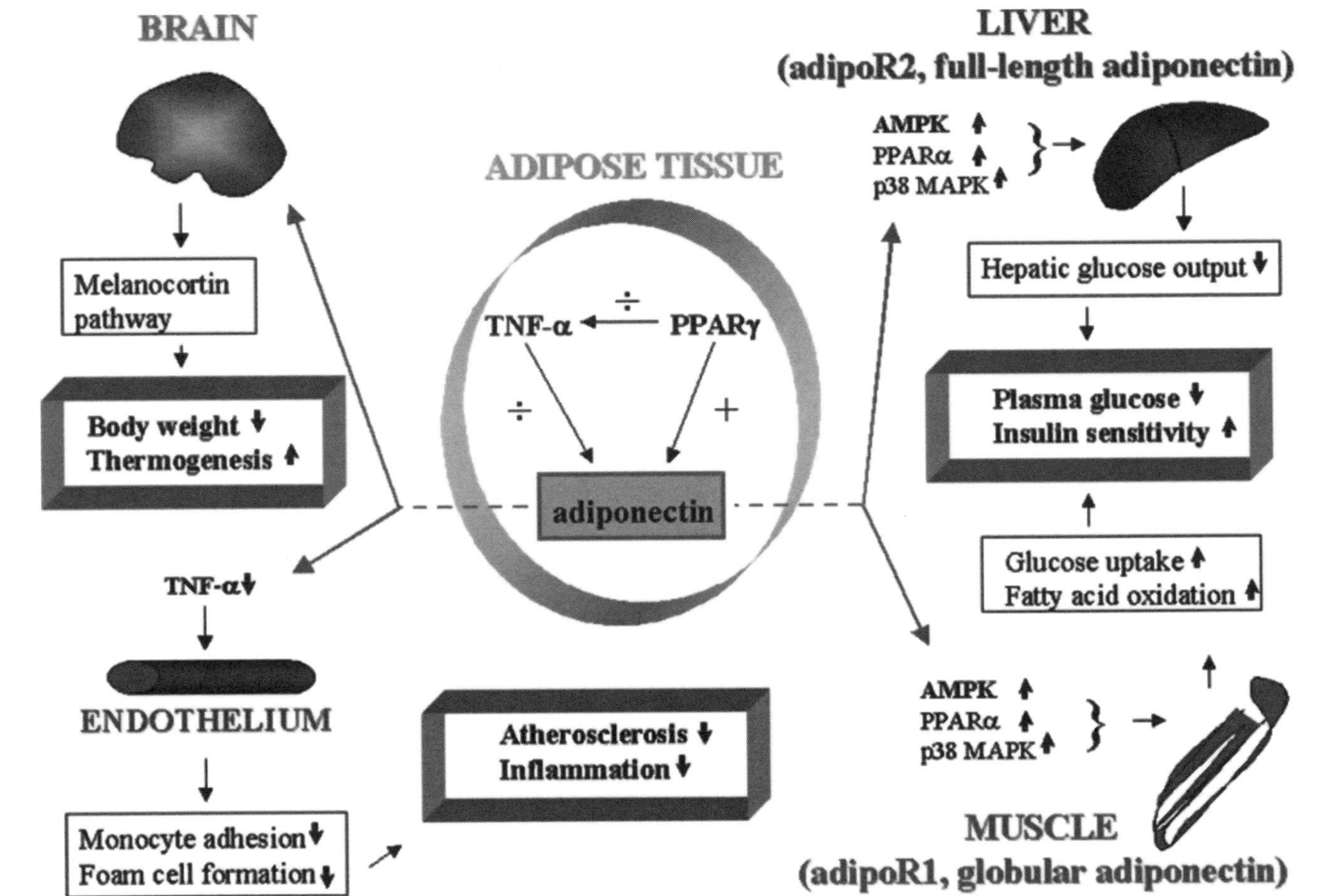

Fig. 6.3 Illustration of target tissues and proposed mode of action and regulation of adiponectin. (Reproduced from Lihn AS et al. Obes Rev 2005;6:13–21.)

Ma et al. also generated adiponectin knockout mice. Their results, however, were quite different from those reported by Maeda et al. Adiponectin-deficient mice were found to have normal body and fat pad weights as well as normal circulating glucose and insulin levels *(72)*. They also responded to a glucose tolerance test in a manner similar to wild-type mice suggesting no overt insulin resistance. High fat feeding for 7 months did not result in any significant differences in weight gain or glucose or insulin tolerance tests between normal and adiponectin-deficient mice *(72)*. Increased β-oxidation in skeletal muscle and liver was the only significant difference found between the adiponectin knockout mice and wild-type mice *(72)*. The reasons for the conflicting results between these studies are unclear; however, a number of possibilities exist, including differences in the generation of the knockout mice as well as the duration and composition of the diet.

REGULATION OF ADIPONECTIN GENE EXPRESSION AND SECRETION

Due to adiponectin's important insulin-sensitizing, antiatherogenic and anti-inflammatory properties, it has become of major interest to identify factors that play a role in the regulation of adiponectin expression and secretion from adipose tissue. Identification of such factors may lead to the identification of potential therapeutic targets aimed at elevating levels of this protein in disease states such as coronary artery disease and type 2 diabetes.

Adiponectin levels are influenced by many factors. Scherer et al. were the first to describe that insulin acutely stimulates secretion of adiponectin from 3T3-L1 adipocytes *(10)*. Longer-term incubation (>16 h) with insulin, however, has been shown to increase or decrease both adiponectin secretion and gene expression *(73)*. Interleukin-6 (IL-6) and TNF-α are cytokines produced from adipose tissue, and levels of these cytokines are increased in insulin resistance and obesity. Both cytokines inhibit adiponectin gene expression and secretion from adipocytes *(74, 75)*. Table 6.1 provides a brief summary of some of the factors involved in the regulation of adiponectin secretion and gene expression.

Other hormonal regulatory factors of adiponectin include insulin-like growth factor (IGF-1), growth hormone, and leptin. IGF-1 increases adiponectin gene expression in adipocytes. Growth hormone increases adiponectin gene expression and secretion. Leptin, another adipokine whose levels are dysregulated in insulin resistance, obesity, and type 2 diabetes has been shown to inhibit adiponectin secretion.

Pharmacologic agents have also been shown to affect adiponectin gene expression and protein secretion. PPAR-γ ligands such as the antidiabetic class of drugs thiazolidinediones (TZDs) are known to enhance insulin sensitivity in insulin-resistant type 2 diabetic animal models as well as insulin-resistant patients. Previously, it was unknown how the TZDs increased insulin sensitivity; however recent studies have shown that TZDs increase adiponectin expression and secretion from adipocytes. Therefore, it is believed that at least a portion of the insulin-sensitizing properties of the TZDs results from increased circulating levels of adiponectin.

Interestingly, there appear to be gender-related differences in the circulating concentrations of adiponectin. Plasma adiponectin levels are 35% lower in human males compared with human females (6.0 μg/ml vs. 9.1 μg/ml) *(76)*. There are no significant

Table 6.1
Factors influencing adiponectin secretion and gene expression

Factor	*Adiponectin gene expression*	*Adiponectin secretion*
Insulin	+/−	+/−
IGF-1	+	Not determined
PPAR-γ ligands/TZDs	+	+
TNF-α	−	−
Glucocorticoids	−	Not determined
β-adrenergic agonists	−	Not determined
cAMP	−	−
Interlukin-6	−	−
Growth hormone	+	+
Exercise	Not determined	+
Leptin	Not determined	−
Free fatty acids	Not determined	−
Weight loss	+	+

Source: Modified from Stefan N. and Stumvoll M. Adiponectin—its role in metabolism and beyond Horm Metab Res 2002;34:469–474.

differences in plasma adiponectin levels between pre- and postmenopausal women *(76)*. This suggests that male sex hormones are a potential regulator of circulating adiponectin levels. Indeed, Nishizawa et al. demonstrated that testosterone decreased adiponectin secretion from 3T3-L1 adipocytes, and castration of male mice increased circulating adiponectin levels compared with noncastrated littermates *(76)*. Interestingly however, Bryzgalova et al. recently reported that estrogen receptor alpha knockout mice (ERKO) had lower serum levels of adiponectin and pronounced insulin resistance, indicating that estrogen (acting through estrogen receptor alpha) may indeed play a role in the regulation of adiponectin secretion *(77)*.

Adiponectin has a relatively long half-life in serum (2.5–6 h), and it was recently determined that adiponectin levels are also determined in part by ultradian patterns *(29, 78)*. In other words, adiponectin is secreted with diurnal variations in less than a 24-h period *(79)*. In normal human males, serum adiponectin was characterized by a nocturnal decline starting in the late evening and reaching its maximum decrease in the early morning (~3 a.m.; $3.56 \pm 0.3\ \mu g/ml$) *(79)*. Serum adiponectin levels were higher during the day with peak levels reached at approximately 11 a.m. ($5.28 \pm 0.3\ \mu g/ml$) *(79)*. Although both adiponectin and leptin exhibit similar variations in diurnal rhythms, these rhythms do not overlap and suggest a possible regulation by one adipokine or the other. Indeed, a recent study suggests that leptin plays a role in the regulation of circulating adiponectin levels. Central leptin gene therapy administered in *ob/ob* and wild-type mice decreased plasma levels of adiponectin without an alteration in TNF-α levels *(80)*. In addition, peripheral administration of leptin also significantly reduced plasma levels of adiponectin in *ob/ob* and wild-type mice *(80)*.

The effects of weight loss and exercise have also been investigated as potential mediators of adiponectin secretion and expression. Obese men ($BMI > 35\ kg/m^2$) were placed on a calorie-restricted diet for 20 weeks. Prior to weight loss, plasma adiponectin levels were 47% lower in obese mean compared with lean individuals; after diet-induced weight loss of approximately 20 kg, plasma adiponectin levels increased by 51% (2.3 ± 0.6 vs. 3.4 ± 0.8 μg/ml) *(81)*. Adiponectin mRNA was collected from adipose tissue biopsies from these patients before and after weight loss, and after weight reduction, adiponectin mRNA levels increased by 45% *(81)*. Plasma adiponectin was also measured in a group of individuals before and after weight loss by gastric partition surgery. Prior to surgery, the patients had a mean BMI of 39.57 ± 5.89 kg/m^2 and an average circulating concentration of adiponectin of 4.53 ± 1.46 μg/ml *(82)*. After gastric partitioning surgery, the subjects lost >20 kg, had an average BMI of 31.22 ± 5.21 kg/m^2 and average circulating concentration of adiponectin of 6.63 ± 2.32 μg/ml *(82)*. In both of these studies, the increases in plasma adiponectin levels were significantly correlated with increases in insulin sensitivity *(81, 82)*

Other studies provide further evidence for the dysregulation of adiponectin in obesity and diabetes. Hu et al. demonstrated that apM1 is dysregulated in obesity *(12)*. A reduction in apM1 mRNA was observed in both obese humans and mice compared with normal controls *(12)*. Arita et al. measured plasma adiponectin from nonobese and obese subjects and found that circulating levels of this protein are significantly reduced in obese subjects (8.9 μg/ml vs. 3.7 μg/ml) *(14)*. Administration of TZDs to obese mice and cultured 3T3-L1 adipocytes increased mRNA expression of apM1 in a dose- and time-dependent manner *(83)*. Administration of TZDs to insulin-resistant humans and mice also increased circulating levels of adiponectin *(83)*.

Although many factors including circulating hormones, therapeutic agents such as PPAR-γ agonists, exercise, and weight loss have been identified as factors playing a role in the regulation of adiponectin secretion and expression, there are many as yet unidentified factors that also play a role in the regulation of adiponectin.

ROLE OF ADIPONECTIN IN HUMAN DISEASE

Even though adiponectin was only recently discovered, studies have demonstrated that it is directly involved in a number of disease states. Originally, it was noted that plasma adiponectin levels and adiponectin gene expression are reduced in obesity and type 2 diabetes. In these patients, adiponectin levels are increased by treatment with TZDs (*22,58,83–85*) and weight loss *(82)*. Adiponectin has also been implicated in cardiovascular health, including identification as a marker for predisposition to hypertension in men *(86)*. In addition, hypoadiponectinemia is a highly sensitive serum marker for the prediction of future cardiovascular events *(5)*. Retrospective case-control studies demonstrate that patients with the highest levels of adiponectin have a dramatically reduced 6-year risk of myocardial infarction compared with case controls with the lowest adiponectin levels, and this relationship persists even when controlling for family history, BMI, alcohol, history of diabetes and hypertension, hemoglobin A1c, C-reactive protein (CRP), and lipoprotein levels *(87)*. Recent studies have also demonstrated that platelet activation is associated with hypoadiponectinemia and carotid atherosclerosis *(88, 89)*. The exact mechanisms of the antiatherosclerotic activity of adiponectin have not been completely elucidated. However, the association between adiponectin levels and cardiovascular risk independent of other variables suggests that adiponectin mediates direct effects on vascular health, as opposed to indirect effects through insulin sensitivity and diabetes *(5)*. A number of studies have shown direct effects of adiponectin on endothelial and vascular smooth muscle cells *(90, 91)*.

Adiponectin levels are decreased in patients with coronary heart disease, and it has been suggested that adiponectin modulates the endothelial inflammatory disease associated with coronary heart disease *(52)*. It has also been hypothesized that adiponectin has inflammatory-modulating activities, and clinical studies have demonstrated inverse associations between adiponectin levels and serum markers of inflammation *(92)*. Although it is not clear how or whether adiponectin itself has anti-inflammatory properties, it is clear that adiponectin production by adipose tissue can be inhibited by systemic inflammation, at least under some circumstances *(5)*. In addition to its possible anti-inflammatory properties and their implications for cardiovascular disease (CVD), it is important to mention the recent demonstration that adiponectin may also have an important role in protecting against cardiac hypertrophy in cardiac overload states such as hypertension, hypertrophic cardiomyopathy, and ischemic heart disease *(93, 94)*. Thus, the decreased levels of this protein in obesity may represent multiple connections to cardiac risk: inflammation-induced cardiovascular insufficiency and direct myocardial insult. However, the mechanism(s) responsible for the hypoadiponectinemia observed in insulin resistance, obesity, and cardiovascular disease has yet to be determined. Therefore, adiponectin may also provide one of the links between obesity and coronary heart disease as well as insulin resistance and type 2 diabetes.

CONCLUSION

Studies have clearly demonstrated that adipokines have a variety of physiologic effects. Adiponectin has anti-inflammatory, antiatherogenic, and insulin-sensitizing effects. The metabolic effects of adiponectin are primarily regulated through effects on the liver and skeletal muscle. A number of compounds have been implicated in the regulation of adiponectin secretion. A more complete understanding of the synthesis and regulation of adiponectin secretion will likely lead to better approaches for the management of obesity, type 2 diabetes, atherosclerosis, and cardiovascular disease.

REFERENCES

1. Fruhbeck G, Gomez-Ambrosi J, Muruzabal FJ, Burrell MA. The adipocyte: a model for integration of endocrine and metabolic signaling in energy metabolism regulation. Am J Physiol Endocrinol Metab 2001;280:E827–E847.
2. Trayhurn P. Endocrine and signalling role of adipose tissue: new perspectives on fat. Acta Physiol Scand 2005;184:285–293.
3. Havel PJ. Update on adipocyte hormones: regulation of energy balance and carbohydrate/lipid metabolism. Diabetes 2004;53(Suppl 1):S143–S151.
4. Rajala MW, Scherer PE. Minireview: The adipocyte—at the crossroads of energy homeostasis, inflammation, and atherosclerosis. Endocrinology 2003;144:3765–3773.
5. Berg AH, Scherer PE. Adipose tissue, inflammation, and cardiovascular disease. Circ Res 2005;96:939–949.
6. Okamoto Y, Kihara S, Ouchi N, et al. Adiponectin reduces atherosclerosis in apolipoprotein E-deficient mice. Circulation 2002;106:2767–2770.
7. Kubota N, Terauchi Y, Yamauchi T, et al. Disruption of adiponectin causes insulin resistance and neointimal formation. J Biol Chem 2002;277:25863–25866.
8. Wang B, Jenkins JR, Trayhurn P. Expression and secretion of inflammation-related adipokines by human adipocytes differentiated in culture: integrated response to TNF-alpha. Am J Physiol Endocrinol Metab 2005;288:E731–E740.

9. Shimada K, Miyazaki T, Daida H. Adiponectin and atherosclerotic disease. Clin Chim Acta 2004;344:1–12.
10. Scherer PE, Williams S, Fogliano M, Baldini G, Lodish HF. A novel serum protein similar to C1q, produced exclusively in adipocytes. J Biol Chem 1995;270:26746–26749.
11. Bogan JS, Lodish HF. Two compartments for insulin-stimulated exocytosis in 3T3-L1 adipocytes defined by endogenous ACRP30 and GLUT4. J Cell Biol 1999;146:609–620.
12. Hu E, Liang P, Spiegelman BM. AdipoQ is a novel adipose-specific gene dysregulated in obesity. J Biol Chem 1996;271:10697–10703.
13. Yamauchi T, Kamon J, Waki H, et al. The fat-derived hormone adiponectin reverses insulin resistance associated with both lipoatrophy and obesity. Nat Med 2001;7:941–946.
14. Arita Y, Kihara S, Ouchi N, et al. Paradoxical decrease of an adipose-specific protein, adiponectin, in obesity. Biochem Biophys Res Commun 1999;257:79–83.
15. Fruebis J, Tsao TS, Javorschi S, et al. Proteolytic cleavage product of 30-kDa adipocyte complement-related protein increases fatty acid oxidation in muscle and causes weight loss in mice. Proc Natl Acad Sci USA 2001;98:2005–2010.
16. Berg AH, Combs TP, Du X, Brownlee M, Scherer PE. The adipocyte-secreted protein Acrp30 enhances hepatic insulin action. Nat Med 2001;7:947–953.
17. Suganami T, Nishida J, Ogawa Y. A paracrine loop between adipocytes and macrophages aggravates inflammatory changes: role of free fatty acids and tumor necrosis factor alpha. Arterioscler Thromb Vasc Biol 2005;25:2062–2068.
18. Kern PA, Di Gregorio GB, Lu T, Rassouli N, Ranganathan G. Adiponectin expression from human adipose tissue: relation to obesity, insulin resistance, and tumor necrosis factor-alpha expression. Diabetes 2003;52:1779–1785.
19. Yilmaz MI, Sonmez A, Caglar K, et al. Peroxisome proliferator-activated receptor gamma (PPAR-gamma) agonist increases plasma adiponectin levels in type 2 diabetic patients with proteinuria. Endocrine 2004;25:207–214.
20. Osei K, Gaillard T, Kaplow J, Bullock M, Schuster D. Effects of rosglitazone on plasma adiponectin, insulin sensitivity, and insulin secretion in high-risk African Americans with impaired glucose tolerance test and type 2 diabetes. Metabolism 2004;53:1552–1557.
21. Phillips SA, Ciaraldi TP, Kong AP, et al. Modulation of circulating and adipose tissue adiponectin levels by antidiabetic therapy. Diabetes 2003;52:667–674.
22. Yu JG, Javorschi S, Hevener AL, Kruszynska YT, Norman RA, Sinha M, Olefsky JM. The effect of thiazolidinediones on plasma adiponectin levels in normal, obese, and type 2 diabetic subjects. Diabetes 2002;51:2968–2974.
23. Koerner A, Kratzsch J, Kiess W. Adipocytokines: leptin—the classical, resistin—the controversical, adiponectin—the promising, and more to come. Best Pract Res Clin Endocrinol Metab 2005;19:525–546.
24. Maeda K, Okubo K, Shimomura I, Funahashi T, Matsuzawa Y, Matsubara K. cDNA cloning and expression of a novel adipose specific collagen-like factor, apM1 (AdiPose Most abundant Gene transcript 1). Biochem Biophys Res Commun 1996;221:286–289.
25. Nakano Y, Tobe T, Choi-Miura NH, Mazda T, Tomita M. Isolation and characterization of GBP28, a novel gelatin-binding protein purified from human plasma. J Biochem (Tokyo) 1996;120:803–812.
26. Wang Y, Xu A, Knight C, Xu LY, Cooper GJ. Hydroxylation and glycosylation of the four conserved lysine residues in the collagenous domain of adiponectin. Potential role in the modulation of its insulin-sensitizing activity. J Biol Chem 2002;277:19521–19529.
27. Wang Y, Lu G, Wong WP, et al. Proteomic and functional characterization of endogenous adiponectin purified from fetal bovine serum. Proteomics 2004;4:3933–3942.
28. Berg AH, Combs TP, Scherer PE. ACRP30/adiponectin: an adipokine regulating glucose and lipid metabolism. Trends Endocrinol Metab 2002;13:84–89.

29. Pajvani UB, Du X, Combs TP, et al. Structure-function studies of the adipocyte-secreted hormone Acrp30/adiponectin. Implications fpr metabolic regulation and bioactivity. J Biol Chem 2003;278:9073–9085.
30. Hug C, Lodish HF. Diabetes, obesity, and Acrp30/adiponectin. Biotechniques 2002;33:654, 656, 658.
31. Chandran M, Phillips SA, Ciaraldi T, Henry RR. Adiponectin: more than just another fat cell hormone? Diabetes Care 2003;26:2442–2450.
32. Waki H, Yamauchi T, Kamon J, et al. Generation of globular fragment of adiponectin by leukocyte elastase secreted by monocytic cell line THP-1. Endocrinology 2005;146:790–796.
33. Pajvani UB, Hawkins M, Combs TP, et al. Complex distribution, not absolute amount of adiponectin, correlates with thiazolidinedione-mediated improvement in insulin sensitivity. J Biol Chem 2004;279:12152–12162.
34. Vionnet N, Hani E, Dupont S, et al. Genomewide search for type 2 diabetes-susceptibility genes in French whites: evidence for a novel susceptibility locus for early-onset diabetes on chromosome 3q27-qter and independent replication of a type 2-diabetes locus on chromosome 1q21–q24. Am J Hum Genet 2000;67:1470–1480.
35. Takahashi M, Arita Y, Yamagata K, et al. Genomic structure and mutations in adipose-specific gene, adiponectin. Int J Obes Relat Metab Disord 2000;24:861–868.
36. Kondo H, Shimomura I, Matsukawa Y, et al. Association of adiponectin mutation with type 2 diabetes: a candidate gene for the insulin resistance syndrome. Diabetes 2002;51:2325–2328.
37. Vasseur F, Lepretre F, Lacquemant C, Froguel P. The genetics of adiponectin. Curr Diab Rep 2003;3:151–158.
38. Vozarova de Court, Hanson RL, Funahashi T, et al. Common polymorphisms in the adiponectin gene ACDC are not associated with diabetes in Pima Indians. Diabetes 2005;54:284–289.
39. Stumvoll M, Tschritter O, Fritsche A, et al. Association of the T-G polymorphism in adiponectin (exon 2) with obesity and insulin sensitivity: interaction with family history of type 2 diabetes. Diabetes 2002;51:37–41.
40. Bouatia-Naji N, Meyre D, Lobbens S, et al. ACDC/Adiponectin polymorphisms are associated with severe childhood and adult obesity. Diabetes 2006;55:545–550.
41. Yamauchi T, Kamon J, Ito Y, et al. Cloning of adiponectin receptors that mediate antidiabetic metabolic effects. Nature 2003;423:762–769.
42. Yamauchi T, Kamon J, Minokoshi Y, et al. Adiponectin stimulates glucose utilization and fatty-acid oxidation by activating AMP-activated protein kinase. Nat Med 2002;8:1288–1295.
43. Civitarese AE, Jenkinson CP, Richardson D, et al. Adiponectin receptors gene expression and insulin sensitivity in non-diabetic Mexican Americans with or without a family history of type 2 diabetes. Diabetologia 2004;47:816–820.
44. Debard C, Laville M, Berbe V, et al. Expression of key genes of fatty acid oxidation, including adiponectin receptors, in skeletal muscle of Type 2 diabetic patients. Diabetologia 2004;47: 917–925.
45. Staiger H, Kaltenbach S, Staiger K, et al. Expression of adiponectin receptor mRNA in human skeletal muscle cells is related to in vivo parameters of glucose and lipid metabolism. Diabetes 2004;53:2195–2201.
46. Tsuchida A, Yamauchi T, Ito Y, et al. Insulin/Foxo1 pathway regulates expression levels of adiponectin receptors and adiponectin sensitivity. J Biol Chem 2004;279:30817–30822.
47. Beylot M, Pinteur C, Peroni O. Expression of the adiponectin receptors AdipoR1 and AdipoR2 in lean rats and in obese Zucker rats. Metabolism 2006;55:396–401.
48. Hug C, Wang J, Ahmad NS, Bogan JS, Tsao TS, Lodish HF. T-cadherin is a receptor for hexameric and high-molecular-weight forms of Acrp30/adiponectin. Proc Natl Acad Sci USA 2004;101: 10308–10313.

49. Ouchi N, Kihara S, Arita Y, et al. Adiponectin, an adipocyte-derived plasma protein, inhibits endothelial NF-kappaB signaling through a cAMP-dependent pathway. Circulation 2000;102: 1296–1301.
50. Tsuchihashi H, Yamamoto H, Maeda K, et al. Circulating concentrations of adiponectin, an endogenous lipopolysaccharide neutralizing protein, decrease in rats with polymicrobial sepsis. J Surg Res 2006;134:348–353.
51. Peake PW, Shen Y, Campbell LV, Charlesworth JA. Human adiponectin binds to bacterial lipopolysaccharide. Biochem Biophys Res Commun 2006;341:108–115.
52. Ouchi N, Kihara S, Arita Y, et al. Novel modulator for endothelial adhesion molecules: adipocyte-derived plasma protein adiponectin. Circulation 1999;100:2473–2476.
53. Hotta K, Funahashi T, Arita Y, et al. Plasma concentrations of a novel, adipose-specific protein, adiponectin, in type 2 diabetic patients. Arterioscler Thromb Vasc Biol 2000;20:1595–1599.
54. Chan KC, Chou HH, Wu DJ, Wu YL, Huang CN. Diabetes mellitus has an additional effect on coronary artery disease. Jpn Heart J 2004;45:921–927.
55. Matsubara M, Maruoka S, Katayose S. Inverse relationship between plasma adiponectin and leptin concentrations in normal-weight and obese women. Eur J Endocrinol 2002;147:173–180.
56. Staiger H, Tschritter O, Machann J, et al. Relationship of serum adiponectin and leptin concentrations with body fat distribution in humans. Obes Res 2003;11:368–372.
57. Park KG, Park KS, Kim MJ, et al. Relationship between serum adiponectin and leptin concentrations and body fat distribution. Diabetes Res Clin Pract 2004;63:135–142.
58. Motoshima H, Wu X, Sinha MK, et al. Differential regulation of adiponectin secretion from cultured human omental and subcutaneous adipocytes: effects of insulin and rosiglitazone. J Clin Endocrinol Metab 2002;87:5662–5667.
59. Cnop M, Havel PJ, Utzschneider KM, et al. Relationship of adiponectin to body fat distribution, insulin sensitivity and plasma lipoproteins: evidence for independent roles of age and sex. Diabetologia 2003;46:459–469.
60. Stefan N, Bunt JC, Salbe AD, Funahashi T, Matsuzawa Y, Tataranni PA. Plasma adiponectin concentrations in children: relationships with obesity and insulinemia. J Clin Endocrinol Metab 2002;87:4652–4656.
61. Weyer C, Funahashi T, Tanaka S, Hotta K, Matsuzawa Y, Pratley RE, Tataranni PA. Hypoadiponectinemia in obesity and type 2 diabetes: close association with insulin resistance and hyperinsulinemia. J Clin Endocrinol Metab 2001;86:1930–1935.
62. Lindsay RS, Funahashi T, Hanson RL, et al. Adiponectin and development of type 2 diabetes in the Pima Indian population. Lancet 2002;360:57–58.
63. Gil-Campos M, Canete R, Gil A. Hormones regulating lipid metabolism and plasma lipids in childhood obesity. Int J Obes Relat Metab Disord 2004;28(Suppl 3):S75–S80.
64. Yamauchi T, Waki H, Kamon J, et al. Inhibition of RXR and PPARgamma ameliorates diet-induced obesity and type 2 diabetes. J Clin Invest 2001;108:1001–1013.
65. Ferre P. The biology of peroxisome proliferator-activated receptors: relationship with lipid metabolism and insulin sensitivity. Diabetes 2004;53(Suppl 1):S43–S50.
66. Combs TP, Berg AH, Obici S, Scherer PE, Rossetti L. Endogenous glucose production is inhibited by the adipose-derived protein Acrp30. J Clin Invest 2001;108:1875–1881.
67. Qi Y, Takahashi N, Hileman SM, et al. Adiponectin acts in the brain to decrease body weight. Nat Med 2004;10:524–529
68. Spranger J, Verma S, Gohring I, et al. Adiponectin does not cross the blood-brain barrier but modifies cytokine expression of brain endothelial cells. Diabetes 2006;55:141–147.
69. Pan W, Tu H, Kastin AJ: Differential BBB interactions of three ingestive peptides: obestatin, ghrelin, and adiponectin. Exp Neurol 2006;198:222–233.

70. Baskin ML, Ard J, Franklin F, Allison DB. Prevalence of obesity in the United States. Obes Rev 2005;6:5–7.
71. Maeda N, Shimomura I, Kishida K, et al. Diet-induced insulin resistance in mice lacking adiponectin/ACRP30. Nat Med 2002;8:731–737.
72. Ma K, Cabrero A, Saha PK, et al. Increased beta-oxidation but no insulin resistance or glucose intolerance in mice lacking adiponectin. J Biol Chem 2002;277:34658–34661.
73. Halleux CM, Takahashi M, Delporte ML, Detry R, Funahashi T, Matsuzawa Y, Brichard SM. Secretion of adiponectin and regulation of apM1 gene expression in human visceral adipose tissue. Biochem Biophys Res Commun 2001;288:1102–1107.
74. Fasshauer M, Kralisch S, Klier M, Lossner U, Bluher M, Klein J, Paschke R. Adiponectin gene expression and secretion is inhibited by interleukin-6 in 3T3-L1 adipocytes. Biochem Biophys Res Commun 2003;301:1045–1050.
75. Fasshauer M, Klein J, Neumann S, Eszlinger M, Paschke R. Hormonal regulation of adiponectin gene expression in 3T3-L1 adipocytes. Biochem Biophys Res Commun 2002;290:1084–1089.
76. Nishizawa H, Shimomura I, Kishida K, et al. Androgens decrease plasma adiponectin, an insulin-sensitizing adipocyte-derived protein. Diabetes 2002;51:2734–2741.
77. Bryzgalova G, Gao H, Ahren B, et al. Evidence that oestrogen receptor-alpha plays an important role in the regulation of glucose homeostasis in mice: insulin sensitivity in the liver. Diabetologia 2006;49:588–597.
78. Hoffstedt J, Arvidsson E, Sjolin E, Wahlen K, Arner P. Adipose tissue adiponectin production and adiponectin serum concentration in human obesity and insulin resistance. J Clin Endocrinol Metab 2004;89:1391–1396.
79. Gavrila A, Peng CK, Chan JL, Mietus JE, Goldberger AL, Mantzoros CS. Diurnal and ultradian dynamics of serum adiponectin in healthy men: comparison with leptin, circulating soluble leptin receptor, and cortisol patterns. J Clin Endocrinol Metab 2003;88:2838–2843.
80. Ueno N, Dube MG, Inui A, Kalra PS, Kalra SP. Leptin modulates orexigenic effects of ghrelin and attenuates adiponectin and insulin levels and selectively the dark-phase feeding as revealed by central leptin gene therapy. Endocrinology 2004;145:4176–4184.
81. Bruun JM, Lihn AS, Verdich C, Pedersen SB, Toubro S, Astrup A, Richelsen B. Regulation of adiponectin by adipose tissue-derived cytokines: in vivo and in vitro investigations in humans. Am J Physiol Endocrinol Metab 2003;285:E527–E533.
82. Yang WS, Lee WJ, Funahashi T, et al. Weight reduction increases plasma levels of an adipose-derived anti-inflammatory protein, adiponectin. J Clin Endocrinol Metab 2001;86:3815–3819.
83. Maeda N, Takahashi M, Funahashi T, et al. PPARgamma ligands increase expression and plasma concentrations of adiponectin, an adipose-derived protein. Diabetes 2001;50:2094–2099.
84. Combs TP, Wagner JA, Berger J, et al. Induction of adipocyte complement-related protein of 30 kilodaltons by PPARgamma agonists: a potential mechanism of insulin sensitization. Endocrinology 2002;143:998–1007.
85. Yang WS, Jeng CY, Wu TJ, et al. Synthetic peroxisome proliferator-activated receptor-gamma agonist, rosiglitazone, increases plasma levels of adiponectin in type 2 diabetic patients. Diabetes Care 2002;25:376–380.
86. Iwashima Y, Katsuya T, Ishikawa K, et al. Hypoadiponectinemia is an independent risk factor for hypertension. Hypertension 2004;43:1318–1323.
87. Pischon T, Girman CJ, Hotamisligil GS, Rifai N, Hu FB, Rimm EB. Plasma adiponectin levels and risk of myocardial infarction in men. JAMA 2004;291:1730–1737.
88. Shoji T, Koyama H, Fukumoto S, et al. Platelet activation is associated with hypoadiponectinemia and carotid atherosclerosis. Atherosclerosis 2006;188:190–195.
89. Iwashima Y, Horio T, Suzuki Y, et al. Adiponectin and inflammatory markers in peripheral arterial occlusive disease. Atherosclerosis 2006;188:384–390.

90. Goldstein BJ, Scalia R. Adiponectin: a novel adipokine linking adipocytes and vascular function. J Clin Endocrinol Metab 2004;89:2563–2568.
91. Halperin F, Beckman JA, Patti ME, et al. The role of total and high-molecular-weight complex of adiponectin in vascular function in offspring whose parents both had type 2 diabetes. Diabetologia 2005;48:2147–2154.
92. Ouchi N, Kihara S, Funahashi T, et al. Reciprocal association of C-reactive protein with adiponectin in blood stream and adipose tissue. Circulation 2003;107:671–674.
93. Liao Y, Takashima S, Maeda N, et al. Exacerbation of heart failure in adiponectin-deficient mice due to impaired regulation of AMPK and glucose metabolism. Cardiovasc Res 2005;67:705–713.
94. Shibata R, Ouchi N, Ito M, et al. Adiponectin-mediated modulation of hypertrophic signals in the heart. Nat Med 2004;10:1384–1389.

7 The Role of the Gastrointestinal Hormones Ghrelin, Peptide YY, and Glucagon-like Peptide-1 in the Regulation of Energy Balance

Ruben Nogueiras, Hilary Wilson, Diego Perez-Tilve, and Matthias H. Tschöp

CONTENTS

INTRODUCTION

The gastrointestinal tract secretes hormones into the bloodstream to activate defined circuits of the central nervous system that regulate energy homeostasis. The story behind this intriguing model began more than 100 years ago, when a hormone named secretin was isolated from duodenal mucosa *(1)*. Since the isolation of secretin, the past century has generated the discovery of many other hormones, some of them discovered in the past decade. The mechanisms of action of those hormones and their possible uses in pharmaceutical therapies have recently become a focus of many research groups around the world.

GHRELIN

One of the major players among gut hormones in the regulation of food intake is the only known circulating hormone that stimulates food intake: ghrelin. In 1999, ghrelin was identified as the endogenous ligand of the growth hormone secretagogue receptor

From: *Contemporary Endocrinology: Energy Metabolism and Obesity: Research and Clinical Applications*
Edited by: P. A. Donohoue © Humana Press Inc., Totowa, NJ

(GHSR) *(2)*, with the highest activation in stomach extracts *(2)*. The ligand took this name from the proto-Indo-European word *ghre*, which means "grow," and from *relin*, relating to its GH-releasing activities. Some months after ghrelin was discovered, an independent group identified this same peptide from the stomach, but named it motilin-related peptide *(3)*. Prior to this, in 1998, a similar sequence was submitted under the name of motilin-homologue *(4)*. These three peptides have a very high homology, and because of their similarities in the structure and actions, motilin-related peptide, ghrelin, and motilin-homologue can be considered as a novel gastrointestinal hormone family.

The ghrelin precursor preproghrelin possesses 117 amino acids and results in the ghrelin peptide, consisting of 28 amino acids with an *n*-octanoylated serine in position 3. After the discovery of the 28-amino-acid ghrelin, several other isoforms produced by alternative splicing of the ghrelin gene were found, the main circulating form being des-acylated [des-(Gln14)] ghrelin, constituting about 80–90% of total ghrelin. Des-acyl-ghrelin cannot activate GHSR-1a and therefore does not share endocrine activities of octanoylated ghrelin. However, des-acyl-ghrelin seems to have cardio-protective, antiproliferative, and adipogenic properties and can antagonize octanoyl-ghrelin–induced effects on insulin secretion and blood glucose levels in humans *(5)*.

Although present elsewhere in the body, ghrelin is produced primarily in the stomach (around 65% of plasma ghrelin levels arise from the stomach) by the X/A-like cells within the oxyntic glands of the gastric fundus mucosa. The small intestine, brain, pituitary, pancreas, kidney, lymphocytes, lung, placenta, testis, and ovary also express detectable amounts of ghrelin *(6)*.

Ghrelin and Energy Balance

Ghrelin is the first and only gut peptide proven to have substantial orexigenic properties. It potently stimulates food intake in humans and rodents after peripheral administration. Central administration of ghrelin directly into the CNS of rodents rapidly increases food intake, and centrally administered ghrelin is equipotent when compared to all other known orexigenic factors *(7)*. Endogenous ghrelin levels are closely related to meal patterns, rising before meals and falling within 1 h after eating *(8)*. Ghrelin peaks of similar magnitude are observed before each meal of the day, suggesting that ghrelin may be involved in meal initiation *(8)* or meal preparation. In addition, the postprandial ghrelin reduction is proportional to the ingested calorie load *(9)*. Circulating ghrelin levels are highest in the fasting state and are elevated in patients with anorexia nervosa, as well as in animals in states of cachexia *(10)*. Conversely, ghrelin levels are decreased in human and rodent obesity *(11, 12)*; moreover, subjects with a low body mass index (BMI) have higher ghrelin levels than lean subjects *(13, 14)*. An exception is patients with Prader-Willi syndrome, which are hyperphagic, obese, and GH deficient. Whereas all other studied obese subjects have low ghrelin levels, patients with Prader-Willi syndrome have high ghrelin levels *(15)*, which could result from the hypothalamic damage observed in these subjects *(16)*.

Several studies have suggested that orexigenic effects of ghrelin are mediated via leptin-responsive neurons in the hypothalamus (*17–20*). Within the hypothalamus, specific nuclei containing leptin and/or ghrelin receptor–expressing neurons are known to be critical sites of integration for leptin and ghrelin pathways and are consequently important in the regulation of energy balance. The most relevant nucleus is probably the arcuate nucleus (Arc), where two distinct leptin- and ghrelin-responsive cell groups exist. Neuropeptide Y (NPY) and agouti-related peptide (AgRP) are potent stimulators of food intake, while an adjacent set of Arc neurons coexpress POMC and cocaine and amphetamine regulated transcript (CART), which suppress food intake. Leptin stimulates POMC/CART neurons and inhibits NPY/AgRP neurons, resulting in inhibition of feeding and an increase in energy expenditure. Conversely, ghrelin activates NPY/AgRP neurons, which in turn inhibit POMC neurons. Thereby, ghrelin stimulates feeding and decreases energy expenditure *(20)*. Interestingly, it was observed that ablation of the Arc with monosodium glutamate significantly diminishes the central effects of ghrelin on food intake *(21)*. In addition to the Arc, the hindbrain has also been shown to mediate orexigenic effects of ghrelin *(22)*. Consistent with such findings, the administration of ghrelin in the fourth ventricle or directly on the dorsal vagal complex results in a hyperphagic response similar to that obtained with administration into the third ventricle *(22)*.

In addition to the central pathways, ghrelin may also act on peripheral sites such as the gastric vagus nerve, but its effectson food intake after peripheral administration are less potent and appear to be more temporary *(23)*. In vitro studies show that ghrelin can stimulate the expression of peroxisome proliferator-activated receptor (PPAR)-γ2, thus indicating that ghrelin could act directly on adipocytes to stimulate adipogenesis *(24)*. The administration of both ghrelin and desoctanoyl ghrelin in the bone marrow also stimulate adipogenesis *(25)*. Ghrelin also has direct effects on brown adipose tissue, decreasing adiponectin expression *(26)*. It remains unclear however if such effects are physiologically relevant and if a ghrelin-responsive receptor can be identified in adipose tissue.

In addition to its functions on food intake and energy balance, ghrelin increases gastric acid secretion and gastric motility in rats *(27, 28)*, and these effects are abolished by pretreatment with either atropine or bilateral cervical vagotomy. Ghrelin also stimulates gastric emptying *(29)* and gastrin release *(30)*. Ghrelin-induced changes in gastric emptying could again modulate food intake in an indirect manner, but that hypothesis has not yet been scientifically tested.

Ghrelin and Glucose Homeostasis

The fact that gastric absorption of carbohydrates, especially glucose, decreases ghrelin secretion implies that ghrelin may interact with components of glucose homeostasis. Indeed, in vitro and in vivo experiments show that ghrelin influences insulin secretion *(31)*, and plasma ghrelin levels decrease after oral and intravenous glucose administration *(14)*. Human and animal studies have demonstrated a negative correlation between circulating ghrelin concentrations and insulin secretion (*32–35*). It is important to note that most of these studies used hyperinsulinemic euglycemic clamp conditions as a tool, and therefore changes in ghrelin level may be secondary to the supraphysiologic duration or extent of hyperinsulinemia. Furthermore, data from different studies paint a somewhat inconsistent picture. However, the current opinion still is that both insulin and glucose are likely to have a suppressive impact on ghrelin secretion. Regarding ghrelin's impact on glucose homeostasis, ghrelin levels in a physiologic range decreased insulin secretion, whereas higher levels had either no effect or increased insulin secretion. In most studies, ghrelin action leads to a modestly hyperglycemic glucose concentration *(36)*. Date et al. reported stimulation of insulin secretion in isolated rat pancreatic islets by ghrelin in the presence of only slight hyperglycemia *(37)*. It was suggested that ghrelin may influence insulin secretion by acting directly on insulin producing β-cells of the pancreas *(37)*, as the ghrelin receptor GHSR-1a is expressed in pancreatic islets *(38)*. Consistent with a ghrelin-insulin interaction, another study described lower ghrelin levels in patients with PCOS, a syndrome characterized in part by decreased insulin sensitivity *(39)*. However, it was demonstrated in normal lean subjects that only prolonged hyperinsulinemia results in suppressed plasma ghrelin levels *(40)*, suggesting that physiologic postprandial peaks of insulin are unlikely to be responsible for a postmeal suppression of ghrelin levels in the healthy lean subjects *(40)*.

Ghrelin and Ghrelin Receptor Knockout Mice

Initial reports of ghrelin-null and GHSR-null mice did not describe the expected significant impairments in energy balance or growth *(41,42)*. Furthermore, in contrast withsuggestions that ghrelin may influence leptin and insulin secretion, fasting serum levels of leptin and insulin were identical between wild-type and GHSR-null mice or ghrelin-null mice. Possibly, compensatory mechanisms during embryonic or early postnatal development are acting to develop and maintain a normal phenotype and balanced energy metabolism in ghrelin-null or GHSR-null mice. Such an explanatory construct has also been used by obesity researchers to explain the lack of a striking phenotype of other knockout models of orexigenic agents, such as NPY *(43)* or AgRP *(44)*. However, actual evidence for this explanation, such as compensatory up- or downregulation of other energy balance regulatory genes, remains to be identified. Although missing the lipodystrophic, cachectic, or small phenotype, ghrelin-null mice exhibit a lower respiratory quotient (on a high-fat diet), which indicates increased fat oxidation in the absence of ghrelin, suggesting that ghrelin may after all play an endogenous role regarding the choice of metabolic fuels *(45)*.

New light was shed on ghrelin's role in energy metabolism, and enthusiasm was renewed for ghrelin as a possible drug target for the treatment of obesity when two recent reports showed that ghrelin-null as well as GHSR-null mice were protected against the development of diet-induced obesity *(46)*. Extending first reports, it was shown that female GHSR-null mice fed a standard diet gained less body weight and had less fat mass than the wild-type mice. In addition, the authors reported improved glucose tolerance in male GHSR-null mice maintained under standard diet, which points to an adiposity-independent effect of ghrelin on glucose homeostasis, as male null mice had similar body weights to their wild-type littermates on standard chow.

A follow up report on ghrelin-null mice also reveals a gender-specific effect on body weight gain. When fed a high-fat diet from 6 weeks of age for up to 16 weeks, male ghrelin-null mice exhibit attenuated body weight gain and lower body fat associated with decreased feeding efficiency and increased energy expenditure. Also, plasma levels of lipids, glucose, leptin, and insulin were lower than in wild-type controls on chronic high-fat diet, likely as a result of protection against increased adiposity. Considering the gender-specific differences in the body weight development of ghrelin-

and GHSR-null mice, it was suggested that sex hormones such as estradiol and testosterone may play a role by modulating neuronal excitability of ghrelin's target neurons in the hypothalamic arcuate nucleus *(47)*.

Apart from the above-described model of complete lack of GHSR as a result of targeted mouse mutagenesis, one study performed in rats showed selective attenuation of GHSR protein expression in the arcuate nucleus of rats to cause a decrease in body weight and adipose tissue. Daily food intake in such rats lacking GHSR only in the hypothalamic arcuate nucleus was reduced, and the stimulatory effect of GHS treatment on feeding was abolished. These findings suggest that the expression of GHSR in this particular nucleus is significantly involved in the regulation of food intake and adiposity levels *(48)*.

Finally, in an opposite genetic approach, transgenic mice overexpressing human GHSR in GHRH neurons appear to have similar body weights in adulthood in comparison with wild-type mice. However, adipose mass was surprisingly reduced, particularly in females *(49)*. Organ and muscle weights of transgenic mice were increased despite chronic exposure to a high-fat diet. Food intake and adipose tissue responses to high-fat diet were unaffected, as were locomotor and anxiety behaviors, although GHRH/GHSR mice remained significantly leaner than wild-type littermates. Interestingly, GHSR transgenic mice did not show an increased sensitivity for the treatment with exogenous GHS ligands. One must conclude that constitutive overexpression of GHSR can reduce adiposity without affecting other GHSR-mediated signals. However, several issues remain unclear, for example how overexpression specifically in GHRH neurons relates to the very different physiologic expression pattern, which subtypes of ghrelin peptide or GHSR were exactly expressed, and how complex processes such as the acylation of cleaved ghrelin peptide or the constitutive activity of GHSR function given the highly artificial situation of this model.

Obestatin

Recently, Zhang et al. *(50)* identified a novel ghrelin-associated peptide on the basis of bioinformatic searches of putative hormones derived from the prepropeptides of known peptide hormones. This peptide is encoded by 23 amino acids, with a flanking conserved glycine residue at the C-terminus, and is named obestatin. Obestatin has been reported to show a high affinity for GPR39, whereas ghrelin, motilin, neurotensin, or neuromedin U were unable to bind to this receptor in this first study. Furthermore, nonamidated obestatin and truncated (des1-10) obestatin were shown in the same report to have a lower binding affinity for GPR39 than did obestatin. Parallel in vitro binding studies suggested that obestatin binding can be observed at the pituitary, stomach, ileum, and hypothalamus.

Regarding the physiologic effects of obestatin, these studies suggested that obestatin can antagonize ghrelin's effects on food intake, body weight, and gastric emptying but has no effect on growth hormone levels. Zhang et al. showed that intraperitoneal injection of obestatin suppresses food intake in a time- and dose-dependent manner, and intracerebroventricular treatment with obestatin also decreases food intake, similar to the anorexigenic effect of the synthetic melanocortin agonist MTII. In contrast, treatment with the nonamidated obestatin was less effective in creating a negative energy balance, suggesting that similar to ghrelin, a posttranslational modification is crucial for the peptide's bioactivity. Furthermore, treatment with obestatin led to a sustained suppression of gastric emptying activity. In vitro, isometric force measurement demonstrated that obestatin treatment decreased the contractile activity of jejunum and antagonized the stimulatory effect of ghrelin. In summary, after both central and peripheral administration, obestatin seems to antagonize ghrelin actions when both hormones were administered together. The fact that the same precursor leads to two different peptides with orexigenic and anorexigenic actions is reminiscent of some other cases such as POMC, which as a precursor peptide is also fragmented into several peptides with partially opposing effects on food intake. Mechanisms such as these, displaying an apparent biological contradiction, demonstrate that energy balance regulation depends not only on the expression of different genes, but also on the rate of transcription from the precursor to specific gene products as well as the posttranslational modification of such products. Intriguingly, the discovery of obestatin might explain why ghrelin-null mice, which would be lacking an orexigenic as well as an anorexigenic factor, do not show the expected strong phenotype. As it is typical when a new discovery appears, numerous unanswered questions arise, and further studies will be necessary to find those answers. Although obestatin decreased food intake and body weight in rodents, serum leptin levels were not affected after treatment with obestatin, suggesting minimal modulation of body-fat content. Moreover, fasting did not change serum obestatin levels, and circulating levels of obestatin are much lower than ghrelin, thus the relevance of endogenous obestatin remains unclear. Future studies have to address whether obestatin is able to exert an anorexigenic effect in obese animal models or simply suppress appetite by triggering nausea or visceral illness. Finally, one of the most interesting points will be to examine the significance of this hormone in humans. Obviously, the development of synthetic agonists for obestatin may exert enhanced potency and provide orally active agents, but at this point the available information does not allow us to judge if obestatin may represent a valuable drug target for the treatment of obesity. So far, there have been no reports confirming the results published by Zhang et al., and numerous future studies are necessary to confirm the role of obestatin in the control of energy balance and metabolism and explain the respective mechanisms of action.

PEPTIDE YY

Peptide YY (PYY) is a 36-amino-acid peptide originally isolated from porcine intestine *(51)* that belongs to the family of NPY. PYY is also expressed in the open-ended L-type endocrine cells of the terminal ileum and colon in the rat, dog, and human (*52–54*) and in cells along the periphery of pancreatic islets. But there are important structural differences among the members of this family. PYY levels decrease in the fasting state and increase in response to food intake, acting to inhibit gastric motility, gastric acid, and insulin secretion *(55)*. PYY release is dependent on the number of calories ingested and the composition of the food consumed, fat increasing PYY levels more potently than proteins or carbohydrates. In addition to its expression in the gastrointestinal tract, PYY is also produced in the hypothalamus and hindbrain regions *(56)*, and PYY receptors exhibit dense localizations in thalamic, limbic, and hindbrain nuclei (*57–59*). PYY_{1-36} and PYY_{3-36} are the two predominant molecular forms of PYY in the blood *(60)*, PYY_{3-36} being the truncated form created by cleavage of the N-terminus Tyr-Pro residues by dipeptidyl peptidase IV *(61)*. PYY_{1-36} and PYY_{3-36} show somewhat selective affinity to Y1 and Y2 receptors, respectively, and PYY_{3-36} potently activates Y1 and Y5 receptors.

Central Effects Versus Peripheral Effects

PYY shows very different actions depending on administration at the central or the peripheral level. Centrally administered PYY increases food intake even more potently than NPY. Along with ghrelin and melanocortin receptor 4 inverse agonists, PYY is one of the most potent acute stimulators of food intake when directly administered into the central nervous system (CNS). PYY produces massive hyperphagia if injected into the lateral or third cerebral ventricles, into the periventricular nucleus, or into the hippocampus, which is not usually associated with strong and immediate orexigenic responses.

Contrary to its central effects, several reports from one study group have shown that peripheral administration of PYY_{3-36} may reduce food intake in rodents, primates, and humans (*64–66*). Consistent with those findings, it has been speculated that elevated systemic levels of PYY_{3-36} resulting from gastric bypass surgery may be leading to a reduction of food intake, thereby contributing to the procedure's beneficial effects *(63)*. In rodents, it has been reported that a single dose of peripherally administered PYY_{3-36} suppressed food intake in a transient manner. Furthermore, PYY_{3-36} seems to inhibit food intake dose-dependently when administered by continuous intravenous infusion to non-food-deprived rats. PYY_{1-36}, if at all anorexigenic, is reported to be less potent than PYY_{3-36} in decreasing food intake, while PYY_{3-36} has been suggested to reduce food intake by decreasing meal size and increasing the satiety ratio (postmeal interval per meal size). PYY_{3-36} also appears to inhibit food intake in sham-feeding rats, indicating that this hormone can reduce food intake independently of its inhibitory action on gastric emptying *(67)*.

In humans, infusion of PYY_{3-36} has been reported to cause an equivalent inhibition of appetite and food intake in the obese and lean groups, suggesting that obesity is not associated with PYY resistance. Fasting PYY levels have been shown to be lower in the obese group than in the lean group, and there was a negative correlation between fasting PYY levels and BMI. Furthermore, postprandial PYY release was lower in obese than in lean subjects *(65)* overall, suggesting that PYY deficiency could be the cause for obesity and PYY replacement therapy may be a simple way to cure this rapidly spreading disease.

However, a substantial number of independent laboratories have been unable to reproduce the anorexigenic or the body-weight-lowering effects of PYY_{3-36} in rodents *(68)*. These groups only detected a transient decrease in body weight in *ob/ob* mice when using continuous administration and implanted osmotic minipumps. In fact, they observed a significant reduction in locomotor activity and rearing and sniffing behavior after PYY_{3-36} administration, while energy expenditure tended to decrease, even though the reduction was not significant. Thus, these findings do not support the suggestion that PYY_{3-36} treatment produced a negative energy balance.

One possible explanation for such controversial findings could be that without a proper habituation of the mice, the action of PYY_{3-36} is not evident due to the interference of stress caused by handling the animals *(69)*. However, extensive habituation and acclimatization was part of the protocols that led to negative findings *(68)*, and no signs of stress were detected based on those protocols including changes in plasma corticosteroids, in hypothalamic c-fos expression in the paraventricular nucleus area, or by monitoring feeding and baseline conditions or other stress-sensitive behaviors. Basically, the issue remains unresolved with laboratories finding few, none, opposite, or similar effects since the original reports were published. Most likely, various conditions and models are necessary to see the anorectic effects of PYY, which also might be less potent than originally thought.

Mechanism of Action

PYY_{3-36} has been shown to act at the hypothalamic level. Consistent with the possible opposing effects of ghrelin and PYY on food intake, a high percentage (50%) of Arc neurons have been reported to be activated by ghrelin and inhibited by PYY. Moreover, peripherally injected PYY partly reversed fasting-induced c-Fos expression in Arc neurons of mice *(70)*. Finally, immunohistochemical studies demonstrated that peripherally administered PYY_{3-36} induced c-Fos expression in Arc neurons expressing POMC.

PYY_{3-36} acts as an agonist at the Y2-R thereby triggering a negative autofeedback loop on NPY neurons and in doing so causes removal of the tonic inhibition on adjacent POMC neurons. In one study in Y2-R knockout mice, PYY_{3-36} did not reduce food intake, indicating that this receptor may play a key role in the controversially discussed anorectic effects of PYY_{3-36}. Furthermore, the effects of PYY_{3-36} are associated with an increase in POMC mRNA and a decrease in NPY mRNA expression levels in the Arc *(71)*. Currently available evidence suggests that melanocortin 4 receptors (MC4Rs) are the most important melanocortin receptor subtypes for the regulation of food intake. MC4Rs are also believed to be the very core of molecular body weight control in humans. However, more recent studies have demonstrated that both MC4R and POMC knockout mice are responsive to the anorexigenic effects of PYY_{3-36} *(69, 72, 73)*, suggesting that these factors are not essential for PYY_{3-36} actions.

In parallel, recent data showed by double immunostaining that approximately 20% of melanocyte stimulating hormone (MSH) expressing neurons of the Arc were activated by peripheral administration of PYY_{3-36} *(74)*. Colocalization in Arc neurons of CART and MSH, a cleavage product of the POMC gene, suggests that CART, which suppresses feeding independently of the MC4R system when administered intracerebroventricularly *(75)*, may play a role as a PYY_{3-36} target. Interestingly, it was observed that PYY_{3-36} appears to achieve at least part of its controversially discussed effects on feeding via the afferent vagus nerve, as it was observed that PYY_{3-36} had no effect on food intake in vagotomized rats or in rats with bilateral midbrain transactions in which the efferent fibers ascending from the nucleus of the solitary tract (NTS; a crucial component of the afferent vagal pathway) are ablated *(74)*. Finally, an in-depth neuroanatomy and electrophysiology study showed that peripherally administered PYY_{3-36} powerfully activates neurons in the area postrema and NTS, brain-stem areas known to be activated with visceral illness and taste aversion. These authors also demonstrated using classic behavioral tests that peripheral administration of PYY_{3-36} causes conditioned taste aversion in mice. In this report, extensive electrophysiologic studies also reveal that contrary to initial belief, PYY does not increase firing rate of satiety promoting POMC neurons but rather decreases their activity. In summary, inhibitory effects of PYY on food intake by PYY_{3-36} are a rather elusive phenomenon, which may in part result from induction of visceral illness *(76)*.

GLUCAGON-LIKE PEPTIDES

Glucagon-like peptide (GLP)-1 and GLP-2 are two gut hormones derived from posttranslational modification of the larger precursor molecule proglucagon *(77)*. Proglucagon is synthesized within the enteroendocrine L-cells in the intestines, primarily the ileum and colon. Both peptides have previously been implicated in energy balance regulation. GLP-1 is mainly known for its beneficial effects on glucose homeostasis. GLP-1 administration affects blood glucose levels through stimulation of glucose-dependent insulin secretion and the inhibition of glucagon secretion, gastric emptying, and food intake *(78)*. GLP-2 is a 33-amino-acid peptide that seems to regulate energy homeostasis via acute and chronic effects on gut motility, as well as via effects on nutrient ingestion and absorption *(78)*.

The major stimulus for GLP-1 and GLP-2 secretion is the ingestion of nutrients, including glucose, fatty acids, and dietary fiber *(79)*. When nutrients are ingested, the release of GLP-1 and GLP-2 into the circulation occurs in a biphasic manner, consisting of a rapid (within 10–15 min) early phase followed by a more prolonged (within 30–60 min) second phase *(80)*. Two different mechanisms are responsible for this biphasic pattern: the vagus nerve, the neurotransmitter gastrin-releasing peptide, and the hormone glucose-dependent insulinotropic peptide (GIP) contribute to the rapid release of GLP-1 and GLP-2 from distal L-cells in response to nutritional stimuli *(79)*. In contrast, direct stimulation of the L-cells by digested nutrients is responsible for the second phase of peptide release *(81)*. GLP-1 is secreted as GLP-1_{7-37} and GLP-1_{7-36}, but the half-life of its bioactive forms is very short (less than 2 min) *(82)*, whereas GLP-2 is slightly more stable, with a half-life of approximately 5–7 min *(83)*. The enzyme mainly responsible for the rapid degradation of both GLP-1 and GLP-2 is dipeptidyl-peptidase IV (DPP-IV), which produces the inactive peptides GLP-1_{9-37} and GLP-2_{3-33}.

Biological Effects on Food Intake and Mechanisms of Action

Central or peripheral administration of GLP-1R agonists leads to the inhibition of food intake and reduction in body weight in rodents *(84, 85)*. GLP-1 also inhibits food intake and promotes satiety in normal, obese, and diabetic humans (*86–88*). One hypothesis is that similar to recent reports on PYY, GLP-1 achieves suppression of food intake by inducing nausea, taste aversion, and visceral illness. This hypothesis is supported by increasing amounts of evidence from a series of elaborate studies (*89–92*). However, recent results from clinical studies indicate that activation by the GLP-1 receptor with the GLP-1 analogue exendin only transiently causes nausea in humans, while appetite and body weight lowering effects are sustained chronically *(93)*. It has also been proposed that the inhibitory effects of GLP-1 on food intake can be mediated indirectly by its ability to slow gastric emptying, thereby promoting gastric distension and a sensation of satiety. In addition, neurons that express GLP-1 are located in the hypothalamus and NTS, CNS regions that are thought to be important for regulating appetite and satiety *(94, 95)*.

In rats, central administration of GLP-1 dose-dependently reduces food intake (*96–99*), an effect that is reversed by coadministration of the GLP-1 receptor antagonist exendin$_{9-39}$ *(99)*. GLP-1 receptors in the hypothalamus likely mediate the reduction of food intake by activating and blocking the pathways known to control energy balance (*89–92*, *95*,*100–102*), whereas GLP-1 receptors in the amygdala appear to comediate the reduction of food intake by the activation of aversive signaling pathways that produce visceral illness (*89–92*).

Peripherally administered GLP-1 also has an anorexigenic effect on healthy *(88)*, obese *(87)*, and diabetic humans *(88, 102)*. Because the half-life of active GLP-1 is very short, the reduction of food intake is probably due to the result of GLP-1 inhibitory effects on the gastrointestinal transit and reduced gastric emptying *(100)*. However, peripherally administered GLP-1 can cross the blood-brain barrier *(101)*; thus, its role and activity within the CNS regarding food intake regulation deserves further detailed studies. Interestingly, GLP-1R-/- mice exhibit normal feeding behavior and body weight *(102)*, indicating either the existence of another relevant receptor for GLP-1 and its analogues or again reflecting a compensatory mechanism preventing an imbalance during early development of the knockout mouse model.

GLP-2 has beneficial effects on intestinal growth *(106, 107)*, and its actions are mediated by a specific receptor (GLP-2R) *(108)*. In rats, the infusion of GLP-2 prevented the development of small bowel mucosal villous hypoplasia *(109)* and has also produced beneficial effects on the gastrointestinal epithelium of rodents *(110)*. However, there is limited evidence that GLP-2 has trophic effects on the stomach, pancreas, or even any peripheral organs. Although GLP-2 is structurally very similar to GLP-1, its role in food intake is less clear; some studies have found that central administration of GLP-2 in rats decreases food intake *(111)*, whereas a study in mice treated with GLP-2 for 9 days found no effect on food intake or weight gain *(112)*. In humans, no effect has been observed on food intake or weight gain using GLP-2 *(113, 114)*.

Oxyntomodulin

Oxyntomodulin (oxm) is a 37-amino-acid peptide that is also produced by posttranslational processing of preproglucagon in the intestine and in the CNS. Similar to GLP-1, oxm is rapidly released from the L-cells of the distal small intestine after food ingestion in proportion to the amount of calories ingested with a meal. In rats, intracerebro ventricular administration of oxm is reported to inhibit food intake with greater potency than GLP-1 *(112)*, and oxm appears to act via GLP-1R or via a GLP-1-like receptor. Oxm action leads to increased cAMP accumulation and somatostatin secretion as well as H^+ production in cell preparations *(113, 114)*. Moreover, anorectic actions of oxm are blocked by coadministration of the GLP-1 receptor antagonist exendin$_{9-39}$ *(115)*. However, the affinity of oxm for the GLP-1R is lower than that of GLP-1 in spite of its more potent effect on food intake, suggesting that the potent action of oxm on food intake could also be mediated by another receptor. Another finding that supports the hypothesis of the existence and functional role of a currently unknown second receptor is the stimulation of different areas of the brain by oxm and GLP-1. GLP-1 activates cells in the brain stem and other central autonomic control sites *(116)*, whereas oxm-mediated stimulation is predominately restricted to the hypothalamic arcuate nucleus *(117)*. Thus, the precise molecular mechanisms by which oxm achieves its biological actions, including inhibition of food intake, remain inconclusive to date. Recently, it was shown that oxm is also a potent inhibitor of food intake when administered intraperitoneally to rats *(117)*. Furthermore, in humans, intravenous infusion of oxm significantly reduced food intake and cumulative 12-h caloric intake, but it did not affect cumulative 24-h energy intake. Oxm was able to decrease circulating levels of the orexigenic hormone ghrelin by 44% in human subjects, suggesting that ghrelin might be one possible mediator of oxm actions on energy balance *(118)*. As with GLP-1, in addition to its effects on food intake, oxm has also been shown to augment postprandial insulin secretion, inhibit gastric acid secretion, and reduce gastric motility.

CONCLUSION

A substantial body of data provides solid evidence that gut hormones are involved in the regulation of food intake, energy balance, and body fat mass. However, the exact molecular mechanisms, the interaction between the different players, and the physiologic relevance of the mostly pharmacological observations remain to be elucidated. Nevertheless, clinical studies provide early encouraging results regarding the treatment of human obesity with gut hormones or their analogues, suggesting that even without a complete understanding of molecular targets and hormonal cross-talk, safe and effective drug candidates may be developed. Imbalances in gut hormone production or secretion being causally involved in the pathogenesis of obesity and diabetes cannot be concluded based on the currently available scientific evidence.

REFERENCES

1. Bayliss WM, Starling EH. The mechanism of pancreatic secretion. J Physiol 1902;28:325.
2. Kojima M, Hosoda H, Date Y, Nakazato M, Matsuo H, Kangawa K. Ghrelin is a growth-hormone-releasing acylated peptide from stomach. Nature 1999;402:656–660.
3. Tomasetto C, Karam SM, Ribieras S, et al. Identification and characterization of a novel gastric peptide hormone: the motilin-related peptide. Gastroenterology 2000;119:395–405.
4. Sheppard P, Deisher T. Patent application 1998;WO 98/42840, 01.10.
5. Hosoda H, Kojima M, Matsuo H, Kangawa K. Purification and characterization of rat des-Gln14-Ghrelin, a second endogenous ligand for the growth hormone secretagogue receptor. J Biol Chem 2000;275:21995–22000.
6. Gualillo O, Lago F, Gomez-Reino J, Casanueva FF, Dieguez C. Ghrelin, a widespread hormone: insights into molecular and cellular regulation of its expression and mechanism of action. FEBS Lett 2003;552:105–109.
7. Wren AM, Small CJ, Ward HL, et al. The novel hypothalamic peptide ghrelin stimulates food intake and growth hormone secretion. Endocrinology 2000;141:4325–4328.
8. Cummings DE, Purnell JQ, Frayo RS, Schmidova K, Wisse BE, Weigle DS. A preprandial rise in plasma ghrelin levels suggests a role in meal initiation in humans. Diabetes 2001;50:1714–1719.

9. Callahan HS, Cummings DE, Pepe MS, Breen PA, Matthys CC, Weigle DS. Postprandial suppression of plasma ghrelin level is proportional to ingested caloric load but does not predict intermeal interval in humans. J Clin Endocrinol Metab 2004;89:1319–1324.
10. Otto B, Cuntz U, Fruehauf E, et al. Weight gain decreases elevated plasma ghrelin concentrations of patients with anorexia nervosa. Eur J Endocrinol 2001;145:669–673.
11. Tschop M, Weyer C, Tataranni PA, Devanarayan V, Ravussin E, Heiman ML. Circulating ghrelin levels are decreased in human obesity. Diabetes 2001;50:707–709.
12. Nagaya N, Kojima M, Uematsu M, et al. Hemodynamic and hormonal effects of human ghrelin in healthy volunteers. Am J Physiol Regul Integr Comp Physiol 2001;280:R1483–R1487.
13. Ariyasu H, Takaya K, Tagami T, et al. Stomach is a major source of circulating ghrelin, and feeding state determines plasma ghrelin-like immunoreactivity levels in humans. J Clin Endocrinol Metab 2001;86:4753–4758.
14. Shiiya T, Nakazato M, Mizuta M, et al. Plasma ghrelin levels in lean and obese humans and the effect of glucose on ghrelin secretion. J Clin Endocrinol Metab 2002;87:240–244.
15. Cummings DE, Clement K, Purnell JQ, et al. Elevated plasma ghrelin levels in Prader Willi syndrome. Nat Med 2002;8:643–644.
16. Korbonits M, Grossman AB. Ghrelin: update on a novel hormonal system. Eur J Endocrinol 2004;151:S67–70.
17. Kamegai J, Tamura H, Shimizu T, Ishii S, Sugihara H, Wakabayashi I. Central effect of ghrelin, an endogenous growth hormone secretagogue, on hypothalamic peptide gene expression. Endocrinology 2000;141:4797–4800.
18. Nakazato M, Murakami N, Date Y, Kojima M, Matsuo H, Kangawa K, Matsukura S. A role for ghrelin in the central regulation of feeding. Nature 2001;409:194–198.
19. Horvath TL, Diano S, Sotonyi P, Heiman M, Tschop M. Minireview: ghrelin and the regulation of energy balance—a hypothalamic perspective. Endocrinology 2001;142:4163–4169.
20. Zigman JM, Elmquist JK. Minireview: from anorexia to obesity—the yin and yang of body weight control. Endocrinology 2003;144:3749–3756.
21. Tamura H, Kamegai J, Shimizu T, Ishii S, Sugihara H, Oikawa S. Ghrelin stimulates GH but not food intake in arcuate nucleus ablated rats. Endocrinology 2002;143:3268–3275.
22. Faulconbridge LF, Cummings DE, Kaplan JM, Grill HJ. Hyperphagic effects of brainstem ghrelin administration. Diabetes 2003;52:2260–2265.
23. Tschop M, Statnick MA, Suter TM, Heiman ML. GH-releasing peptide-2 increases fat mass in mice lacking NPY: indication for a crucial mediating role of hypothalamic agouti-related protein. Endocrinology 2002;143:558–568.
24. Choi K, Roh SG, Hong YH, et al. The role of ghrelin and growth hormone secretagogues receptor on rat adipogenesis. Endocrinology 2003;144:754–759.
25. Thompson NM, Gill DA, Davies R, Loveridge N, Houston PA, Robinson IC, Wells T. Ghrelin and des-octanoyl ghrelin promote adipogenesis directly in vivo by a mechanism independent of the type 1a growth hormone secretagogue receptor. Endocrinology 2004;145:234–242.
26. Otto V, Fasshauer M, Dalski A, Meier B, Perwitz N, Klein HH, Tschop M, Klein J. Direct peripheral effects of ghrelin include suppression of adiponectin expression. Horm Metab Res 2002;34: 640–645.
27. Masuda Y, Tanaka T, Inomata N, et al. Ghrelin stimulates gastric acid secretion and motility in rats. Biochem Biophys Res Commun 2000;276:905–908.
28. Date Y, Nakazato M, Murakami N, Kojima M, Kangawa K, Matsukura S. Ghrelin acts in the central nervous system to stimulate gastric acid secretion. Biochem Biophys Res Commun 2001;280:904–907.
29. Asakawa A, Inui A, Kaga T, et al. Ghrelin is an appetite-stimulatory signal from stomach with structural resemblance to motilin. Gastroenterology 2001;120:337–345.

30. Lee HM, Wang G, Englander EW, Kojima M, Greeley GH Jr. Ghrelin, a new gastrointestinal endocrine peptide that stimulates insulin secretion: enteric distribution, ontogeny, influence of endocrine, and dietary manipulations. Endocrinology 2002;143:185–190.
31. Broglio F, Benso A, Gottero C, et al. Non-acylated ghrelin does not possess the pituitaric and pancreatic endocrine activity of acylated ghrelin in humans. J Endocrinol Invest 2003;26:192–196.
32. McCowen KC, Maykel JA, Bistrian BR, Ling PR. Circulating ghrelin concentrations are lowered by intravenous glucose or hyperinsulinemic euglycemic conditions in rodents. J Endocrinol 2002; 175:R7–11.
33. Mohlig M, Spranger J, Otto B, Ristow M, Tschop M, Pfeiffer AF. Euglycemic hyperinsulinemia, but not lipid infusion, decreases circulating ghrelin levels in humans. J Endocrinol Invest 2002; 25:RC36–38.
34. Saad MF, Bernaba B, Hwu CM, Jinagouda S, Fahmi S, Kogosov E, Boyadjian R. Insulin regulates plasma ghrelin concentration. J Clin Endocrinol Metab 2002;87:3997–4000.
35. Flanagan DE, Evans ML, Monsod TP, Rife F, Heptulla RA, Tamborlane WV, Sherwin RS. The influence of insulin on circulating ghrelin. Am J Physiol Endocrinol Metab 2003;284:E313–316.
36. Rudovich NN, Dick D, Moehlig M, et al. Ghrelin is not suppressed in hyperglycemic clamps by gastric inhibitory polypeptide and arginine. Regul Pept 2005;127:95–99.
37. Date Y, Nakazato M, Hashiguchi S, et al. Ghrelin is present in pancreatic alpha-cells of humans and rats and stimulates insulin secretion. Diabetes 2002;51:124–129.
38. Volante M, Allia E, Gugliotta P, et al. Expression of ghrelin and of the GH secretagogue receptor by pancreatic islet cells and related endocrine tumors. J Clin Endocrinol Metab 2002;87:1300–1308.
39. Pagotto U, Gambineri A, Vicennati V, Heiman ML, Tschop M, Pasquali R. Plasma ghrelin, obesity, and the polycystic ovary syndrome: correlation with insulin resistance and androgen levels. J Clin Endocrinol Metab 2002;87:5625–5629.
40. Schaller G, Schmidt A, Pleiner J, Woloszczuk W, Wolzt M, Luger A. Plasma ghrelin concentrations are not regulated by glucose or insulin: a double-blind, placebo-controlled crossover clamp study. Diabetes 2003;52:16–20.
41. Sun Y, Wang P, Zheng H, Smith RG. Ghrelin stimulation of growth hormone release and appetite is mediated through the growth hormone secretagogue receptor. Proc Natl Acad Sci U S A 2004;101:4679–4684.
42. Sun Y, Ahmed S, Smith RG. Deletion of ghrelin impairs neither growth nor appetite. Mol Cell Biol 2003;23:7973–7981.
43. Erickson JC, Clegg KE, Palmiter RD. Sensitivity to leptin and susceptibility to seizures of mice lacking neuropeptide Y. Nature 1996;381:415–421.
44. Qian S, Chen H, Weingarth D, et al. Neither agouti-related protein nor neuropeptide Y is critically required for the regulation of energy homeostasis in mice. Mol Cell Biol 2002;22:5027–5035.
45. Wortley KE, Anderson KD, Garcia K, et al. Genetic deletion of ghrelin does not decrease food intake but influences metabolic fuel preference. Proc Natl Acad Sci U S A 2004;101:8227–8232.
46. Zigman JM, Nakano Y, Coppari R, et al. Mice lacking ghrelin receptors resist the development of diet-induced obesity. J Clin Invest 2005;115:3564–3572.
47. Grove KL, Cowley MA. Is ghrelin a signal for the development of metabolic systems? J Clin Invest 2005;115:3393–3397.
48. Shuto Y, Shibasaki T, Otagiri A, et al. Hypothalamic growth hormone secretagogue receptor regulates growth hormone secretion, feeding, and adiposity. J Clin Invest 2002;109:1429–1436.
49. Kamegai J, Wakabayashi I, Miyamoto K, Unterman TG, Kineman RD, Frohman LA. Growth hormone-dependent regulation of pituitary GH secretagogue receptor (GHS-R) mRNA levels in the spontaneous dwarf Rat. Neuroendocrinology 1998;68:312–318.
50. Zhang JV, Ren PG, Avsian-Kretchmer O, Luo CW, Rauch R, Klein C, Hsueh AJ. Obestatin, a peptide encoded by the ghrelin gene, opposes ghrelin's effects on food intake. Science 2005;310:996–999.

51. Tatemoto K, Mutt V. Isolation of two novel candidate hormones using a chemical method for finding naturally occurring polypeptides. Nature 1980;285:417–418.
52. Ali-Rachedi A, Varndell IM, Adrian TE, Gapp DA, Van Noorden S, Bloom SR, Polak JM. Peptide YY (PYY) immunoreactivity is co-stored with glucagon-related immunoreactants in endocrine cells of the gut and pancreas. Histochemistry 1984;80:487–491.
53. El-Salhy M, Wilander E, Juntti-Berggren L, Grimelius L. The distribution and ontogeny of polypeptide YY (PYY)- and pancreatic polypeptide (PP)-immunoreactive cells in the gastrointestinal tract of rat. Histochemistry 1983;78:53–60.
54. Leduque P, Paulin C, Dubois PM. Immunocytochemical evidence for a substance related to the bovine pancreatic polypeptide-peptide YY group of peptides in the human fetal gastrointestinal tract. Regul Pept 1983;6:219–230.
55. Pappas TN, Debas HT, Taylor IL. Peptide YY: metabolism and effect on pancreatic secretion in dogs. Gastroenterology 1985;89:1387–1392.
56. Lundberg JM, Terenius L, Hokfelt T, Tatemoto K. Comparative immunohistochemical and biochemical analysis of pancreatic polypeptide-like peptides with special reference to presence of neuropeptide Y in central and peripheral neurons. J Neurosci 1984;4:2376–2386.
57. Dumont Y, Fournier A, St-Pierre S, Quirion R. Autoradiographic distribution of [125I]Leu31,Pro34] PYY and [125I]PYY3-36 binding sites in the rat brain evaluated with two newly developed Y1 and Y2 receptor radioligands. Synapse 1996;22:139–158.
58. Lynch DR, Walker MW, Miller RJ, Snyder SH. Neuropeptide Y receptor binding sites in rat brain: differential autoradiographic localizations with 125I-peptide YY and 125I-neuropeptide Y imply receptor heterogeneity. J Neurosci 1989;9:2607–2619.
59. Yang H, Li WP, Reeve JR Jr, Rivier J, Tache Y. PYY-preferring receptor in the dorsal vagal complex and its involvement in PYY stimulation of gastric acid secretion in rats. Br J Pharmacol 1998;123:1549–1554.
60. Grandt D, Schimiczek M, Beglinger C, Layer P, Goebell H, Eysselein VE, Reeve JR Jr. Two molecular forms of peptide YY (PYY) are abundant in human blood: characterization of a radioimmunoassay recognizing PYY 1–36 and PYY 3–36. Regul Pept 1994;51:151–159.
61. Eberlein GA, Eysselein VE, Schaeffer M, et al. A new molecular form of PYY: structural characterization of human PYY(3–36) and PYY(1–36). Peptides 1989;10:797–803.
62. Morley JE, Levine AS, Grace M, Kneip J. Peptide YY (PYY), a potent orexigenic agent. Brain Res 1985;341:200–203.
63. Harding RK, McDonald TJ. Identification and characterization of the emetic effects of peptide YY. Peptides 1989;10:21–24.
64. Batterham RL, Cohen MA, Ellis SM, et al. Inhibition of food intake in obese subjects by peptide YY3–36. N Engl J Med 2003;349:941–948.
65. Batterham RL, Cowley MA, Small CJ, et al. Gut hormone PYY(3–36) physiologically inhibits food intake. Nature 2002;418:650–654.
66. Pittner RA, Moore CX, Bhavsar SP, et al. Effects of PYY[3–36] in rodent models of diabetes and obesity. Int J Obes Relat Metab Disord 2004;28:963–971.
67. Chelikani PK, Haver AC, Reidelberger RD. Intravenous infusion of peptide YY(3–36) potently inhibits food intake in rats. Endocrinology 2005;146:879–888.
68. Tschop M, Castaneda TR, Joost HG, et al. Physiology: does gut hormone PYY3–36 decrease food intake in rodents? Nature 2004;430:165.
69. Halatchev IG, Ellacott KL, Fan W, Cone RD. Peptide YY3–36 inhibits food intake in mice through a melanocortin-4 receptor-independent mechanism. Endocrinology 2004;145:2585–2590.
70. Riediger T, Bothe C, Becskei C, Lutz TA. Peptide YY directly inhibits ghrelin-activated neurons of the arcuate nucleus and reverses fasting-induced c-Fos expression. Neuroendocrinology 2004;79:317–326.

71. Challis BG, Pinnock SB, Coll AP, Carter RN, Dickson SL, O'Rahilly S. Acute effects of PYY3–36 on food intake and hypothalamic neuropeptide expression in the mouse. Biochem Biophys Res Commun 2003;311:915–919.
72. Challis BG, Coll AP, Yeo GS, et al. Mice lacking pro-opiomelanocortin are sensitive to high-fat feeding but respond normally to the acute anorectic effects of peptide-YY(3–36). Proc Natl Acad Sci U S A 2004;101:4695–4700.
73. Marsh DJ, Hollopeter G, Huszar D, et al. Response of melanocortin-4 receptor-deficient mice to anorectic and orexigenic peptides. Nat Genet 1999;21:119–122.
74. Koda S, Date Y, Murakami N, et al. The role of the vagal nerve in peripheral PYY3–36-induced feeding reduction in rats. Endocrinology 2005;146:2369–2375.
75. Edwards CM, Abbott CR, Sunter D, et al. Cocaine- and amphetamine-regulated transcript, glucagon-like peptide-1 and corticotrophin releasing factor inhibit feeding via agouti-related protein independent pathways in the rat. Brain Res 2000;866:128–134.
76. Halatchev IG, Cone RD. Peripheral administration of PYY(3–36) produces conditioned taste aversion in mice. Cell Metab 2005;1:159–168.
77. Holst JJ. Enteroglucagon. Annu Rev Physiol 1997;59:257–271.
78. Drucker DJ. Biological actions and therapeutic potential of the glucagon-like peptides. Gastroenterology 2002;122:531–544.
79. Brubaker PL, Anini Y. Direct and indirect mechanisms regulating secretion of glucagon-like peptide-1 and glucagon-like peptide-2. Can J Physiol Pharmacol 2003;81:1005–1012.
80. Herrmann C, Goke R, Richter G, Fehmann HC, Arnold R, Goke B. Glucagon-like peptide-1 and glucose-dependent insulin-releasing polypeptide plasma levels in response to nutrients. Digestion 1995;56:117–126.
81. Roberge JN, Brubaker PL. Regulation of intestinal proglucagon-derived peptide secretion by glucose-dependent insulinotropic peptide in a novel enteroendocrine loop. Endocrinology 1993;133:233–240.
82. Kieffer TJ, McIntosh CH, Pederson RA. Degradation of glucose-dependent insulinotropic polypeptide and truncated glucagon-like peptide 1 in vitro and in vivo by dipeptidyl peptidase IV. Endocrinology 1995;136:3585–3596.
83. Hartmann B, Thulesen J, Kissow H, et al. Dipeptidyl peptidase IV inhibition enhances the intestinotrophic effect of glucagon-like peptide-2 in rats and mice. Endocrinology 2000;141:4013–4020.
84. Turton MD, O'Shea D, Gunn I, et al. A role for glucagon-like peptide-1 in the central regulation of feeding. Nature 1996;379:69–72.
85. Meeran K, O'Shea D, Edwards CM, et al. Repeated intracerebroventricular administration of glucagon-like peptide-1-(7-36) amide or exendin-(9-39) alters body weight in the rat. Endocrinology 1999;140:244–250.
86. Flint A, Raben A, Astrup A, Holst JJ. Glucagon-like peptide 1 promotes satiety and suppresses energy intake in humans. J Clin Invest 1998;101:515–520.
87. Naslund E, Barkeling B, King N, et al. Energy intake and appetite are suppressed by glucagon-like peptide-1 (GLP-1) in obese men. Int J Obes Relat Metab Disord 1999;23:304–311.
88. Gutzwiller JP, Drewe J, Goke B, Schmidt H, Rohrer B, Lareida J, Beglinger C. Glucagon-like peptide-1 promotes satiety and reduces food intake in patients with diabetes mellitus type 2. Am J Physiol 1999;276:R1541–1544.
89. Lachey JL, D'Alessio DA, Rinaman L, Elmquist JK, Drucker DJ, Seeley RJ. The role of central glucagon-like peptide-1 in mediating the effects of visceral illness: differential effects in rats and mice. Endocrinology 2005;146:458–462.
90. Kinzig KP, D'Alessio DA, Seeley RJ. The diverse roles of specific GLP-1 receptors in the control of food intake and the response to visceral illness. J Neurosci 2002;22:10470–10476.

91. Seeley RJ, Blake K, Rushing PA, Benoit S, Eng J, Woods SC, D'Alessio D. The role of CNS glucagon-like peptide-1 (7–36) amide receptors in mediating the visceral illness effects of lithium chloride. J Neurosci 2000;20:1616–1621.
92. Thiele TE, Van Dijk G, Campfield LA, et al. Central infusion of GLP-1, but not leptin, produces conditioned taste aversions in rats. Am J Physiol 1997;272:R726–730.
93. Heine RJ, Van Gaal LF, Johns D, Mihm MJ, Widel MH, Brodows RG; GWAA Study Group. Exenatide versus insulin glargine in patients with suboptimally controlled type 2 diabetes: a randomized trial. Ann Intern Med 2005;143:559–569.
94. Merchenthaler I, Lane M, Shughrue P. Distribution of pre-pro-glucagon and glucagon-like peptide-1 receptor messenger RNAs in the rat central nervous system. J Comp Neurol 1999;403:261–280.
95. Larsen PJ, Tang-Christensen M, Jessop DS. Central administration of glucagon-like peptide-1 activates hypothalamic neuroendocrine neurons in the rat. Endocrinology 1997;138:4445–4455.
96. Van Dijk G, Lindskog S, Holst JJ, Steffens AB, Ahren B. Effects of glucagon-like peptide-I on glucose turnover in rats. Am J Physiol 1996;270:E1015–1021.
97. Hwa JJ, Ghibaudi L, Williams P, Witten MB, Tedesco R, Strader CD. Differential effects of intracerebroventricular glucagon-like peptide-1 on feeding and energy expenditure regulation. Peptides 1998;19:869–875.
98. Tang-Christensen M, Vrang N, Larsen PJ. Glucagon-like peptide 1(7–36) amide's central inhibition of feeding and peripheral inhibition of drinking are abolished by neonatal monosodium glutamate treatment. Diabetes 1998;47:530–537.
99. Tang-Christensen M, Larsen PJ, Goke R, Fink-Jensen A, Jessop DS, Moller M, Sheikh SP. Central administration of GLP-1-(7-36) amide inhibits food and water intake in rats. Am J Physiol 1996;271:R848–856.
100. McMahon LR, Wellman PJ. PVN infusion of GLP-1-(7-36) amide suppresses feeding but does not induce aversion or alter locomotion in rats. Am J Physiol 1998;274:R23–29.
101. McMahon LR, Wellman PJ. Decreased intake of a liquid diet in nonfood-deprived rats following intra-PVN injections of GLP-1 (7-36) amide. Pharmacol Biochem Behav 1997;58:673–677.
102. Toft-Nielsen MB, Madsbad S, Holst JJ. Continuous subcutaneous infusion of glucagon-like peptide 1 lowers plasma glucose and reduces appetite in type 2 diabetic patients. Diabetes Care 1999;22: 1137–1143.
103. Delgado-Aros S, Kim DY, Burton DD, et al. Effect of GLP-1 on gastric volume, emptying, maximum volume ingested, and postprandial symptoms in humans. Am J Physiol Gastrointest Liver Physiol 2002;282:G424–431.
104. Kastin AJ, Akerstrom V, Pan W. Interactions of glucagon-like peptide-1 (GLP-1) with the blood-brain barrier. J Mol Neurosci 2002;18:7–14.
105. Scrocchi LA, Brown TJ, MaClusky N, Brubaker PL, Auerbach AB, Joyner AL, Drucker DJ. Glucose intolerance but normal satiety in mice with a null mutation in the glucagon-like peptide 1 receptor gene. Nat Med 1996;2:1254–1258
106. Drucker DJ. Glucagon-like peptide 2. Trends Endocrinol Metab 1999;10:153–156.
107. Jeppesen PB. Clinical significance of GLP-2 in short-bowel syndrome. J Nutr 2003;133:3721–3724.
108. Munroe DG, Gupta AK, Kooshesh F, et al. Prototypic G protein-coupled receptor for the intestinotrophic factor glucagon-like peptide 2. Proc Natl Acad Sci U S A 1999;96:1569–1573.
109. Chance WT, Foley-Nelson T, Thomas I, Balasubramaniam A. Prevention of parenteral nutrition-induced gut hypoplasia by coinfusion of glucagon-like peptide-2. Am J Physiol 1997;273:G559–563.
110. Tavakkolizadeh A, Shen R, Abraham P, et al. Glucagonlike peptide 2 (glp-2) promotes intestinal recovery following chemotherapy-induced enteritis. Curr Surg 2000;57:502.
111. Tang-Christensen M, Larsen PJ, Thulesen J, Romer J, Vrang N. The proglucagon-derived peptide, glucagon-like peptide-2, is a neurotransmitter involved in the regulation of food intake. Nat Med 2000;6:802–807.

112. Tsai CH, Hill M, Asa SL, Brubaker PL, Drucker DJ. Intestinal growth-promoting properties of glucagon-like peptide-2 in mice. Am J Physiol 1997;273:E77–84.
113. Sorensen LB, Flint A, Raben A, Hartmann B, Holst JJ, Astrup A. No effect of physiological concentrations of glucagon-like peptide-2 on appetite and energy intake in normal weight subjects. Int J Obes Relat Metab Disord 2003;27:450–456.
114. Schmidt PT, Naslund E, Gryback P, Jacobsson H, Hartmann B, Holst JJ, Hellstrom PM. Peripheral administration of GLP-2 to humans has no effect on gastric emptying or satiety. Regul Pept 2003;116:21–25.
115. Dakin CL, Small CJ, Park AJ, Seth A, Ghatei MA, Bloom SR. Repeated ICV administration of oxyntomodulin causes a greater reduction in body weight gain than in pair-fed rats. Am J Physiol Endocrinol Metab 2002;283:E1173–1177.
116. Gros L, Thorens B, Bataille D, Kervran A. Glucagon-like peptide-1-(7-36) amide, oxyntomodulin, and glucagon interact with a common receptor in a somatostatin-secreting cell line. Endocrinology 1993;133:631–638.
117. Schepp W, Dehne K, Riedel T, Schmidtler J, Schaffer K, Classen M. Oxyntomodulin: a cAMP-dependent stimulus of rat parietal cell function via the receptor for glucagon-like peptide-1 (7–36)NH2. Digestion 1996;57:398–405.
118. Dakin CL, Gunn I, Small CJ, et al. Oxyntomodulin inhibits food intake in the rat. Endocrinology 2001;142:4244–4250.
119. Yamamoto H, Lee CE, Marcus JN, et al. Glucagon-like peptide-1 receptor stimulation increases blood pressure and heart rate and activates autonomic regulatory neurons. J Clin Invest 2002;110:43–52.
120. Dakin CL, Small CJ, Batterham RL, et al. Peripheral oxyntomodulin reduces food intake and body weight gain in rats. Endocrinology 2004;145:2687–2695.
121. Cohen MA, Ellis SM, Le Roux CW, et al. Oxyntomodulin suppresses appetite and reduces food intake in humans. J Clin Endocrinol Metab 2003;88:4696–4701.

8 The Role of Growth Hormone Secretagogues and Ghrelin in Feeding and Body Composition

Cyril Y. Bowers, Blandine Laferrère, David L. Hurley, and Johannes D. Veldhuis

Contents

Abstract

In 1984, when it was first demonstrated that growth hormone releasing peptide (GHRP) markedly augmented growth hormone (GH) release in several animal species and increased body weight after daily subcutaneous administration, we postulated that it reflected the activity of a new hypothalamic hypophysiotropic hormone different from growth hormone releasing hormone (GHRH). This implied that it could become valuable clinically to enhance body growth in children via an anabolic nitrogen retention action of GH. A great impetus to develop GHRP/growth hormone secretagogues (GHSs) as therapeutic agents was the cloning of the GHS receptor, GHSR-1a, and identification of the natural hormone ghrelin, which is a unique and novel physiologic regulator of both GH secretion and food intake. Metabolism

From: *Contemporary Endocrinology: Energy Metabolism and Obesity: Research and Clinical Applications*
Edited by: P. A. Donohoue © Humana Press Inc., Totowa, NJ

requires multiple balanced hormonal and cellular actions and interactions of an inordinate complexity, and thus the primary dual action of ghrelin/GHSs on both GH secretion and food intake teleologically seem most reasonable and sound. The fundamental action of these dual effects is underscored in body growth of children and the impaired action of GH in the undernourished, and, thus, this is considered a major principle in the development of the GHSs. Importantly, GHSs and ghrelin have essentially the same actions on GH and food intake, and, when administered continuously to humans for extended time periods, both stimulate the sustained normal physiologic pulsatile secretion of GH. In spite of only small increases in serum pulsatile GH concentrations, both GHSs and ghrelin markedly enhance the increase of serum insulin-like growth factor 1 (IGF-1) and its binding proteins.

The complementary actions of GHSs as well as ghrelin in combination with GHRH again demonstrate that GHSs and ghrelin have the same actions on the GH axis and also demonstrate how ghrelin may act physiologically with GHRH especially as only low amounts of ghrelin as well as GHSs produce these effects. These data support the physiologic actions of both peptides during extended chronic continuous infusion.

The very recent discovery of the new hormone obestatin from the same gene as ghrelin as well as its receptor identification as G-protein orphan receptor 39 (GPR39) bring an outstanding dimension and focus to the role of GHSs/ghrelin in feeding and body composition.

Key Words: Ghrelin, Growth Hormone Secretagogue (GHS), GH/IGF-1, Food Intake, Growth Hormone Releasing Peptide (GHRP-2), Continuous Delivery, Obestatin

INTRODUCTION

A new challenge for clinicians to improve health over the next 10 years will be to help bring together new knowledge on the regulation of the growth hormone (GH) neuroendocrine regulatory system and on the regulation and function of the peripheral GH–insulin-like growth factor (IGF) system in particular via the hypothalamic-pituitary approach (*1–3*). This includes patients with endocrine and nonendocrine disorders and illnesses. Although more subtle in adults, the GH-IGF system is as ubiquitous in actions as insulin but seemingly more complex because of the six IGF binding proteins (IGFBPs), which increase as well as decrease the actions of IGF-1. An impetus facilitating this GH–IGF-1 CNS peripheral approach is the increasing development and improvement of chemical formulations of growth hormone releasing hormone (GHRH), growth hormone secretagogues (GHSs), and, possibly in the future, ghrelin as well as a broad and more in-depth understanding of the basic and clinical aspects of this diffuse endocrine system.

When new hormonal systems are discovered, especially if novel and unique, a cascade of basic and clinical events follows (*4–9*). Leptin of adipose origin and ghrelin mainly of stomach origin are secreted into the peripheral circulation to regulate food intake. They interact on the same neurons of the hypothalamic arcuate nucleus to increase (ghrelin) and decrease (leptin) each other's actions on food intake and, thus, for food intake and GH secretion, ghrelin/GHS can be viewed also as a functional antagonist for leptin and somatotropin release inhibiting factor (SRIF) or somatostatin, respectively. It is notable that ghrelin/GHS regulate GH and food intake and that the actions and interactions of GH and nutrition are well established to be most complementary. More recently, the dramatic discovery of the new hormone obestatin by Zhang et al. as well as identification of its receptor as the G-protein orphan receptor 39 (GPR39; previously ORF39) demonstrates that this peptide decreases food intake without an effect on GH secretion by acting on hypothalamic GPR39 (now designated the obestatin receptor) (Figs. 8.1 and 8.2) *(10)*. Additionally, ghrelin and obestatin

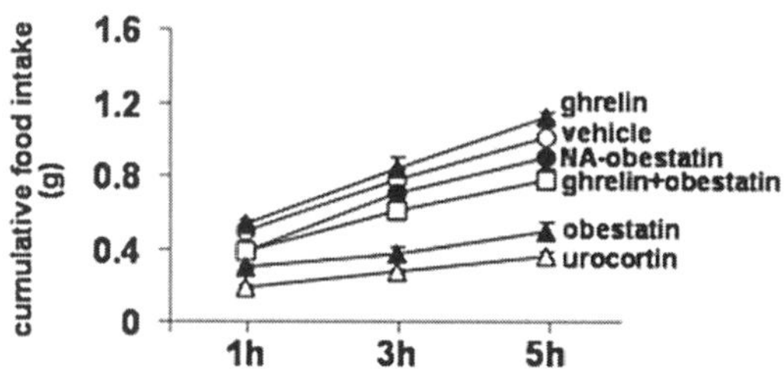

Fig. 8.1 Food intake of adult male mice was decreased by obestatin 1 μmol/kg intracerebroventricularly and 8 nmol/kg intraperitoneally. C-terminal nonamidated obestatin was less effective. (Reproduced from Zhang JV, Ren PG, Avsian-Kretchmer O, Luo CW, Rauch R, Klein C, Hsueh AJW. Obestatin, a peptide encoded by the ghrelin gene, opposes ghrelin's effects on food intake. Science 2005;370:996–999, with permission.).

originate from the same gene, same cell, as well as same preprohormone mainly from the fundus of the stomach. Thus, the principle arises that obestatin and ghrelin may originate at the same various anatomic sites and from the same particular cells/neurons. If this principle is confirmed, the obestatin-ghrelin regulation of food intake will become a major focus.

In need of more immediate understanding are the actions and role of desacyl ghrelin, the presence or absence of ghrelin receptor subtypes, and the high constitutive activity of both the ghrelin and obestatin receptors. In the literature, the word *ghrelin* was not infrequently used without adequately distinguishing it from desacyl ghrelin, which is unfortunate for a number of reasons that sequentially will directly or indirectly eventually become more apparent. Increasing functional actions of GHSs/ghrelin, especially nonendocrine actions, are being revealed that are best explained by effects on yet to be isolated ghrelin subtypes or by other yet to be identified factors.

The above introductory comments underscore some of the current and specific aspects of the still evolving ghrelin system or perhaps the "ghrelin-obestatin" system. Evolutionary findings and the demonstrated biological activity in both animals and humans strongly support the fundamental physiologic and pathophysiologic clinical importance of this complementary interactive network of peptide hormones.

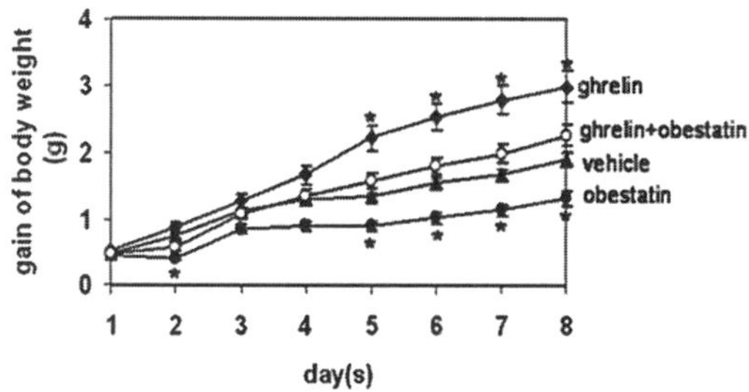

Fig. 8.2 Daily body weight (BW) gain of adult male rats over an 8-day period with 1 μmol/kg obestatin was less than that with 1 μmol/kg BW ghrelin, ghrelin + obestatin, or vehicle treated rats. (Reproduced from Zhang JV, Ren PG, Avsian-Kretchmer O, Luo CW, Rauch R, Klein C, Hsueh AJW. Obestatin, a peptide encoded by the ghrelin gene, opposes ghrelin's effects on food intake. Science 2005;370:996–999, with permission.).

CHEMISTRY AND FUNCTION

In Table 8.1 is recorded the very different amino acid sequences of the growth hormone releasing peptide (GHRP)-2, human(h) ghrelin and human(h) obestatin molecules with 6, 28, and 23 amino acids, respectively. Chemical findings in need of emphasis are the D-amino acid residues of GHRP-2, the eight-carbon-atom straight-chain saturated carboxylic group covalently linked via an ester bond to Ser^3 of ghrelin, and the C-terminal amidation of obestatin because these are important determinants of the biological activity of these three peptides. The active receptor conformation and high-affinity binding of GHRP-2 and ghrelin are determined by the D form of the amino acids and addition of the octanoic acid, respectively, while full activity of obestatin requires terminal amidation. Thus, these specific chemical changes play major roles in the biological activity of these peptides. Without octylation, ghrelin no longer binds to the ghrelin receptor (ghrelin-R). However, increasing evidence is accumulating that the desacyl ghrelin molecule is secreted from sites of de novo synthesis as well as originates as a metabolite of acyl ghrelin and may have other biological activity via an unknown receptor different from the ghrelin-R. The bioactivities of desacyl ghrelin in rats have included adipogenesis in bone marrow after administration of the peptide directly into the bone marrow cavity and enhanced food intake after administration of desacyl ghrelin into the lateral ventricle of the brain but not when administered peripherally *(11, 12)*. A more immediate reason for emphasizing these points is that GHRP-2 would not be expected to induce the activities of the desacyl molecular form of ghrelin while ghrelin itself would because desacyl ghrelin may be derived from exogenous ghrelin. Although the obestatin structure-activity relationships have not been published, its full activity on inhibition of food intake appears to depend on its C-terminal amidation.

Obestatin appears to be a major component of the ghrelin system not only because of its anatomic and molecular origin but also because Zhang et al. have shown that amidated and deamidated obestatin molecular forms circulate in the blood of rats. Amidated obestatin inhibits food intake only after fasting and ghrelin administration, but not in the nonfasted state *(10)*. With regard to GHRP-2, ghrelin, and obestatin, it is reasonable to predict that obestatin will be effective in inhibiting the enhanced food intake of GHRP-2 and ghrelin in humans because both peptides act on the same receptor to increase food intake. The possible inhibitory action of obestatin on the recently described desacyl ghrelin hypothalamic stimulation of food intake is still an unknown.

Table 8.1
Amino acid sequences

GHRP-2
 DAlaDβNalAlaTrpDPheLysNH$_2$

Δh Ghrelin
 O=C(CH/$_2$)$_6$–CH$_3$
 /
 GlySerSerPheLeuSerProGluHisGlnArgValGlnGlnArgLysGluSerLysLysProProAlaLysLeu GlnProArg

h Obestatin
 PheAsnAlaProPheAspValGlyIleLysLeuSerGlyValGlnTyrGlnGlnHisSerGlnAlaLeuNH$_2$

A seemingly enigmatic finding is that ghrelin and obestatin originate from the same gene via the same preprohormone probably by specific convertase enzymes in the intracellular Golgi organelles. This surprising molecular arrangement certainly suggests a stoichiometric relationship in the formation of these two functional opposing hormones and their interactions on food intake. A more indirect relationship evolves from the requirement of the enzymatic octanoylation of ghrelin and C-terminal amidation of obestatin for biological activity. These different molecular requirements along with different intracellular convertases may be reasons for believing these hormones not infrequently could be regulated and secreted differentially rather than in parallel.

A priori, projection of the regulated secretion of ghrelin and obestatin requires consideration that obestatin inhibits the action of ghrelin on food intake but not GH secretion. Although regulation of food intake by numerous hormones reveals its complexity, the inhibition of ghrelin-induced food intake implies a fundamental biological functional aspect of the ghrelin system that is yet to be demonstrated. With regard to the number of peripheral peptide inhibitors of food intake, there are many; however, so far ghrelin is the only peripheral peptide stimulator.

In the absence of ghrelin-R, transgenic female and male mice fed a high-fat diet eat less food, less of the consumed calories are stored, fat is more of the energy substrate, and body weight and body fat are less in these mice than in controls (Fig. 8.3) *(13)*. When the ghrelin-R was absent and mice were fed a normal diet, body weight and body fat were decreased in female but not in male mice. In the absence of the ghrelin hormone, transgenic male mice (female mice not studied) had less rapid body weight gain on a high-fat diet (Fig. 8.4) *(14)*. This was associated with increased energy

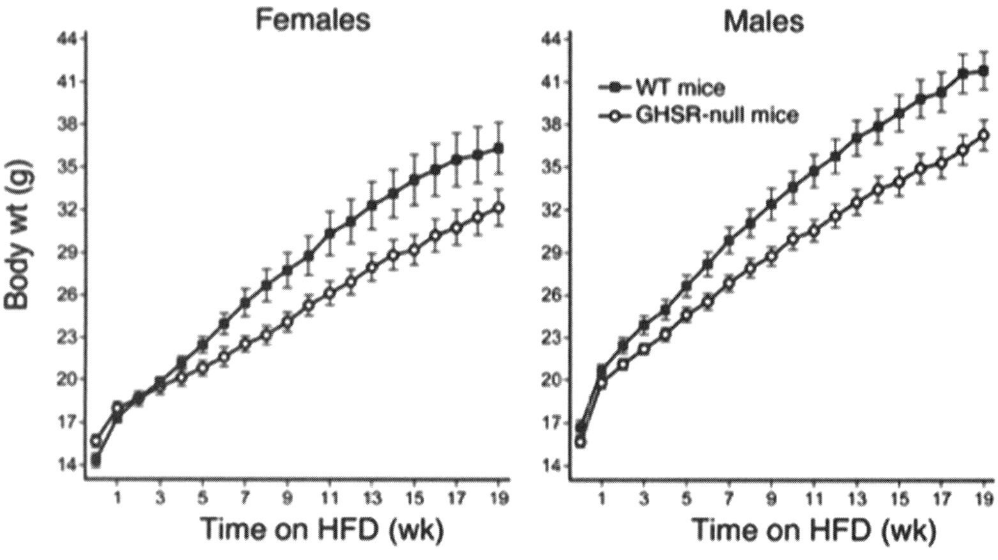

Fig. 8.3 In the absence of ghrelin-R (GHSR-null mice), body weight was less while on a high-fat diet between ages 4 and 19 weeks. Lean mass was unchanged and fat mass was decreased. (Reproduced from Zigman KM, Nakano Y, Coppari R, et al. Mice lacking ghrelin receptors resist the development of diet induced obesity. J Clin Invest 2005;115:3564–3572, with permission.).

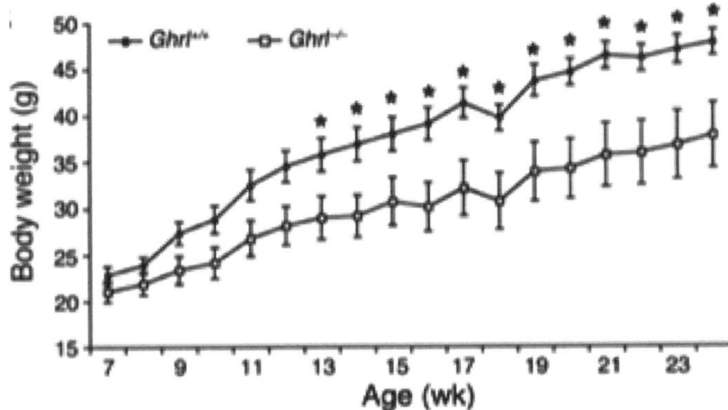

Fig. 8.4 In the absence of the ghrelin hormone (ghrelin-null mice) body weight was less between 13 and 23 weeks on a high-fat diet started 3 weeks postweaning. (Reproduced from Wortley KE, del Rincon JP, Murray JD, Garcia J, Iida K, Thorner MO, Sleeman MW. Absence of ghrelin protects against early-onset obesity. J Clin Invest 2005;115:3573–3578, with permission.).

expenditure and increased locomotive activity as well as decreased adiposity. Both of these studies indicate the ghrelin system is involved in body weight control especially when consuming a high caloric type of obese-inducing diet. In the absence of the ghrelin-R (GHSR-1a), ghrelin no longer increased food intake. Thus, the singularity of this receptor for mediating ghrelin-induced food intake is indicated. Effects of age, sex, diet, body composition, 24-h levels and rhythmic patterns of hormone secretion from the pituitary, thyroid, adrenal, gonads, pancreas, and so forth, will be required in order to appreciate the multifunctional endocrine-metabolic role of the ghrelin system.

Examples of specific actions of ghrelin/GHSs on food intake include increased food intake with subthreshold doses of ghrelin in streptozotocin-treated diabetic-induced rats, which may be explained by low serum leptin and insulin levels *(15)*. Both leptin and insulin inhibit stimulation of the orexigenic neuropeptide Y (NPY) and agouti-related protein (AgRP) hypothalamic arcuate neurons by ghrelin/GHSs and thus ghrelin may be responsible for the hyperphagia of patients with uncontrolled diabetes. Also, because evidence indicates that low-dose GHRP-2 and also ghrelin increase food intake in obese subjects (vide infra), the attenuated postprandial decrease in plasma ghrelin levels that occurs in obese subjects may play a pathophysiologic role in obesity, and a ghrelin receptor antagonist may be of therapeutic value in obesity *(16)*. Large subcutaneous dosages of ghrelin administered to adult male rats had a redistribution effect on tissue levels of fat; muscle fat was decreased, whereas liver fat was increased *(17)*. The authors envision this may be a favorable metabolic adaptation effect that could occur during caloric restriction. Enhancement of body fat in normal mice by chronic administration of the GHSs GHRP-6, ipamorelin, and GHRP-2 is well established *(18)*. This adipogenic effect is not a straightforward uncomplicated subject. Its analysis requires consideration of the lipolytic action of GH and GHSs via its GH releasing action, various endocrine metabolic actions as well as magnitude of the effect on the GH–IGF-1 axis, food intake, serum cortisol and PRL (prolactin) rises and, in addition, protein, fat, and carbohydrate metabolism. Other factors in need of consideration include effects in animals versus humans, effect of GHSs versus ghrelin, and dosage, route, and frequency of administration of these agents. The subject is considered relevant and important in order to understand the actions of the GHSs and to determine their therapeutic applications in order to develop the full spectrum of clinical uses of this new class of agents. Over several years, Van den Berghe et al. have pursued the hypothalamic-pituitary therapeutic approach by assessing the actions and potential therapeutic value of continuous subcutaneous infusion of GHRP-2 alone and together with TRH thyropin releasing hormone and/or LHRH luteinizing hormone releasing hormone in patients with critical illness *(19, 20)*. In these patients, the uniform hypofunction of most of the hypothalamic axes as well as the safety and induction of physiologic hormonal secretion and actions, in particular, GH, IGF-1, IGFBPs, as well as the effects on metabolism are basic reasons for pursuing this approach. On the basis of the Van den Berghe GHRP-2 + TRH studies in critically ill patients in the intensive care unit, De Groot agrees with her that the euthyroid sick syndrome or nonthyroidal illness syndrome (De Groot) is a manifestation of hypothalamic-pituitary dysfunction and from this viewpoint her evidence supports the combined GHRP-2 + TRH treatment approach *(21)*.

RECEPTOR

The ghrelin receptor (ghrelin-R) GHSR-1a belongs to a relatively small family of seven-transmembrane G protein–coupled receptors (Fig. 8.5) *(22)*. Particularly notable

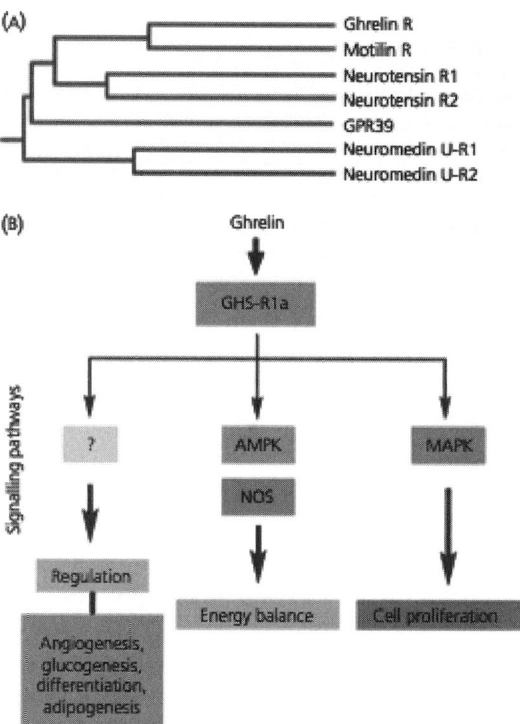

Fig. 8.5 Dendrogram of the ghrelin receptor family and some of the major signaling pathways associated with ghrelin biological activities mediated by the ghrelin-R. (Reproduced from Camina JP. Cell biology of the ghrelin receptor. J Neuroendocrinol 2006;18:65–76, with permission.).

is that the obestatin receptor (obestatin-R; GPR39) and the ghrelin receptor belong to the same family and that both of these receptors function at a high constitutive activity even when unstimulated by their respective hormones. In contrast with ghrelin-R, little is known yet about obestatin-R in respect to the actions of obestatin (see Addendum).

A number of findings demonstrate how the ghrelin-R may uniquely play a role in mediating the actions on GH release and food intake. This includes the ghrelin-R genetics, mutations, structure, intracellular signaling, high constitutive activity, enhancement of the number of hypothalamic ghrelin receptors during starvation, and so forth. Desensitization of the ghrelin-R on GH release by repeated administration of GHSs or ghrelin occurs in both rats and humans but to a much greater degree in rats. Desensitization of the GHS/ghrelin increase in food intake has not been systematically studied but in rats it seems to be less than desensitization of GH secretion. A spectrum of growth and metabolic changes occur in mice as a result of knockout of the ghrelin molecule as well as the ghrelin receptor. Adiposity in mice followed overexpression of the ghrelin receptor in hypothalamic GHRH arcuate neurons, while a small phenotype was induced by overexpression of desacyl ghrelin in transgenic mice presumably via a hypothalamic subtype ghrelin-R *(23)*. Over time, select biological effects of ghrelin/GHSs, especially nonendocrine effects, have been revealed that presumably occur via subtype receptors of ghrelin or perhaps via ghrelin-R with select mutations. Already, evidence indicates binding and activation of the multifunctional CD36 receptor by GHSs. Another noteworthy finding of the ghrelin-R was that under pathophysiologic conditions, the density of this receptor was reported to be five times greater in atherosclerotic coronary arteries *(24)*.

In an outstanding series of studies, Holst et al. characterized the high constitutive activity of the ghrelin-R and other receptors of this evolutionary family. The high constitutive activity of the ghrelin-R as well as the presumed obestatin-R (GPR39) is a particularly remarkable finding. Even without ghrelin or obestatin binding and stimulation of the receptors, these two receptors are markedly turned on at 50 % of their full activity (Fig. 8.6) *(25, 26)*. This obestatin effect is dependent on validation of its binding to GPR39. In the absence of receptor stimulation, elevated levels of intracellular signal transducer inositol triphosphate (IP3) is an indicator of the turned-on receptors. Holst et al. characterized the high constitutively activity of these two receptors. Also, they demonstrated inhibition of the constitutive activity by the [$DArg^1$,$DPhe^5$,$DTrp^{7,9}$,Leu^{11}]-substance P analogue, which has been previously characterized both in vitro and in vivo as a weak competitive receptor antagonist to acute and chronic actions of GHRP-2 and ghrelin. Holst et al. also demonstrated in vitro that this analogue has two types of ghrelin-R inhibiting activities (Fig. 8.6). At a low dose (5 nM, IC_{50}), this substance P analogue is a potent inverse receptor agonist as it decreases elevated intracellular IP3 levels in the absence of ghrelin, but also it is a weak ghrelin GHRP-6 competitive receptor antagonist as high dosages (630 nM, IC_{50}) inhibit receptor binding of both peptides. From results of combined structural-biochemical-mutation studies of the ghrelin-R and the ORF39-R, these authors also proposed the molecular mechanism responsible for the high constitutive activity of these two receptors *(26)*. This consisted of an interactive clustering of the aromatic side chain of three amino acid residues in transmembrane 6 and 7 inducing a tilting of these two transmembrane domains resulting in the turned-on receptor constitutive

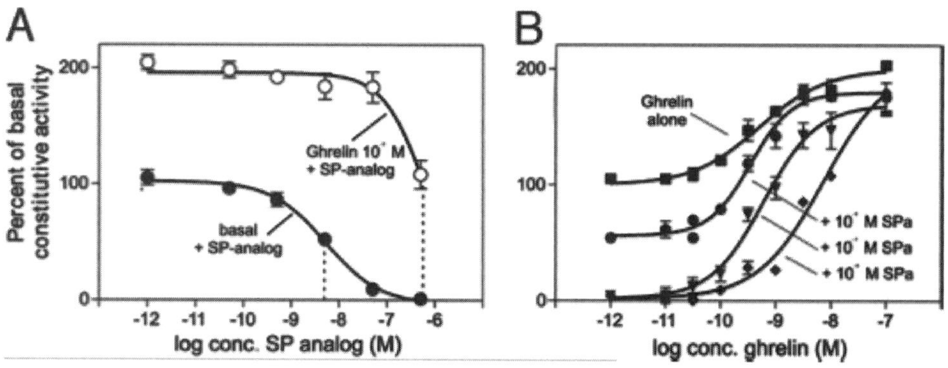

Fig. 8.6 Results in (**A**) and (**B**) demonstrate [DArg[1],DPhe[5],DTrp[7,9],Leu[11]]–substance P is a potent inverse agonist (IC_{50} 5.2 nM) and a weak competitive ghrelin-R antagonist (IC_{50} 630 nM). Changes in IP3 turnover were used to assess the high basal constitutive receptor activity and the ghrelin stimulated receptor activity. (Reproduced from Holst B, Cygankiewicz A, Jensen TH, Ankersen M, Schwartz TW. High constitutive signaling of the ghrelin receptor-identification of a potent inverse agonist. Mol Endocrinol 2003;17 *(11)*:2201–2210, with permission.).

activity. The authors speculated the constitutive turned-on receptor itself may play a role in overeating, and administration of a ghrelin receptor inverse agonist may be effective in treating obesity. There is now a broader spectrum of findings to support the hypothesis that ghrelin and obestatin play a fundamental role in the regulation of food intake at a physiologic and pathophysiologic level. The ghrelin set-point conceptualization proposed by Holst et al. is now further significantly supported and expanded by discovery of obestatin and its receptor. The basis for a potential coupled relationship of ghrelin and obestatin is indeed notable; that is, both hormones originate mainly from the fundus of the stomach, from the same stomach cells, same gene, same preprohormone, and their receptors belong to the same evolutionary family, have the same high constitutive activity, and both regulate food intake but with opposite effects. Obviously, these relationships beg for special explanations.

Petersen et al. very recently reported that continuous intracerebroventricular, 7-day infusion of a very low dose of the substance P ghrelin-R inverse agonist inhibited body weight of male rats *(27)*. This was a dose that would be too low to function as a competitive ghrelin receptor antagonist and thus it was considered to be due to the inverse agonist activity of the substance P analogue. Also, these same investigators published a study with their results and those of Wang et al. and Pantel et al. on structure-function mutational studies of the ghrelin-R (*28–30*). Included are the important genetic studies of Pantel et al. The salient findings of these studies are presented in Figure 8.7. A conclusion from these studies was that the high constitutive activity of the ghrelin-R is a determinant of linear body growth of children and, when inactivated, results in impaired function of the GH–IGF-1 axis. A still unresolved issue to be elucidated is the combination of obesity in a child with a ghrelin receptor mutation that inhibits constitutive activity *(30)*.

Another possible novel functional role of the high constitutive activity of the ghrelin-R in the CNS was proposed in the excellent study by Zigman et al. on the distribution and functional implication of the ghrelin-R in the brain of the rat and

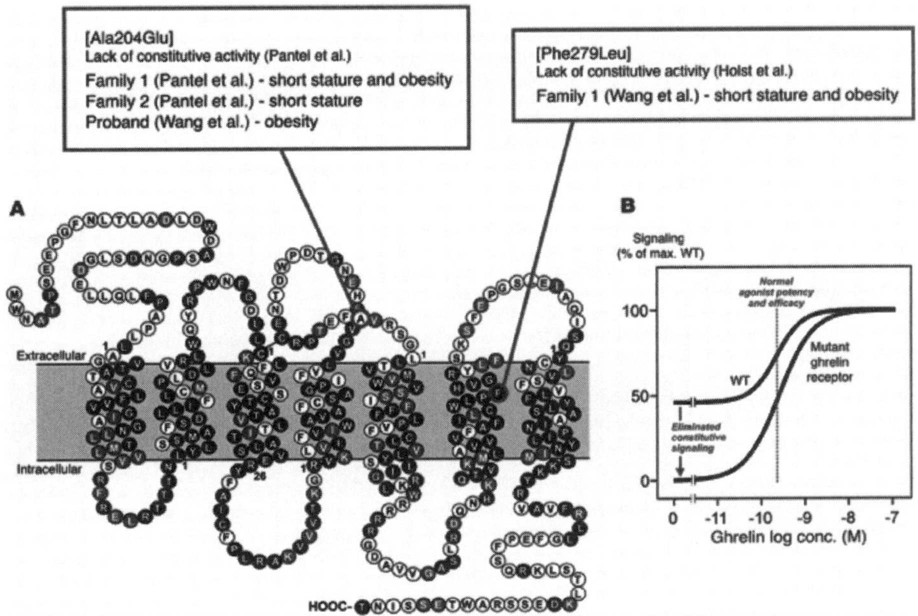

Fig. 8.7 The turned-on constitutive activity of the ghrelin receptor and the genetic phenotype of short stature and obesity meaningfully come together. As recorded in (**B**), the recent publications of Wang et al. and Pantel et al. indicate the single amino acid mutations, Ala204Glu and Phe279Leu (**A**), are associated with both phenotypes and the absence of constitutive activity but importantly with preservation of full potency and efficacy of the ghrelin receptor action. (Reproduced from Holst B, Schwartz TW. Ghrelin receptor mutations-too little height and too much hunger. J Clin Invest 2006;116:637–641, with permission.).

mouse *(31)*. They proposed that the high constitutive activity of the ghrelin-R plays a key functional role at the CNS sites at which the receptor is expressed within the blood-brain barrier and thus does not have immediate access to circulating ghrelin. This is in contrast with the ghrelin-R located in the arcuate nucleus and dorsal vagal complex role. A suggestion of how this may occur is by an increase of the ghrelin-R number. As an example, the ghrelin-R number markedly increased in the rat hypothalamus of the CNS during starvation *(31)*. Besides exogenous ghrelin-R inverse agonist activity, Zigman et al. envisioned the possibility of an endogenous inverse agonist. This is a speculation that can be extended by suggesting that select GHSs, because of their different chemistry, may have ready access to brain sites inaccessible to ghrelin. If this occurs, actions of GHSs at these sites may sensitize and/or desensitize the activity of the CNS ghrelin-R and/or may alter the CNS ghrelin constitutive activity via effects on receptor number and/or activity. Also, receptor modification may be induced at the transcriptional level independent of the ghrelin action.

GHRP-2 CLINICAL STUDIES

The hypothesis was proposed that unnatural GHRPs/GHSs mimic the GH releasing action of the new natural hormone ghrelin and restore normal physiologic function of the GH–IGF-1 axis especially in older men and women *(32)*. Conceptually, our

GHS/ghrelin approach is based on the thesis that GH secretion in normal pulses and patterns over the entire 24-h period is of preeminent and fundamental biological importance in restoring the physiologic secretions, actions, and functions of the IGF-1 system. In these studies, our working approach has been to define the clinical state of decreased GH secretion in normal older men and women as subjects with low serum IGF-1 levels of <125 μg/L. Perhaps there are now more reasons to consider this approach, analogous to an elevated fasting glucose level in the definition of diabetes mellitus.

To raise serum IGF-1 levels and enhance secretion of GH in older men and women, GHRP-2 was administered by continuous subcutaneous infusion via an ambulatory infusion pump *(32)*. Continuous feed-forward stimulation of the hypothalamic-pituitary regulatory sites responsible for synthesis and secretion of GH in turn activate feedback regulation of GH resulting in normal pulsatile secretion. As described by Veldhuis et al., there are a number of interactions of the stimulatory feed-forward effects of GHRP, ghrelin, GHRH, estrogen, and testosterone and the inhibitory feedback effects of GH, IGF-1, and SRIF, together and in various combinations, on the hypothalamic-pituitary unit to regulate pulsatile secretion of GH in humans *(33)*. The synergistic release of GH by intravenous bolus and prolonged continuous subcutaneous administration of combined GHRP + GHRH, regardless of age or gender, support that multiple mechanisms are involved. Preliminary results reveal combined ghrelin + GHRH GH results are the same. In humans, under normal conditions the GH response to GHSs/ghrelin is highly dependent on the synthesis and secretion of GHRH and, under abnormal conditions, the impaired action of GHRH on GH release may be the result of its dependency on endogenous ghrelin.

Another potential future therapeutic approach of the GHSs concerns the increase, decrease, or normalization of the inappropriate actions and/or dysfunctional secretion of ghrelin, which may occur at certain stages of obesity and in undernutrition of older and younger subjects or during chronic illness. It is relevant that both GH and food intake are regulated by ghrelin and the GHSR-1a via each respective interacting feed-forward/feedback network. This makes it possible to project that food intake, like GH secretion, may be normalized by the same extended continuous subcutaneous GHRP-2/GHS approach established to increase pulsatile GH secretion. To develop and evaluate this possible GHS normalization approach will require assessment of various GHSs, route and pattern of administration, as well as dosage and the particular pathophysiology.

A major new challenge is to determine the basic reasons for the dual effect of ghrelin/GHSs on GH and food intake and how this relates to physiology and pathophysiology as well as how this dual action most effectively can be developed therapeutically to alter body composition of humans. Currently, the focus of GHSs in humans has been primarily on food intake. Evidence indicates these two major actions on GH and food intake can be dissociated in both animals and humans. Each action evolves from a different complicated neuroendocrine regulatory system, however, for a still undetermined fundamental reason(s), the major action of ghrelin is on both GH and food intake. Problematic to the detailed understanding of this dual action is the difference among and between animal species, between animals and humans, and, very importantly, in humans as a function of age and sex.

CHILDREN

In reflection, the anabolic effect of an increase in body growth rate in children of short stature that resulted from the chronically administered GHRPs is considered important in principle. Collectively, this represents composite results of a new chemical class of bioactive agents (GHRPs) and a new hormonal system that is complementary to and involves the biological actions of GHRH, GH, and IGF-1, each of which enhances body growth of humans. Recorded in Figure 8.8 are the augmented height velocity levels in short-stature children induced by GHRP administration twice daily or three times daily after intranasal or subcutaneous once-daily administration in different dosages and for different periods of time *(34–36)*. Dosages that acutely release GH in short-stature children were used for each of the studies, however serum IGI-1 levels were only slightly or moderately elevated by the GHSs, and the growth response was less compared with the enhanced catch-up growth response obtained during the first year of recombinant GH therapy. Even high dosages of oral GHRP-2 produce suboptimal therapy for short-stature children *(37)*. A projected more promising clinical approach would be a depot formulation that could be administered once per month or less frequently because evidence indicates this would induce a sustained physiologic pulsatile secretion over the entire 24 h and would result in a much greater elevation of serum IGF-1 level *(38)*. It is probable that the anabolic effect would have been greater

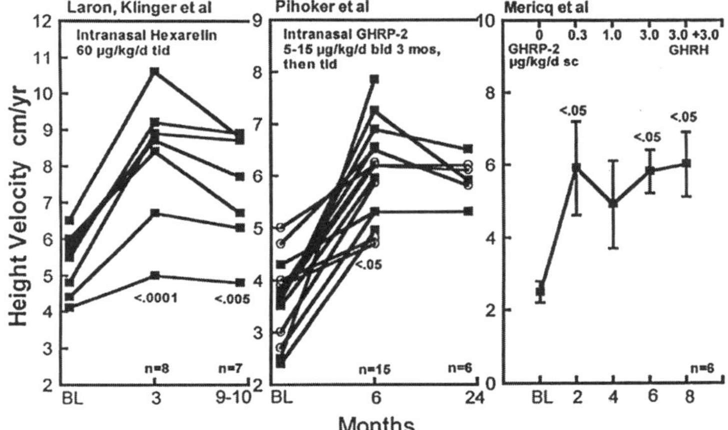

Fig. 8.8 Results of three different investigators demonstrate there is a sustained increased rate of growth in height velocity of short-stature children with varying degrees of GH deficiency by prolonged administration of hexarelin and GHRP-2. In the *left panel* are the results of Klinger and Laron et al. (Eur J Endocrinol 1996;134:715–719); *middle panel*, Pihoker et al. (J Endocrinol 1997;15:79–86); *right panel*, Mericq et al. (J Clin Endocrinol Metab 1998;83:2355–2360). Graphs created from data extracted from text. (Redrawn from Klinger B, Silbergeld A, Deghenghi R, Laron Z. Desensitization from long-term intranasal treatment with hexarelin does not interfere with the biological effects of this growth hormone-releasing peptide in short children. Eur J Endocrinol 1996;134:716–719; Pihoker C, Badger TM, Reynolds GA, Bowers CY. Treatment effects of intranasal growth hormone releasing peptide-2 in children with short stature. J Endocrinol 1997;155:79–86; and Mericq V, Cassorla F, Salazar T, Avila A, Iniguez G, Bowers CY, Merriam GR. Effects of eight months treatment with graded doses of a growth hormone releasing peptide in GH deficient children. J Clin Endocrinol Metab 1998;83:2355–2360.).

if a larger serum IGF-1 level had been achieved by the intermittent GHS approach, which is an effect we believe can now be produced in children as in adults by the GHS continuous delivery approach. Applicable to GHS treatment of short-stature children are a number of projected instructive points about the GHS effect on anabolism and body composition that emerge from analysis of the data obtained from sustained delivery of GHSs in older subjects with low serum IGF-1 levels. With regard to the GHS continuous delivery approach in children, normal physiologic pulsatile secretion of GH probably would be enhanced in normal pattern and amount over the entire 24 h and the GH rise would be sustained as long as the GHS is administered. In humans, the level of GH secretion would not only determine the IGF-1 level and its expected anabolic nitrogen retention action but also body weight presumably via the lipolytic action of GH. When GH is increased, body fat would be unlikely to increase in humans to the degree that has been observed in mice given GHSs. In mice, the adipogenic activity of GHSs may occur because intermittent GHS administration results in high serum GHS levels and because sustained delivery results in desensitization of the GHS-induced GH release, an effect that has not occurred in our studies in humans. Because intermittent rather than sustained GHS administration produces higher GHS levels, this tends to increase cortisol levels transiently and attenuate the circadian secretion of cortisol. The latter would be more expected to occur when GHSs are administered twice daily or three times daily or once per day in the evening rather than the morning. Thus, the therapeutic paradigm would exist in which body fat may be increased or decreased depending on the GHS dose and type of delivery and also its frequency and time-of-day administration. These relationships reveal how a dual complementary action of GHSs on GH–IGF-1 and food intake may come together to produce unique balanced physiologic effects and also to produce imbalance and less efficacious pathophysiologic effects when not administered by 24-h continuous delivery.

NITROGEN RETENTION

As recorded in Figure 8.9, a complementary GHS anabolic action in humans also has been demonstrated by Murthy et al. with oral GHS MK-677 to normal young men during caloric restriction *(39)*. These studies reveal that the GHS nonpeptide MK-677 developed by the Merck group increased nitrogen retention. Over a 7-day period, a single daily oral 25 mg dose of MK-677 at bedtime increased GH secretion in conjunction with a limited increase of serum IGF-1, IGFBP-3, and nitrogen retention. These studies support the anabolic nitrogen retention action of GHSs in normal subjects, however, in unhealthy patients or in patients with hypofunction of the hypothalamic-pituitary axis, these effects would require larger and more frequent GHS dosages, which in turn would produce unwanted pharmacologic effects because GHSs and ghrelin have multifunctional actions. Serum cortisol was not increased in this study but the levels were not acutely determined shortly after the MK-677 dose and the circadian secretion of cortisol was not assessed. Cortisol rises acutely after GHS administration due to the release of ACTH (adrenocortitotropin) by a hypothalamic rather than pituitary action. In addition, serum cortisol levels are greater in the morning than in the evening and thus the GHS/ghrelin tends to increase less cortisol rise when administered in the morning.

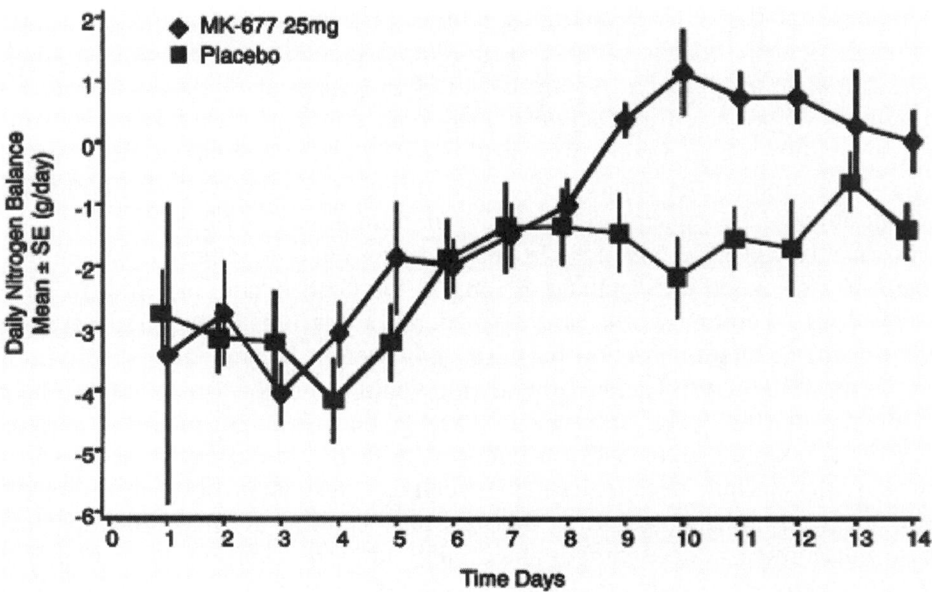

Fig. 8.9 A single oral 25 mg dose of MK-677 increased nitrogen retention (urea and ammonia nitrogen) in 24-h urine collections of normal young men (n = 8) while on a caloric-restricted diet (18 kcal kg^{-1} day^{-1}). Study design was a crossover with caloric-restricted diet and placebo. (Reproduced from Murthy MG, Plunkett LM, Gertz BJ, Wittreich J, Polvino WM, Clemmons DR. MK-677, an orally active growth hormone secretagogue, reverses diet induced catabolism. J Clin Endocrinol Metab 1998;83:320–325, with permission.).

The potential therapeutic value of the GHSs as an activator of the GH–IGF-1 axis is strongly supported by the results of Svensson et al. *(40)*. Although limited in degree, favorable biological effects without major adverse effects were demonstrated in this well-designed, carefully controlled clinical study with MK-677 in normal obese men with a mean age of 37 and BMI of 32. As recorded in Figure 8.10a and b, fat-free mass by DEXA (dual-energy x-ray absorptiometry) was significantly increased by 25 mg daily MK-677 in the morning whereas body fat was unaffected. Also utilizing four-compartment model derived values, MK-677 increased body cell mass without a change in body fat (Fig. 8.10c and d). Before starting MK-677, serum IGF-1 levels were decreased when visceral fat was increased (Fig. 8.11a). At the end of the 2-month MK-677 study, the percent increase in serum IGF-1 levels was associated with the percent decrease in visceral fat volume (Fig. 8.11b). Neither the total amount of visceral nor subcutaneous fat was changed by MK-677 but this may be a function of the GHS approach, duration of administration, type and subpopulation of subjects, as well as age and sex.

A series of preliminary clinical results increasingly support the possibility that ghrelin/GHSs can be effectively developed as therapy for nonendocrine illnesses as well as endocrine disorders via the multifunctional actions of this new therapeutic class of agents. The nonendocrine illnesses include cardiac, vascular, pulmonary, renal, and metabolic disorders/diseases and possibly those of the brain. In particular, the success of this new therapy will depend on the GHS dosage and administration method

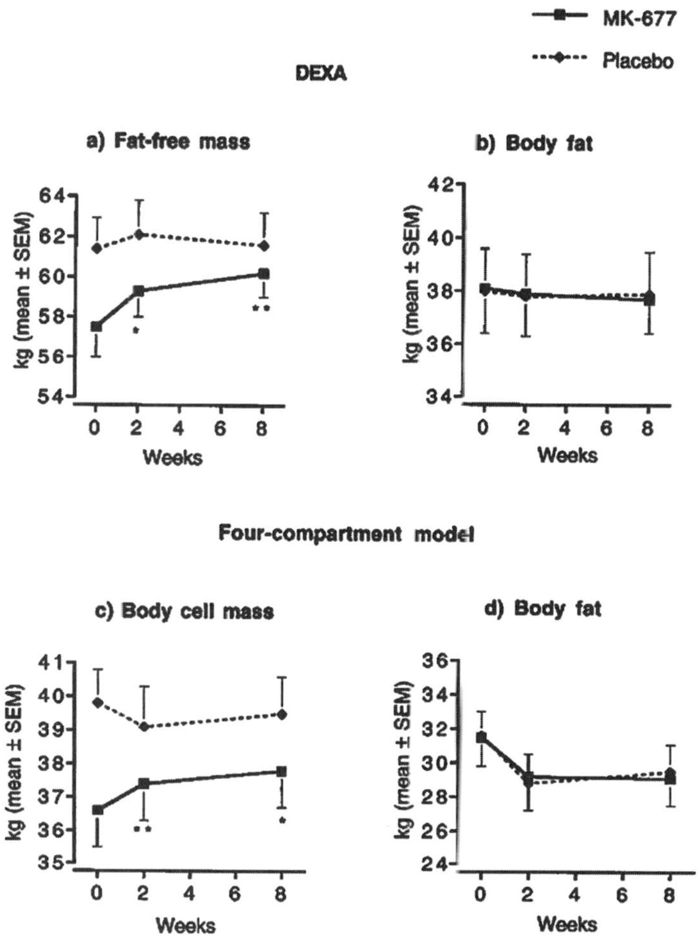

Fig. 8.10 MK-677 25mg/day orally for 8 weeks induced sustained increases of GH and IGF-1 in 12 normal obese men compared with 12 normal obese men given placebo. MK-677 also increased fat-free mass while total fat and visceral fat were unchanged. The mean age, BMI, IGF-1 (μg/L) of the men in the MK-677 versus the placebo group were 36.8 versus 39, 32 versus 32.5, and 150.3 versus 156, respectively. $^{*}p < 0.05$; $^{**}p < 0.01$. (Reproduced from Svensson J. Two month treatment of obese subjects with the oral growth hormone (GH) secretagogue MK-677 increases GH secretion, fat mass, and energy expenditure. J Clin Endocrinol Metab 1998;83:362–369, with permission.).

such as continuous delivery via long-acting formulations. When cachexia with body weight loss and muscle weakness occurs in patients with congestive heart failure (CHF) and also chronic pulmonary obstructive disease (COPD), the mortality is significantly higher in both disorders indicating the possible therapeutic value of reversing or preventing body weight decrease of these patients. Nagaya et al. have treated these two types of patients with intravenous infusion of ghrelin in a large dose (2 μg/kg) over a 30-min period twice per day for 3 weeks, which produced favorable effects on cardiovascular and pulmonary function tests *(41, 42)*. In both studies, food intake, body weight (COPD only), DEXA lean body mass, and hand grip strength (COPD) were evaluated and found to be impaired. In these CHF and COPD patients, there was an acute peak

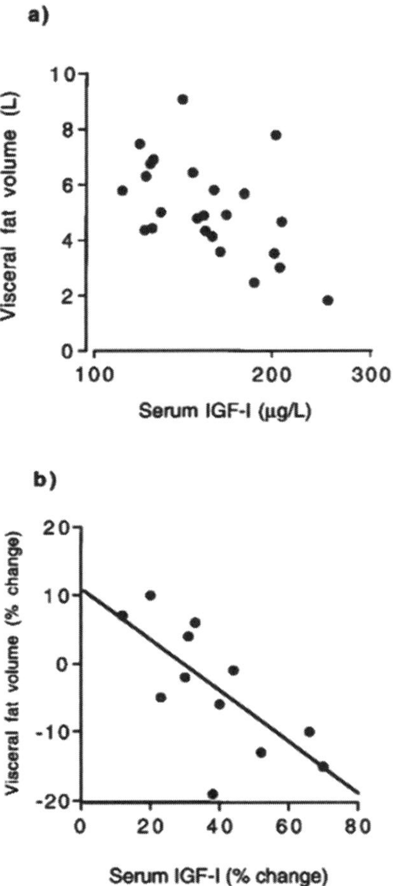

Fig. 8.11 At baseline, correlation of visceral fat volume (L) and serum IGF-1 (μg/L) are recorded in (**a**) ($r = -0.5$; $p < 0.01$), and in (**b**) is the percent change in serum IGF-1 and visceral fat volume at the end of MK-677 treatment ($r = -0.7$; $p < 0.01$). (Reproduced from Svensson J. Two month treatment of obese subjects with the oral growth hormone (GH) secretagogue MK-677 increases GH secretion, fat mass, and energy expenditure. J Clin Endocrinol Metab 1998;83:362–369, with permission.).

rise of GH ~20–25 µg/L at the beginning of the study, but this was not evaluated at the end of the study. Somewhat surprising was that the improved anabolic/metabolic and cardiopulmonary effects occurred without any long-term changes in basal levels of GH and IGF-1 after the 3 weeks of ghrelin administration. This may indicate acute transient effects on the GH–IGF-1 axis as well as the possibility of nonendocrine effects via peripheral ghrelin receptors/subtype receptors, and/or multifunctional CD36 receptors may be responsible for some of the beneficial ghrelin actions in these patients. With regard to activation of the GH–IGF-1 axis, continuous delivery would have been much more effective via sustained 24-h elevated serum levels of the peptide and subsequent increased pulsatile serum GH and IGF-1 levels.

FOOD INTAKE

A definite enhancement of food intake has been achieved by short-term GHS and ghrelin administration in humans and in long-term studies in animals. All routes of administration (intravenous, subcutaneous, intranasal, and oral) are theoretically possible to increase food intake because GHSs effectively release GH by each approach and the same ghrelin-R mediates the GHS actions on GH and food intake. Additionally, sustained GHS delivery in rats produces increased food intake but a small increase of GH. The choice between premeal delivery and continuous delivery of GHS will need specific evaluation and will depend to a degree on an increasing appreciation of how food intake is regulated physiologically and in various pathophysiologic disorders/illnesses.

Studies on the function and role of the ghrelin system are especially noteworthy in exogenous obesity because of decreased GH secretion and enhanced food intake. Some major still deficient details concern the measurement of acyl ghrelin plasma levels after a proper blood collection. This includes the specific measurement of plasma acyl ghrelin levels and reporting in terms of this reference standard as well as determination of the 24-h pattern of acyl ghrelin levels in normal and obese subjects as a function of age, sex, stage of obesity, and nutritional intake *(43)*. How consistently acyl ghrelin rises before meals and how meaningful the degree of the rise is in terms of food intake responsiveness needs critical evaluation in order to better understand the regulation of food intake by ghrelin, especially circulating ghrelin.

Sequential studies performed by Wren et al. convincingly established that ghrelin increases food intake in normal lean subjects and also in normal obese versus lean subjects as reported by Druce et al. *(44,45)*. Results of particular note are that the ghrelin sensitivity on food intake was greater in obese than in lean subjects but the ghrelin GH responsiveness was less in the obese than in the lean subjects. As discussed below, this decreased responsiveness in obese subjects is considered to be secondary to the impaired action of GHRH on the pituitary and is not due to decreased ghrelin secretion.

In the GHRP-2 studies of Laferrère et al. *(46)* demonstrated in Figure 8.12, both food intake (left panel) and GH (right panel) were increased significantly by the same GHS dosage. Even a low dose of GHRP-2 increased food intake indicating obese are not insensitive to orexigenic actions of GHS or presumably ghrelin (Fig. 8.13) *(47)*. Because of the high effectiveness of GHRP-2 in increasing food intake and the possibility of attenuated inhibition of plasma acyl ghrelin levels in obese subjects during the immediate postmeal time period, ghrelin effects on food intake may play a pathophysiologic role in maintaining excess food intake in obese subjects even when body weight is increased at a stable steady state excess level. If this is correct, a ghrelin/GHS receptor antagonist should be effective in reducing body weight in obese subjects.

In other studies on the GH releasing action of GHRP-2 and GHRH alone and together, we showed that obese subjects were insensitive to even large dosages of GHRH, which was reversed by a very low dosage of GHRP-2 when the two peptides were given together *(48)*. From these results, we concluded the pathophysiology of decreased secretion of GH in obesity is due to a yet to be explained impaired pituitary action of GHRH and not due to a decreased action of ghrelin. Also concluded was that excess SRIF secretion or action, which very effectively inhibits the pituitary action of

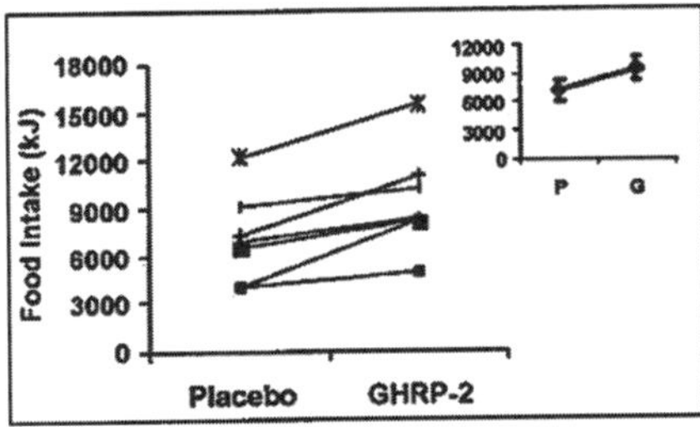

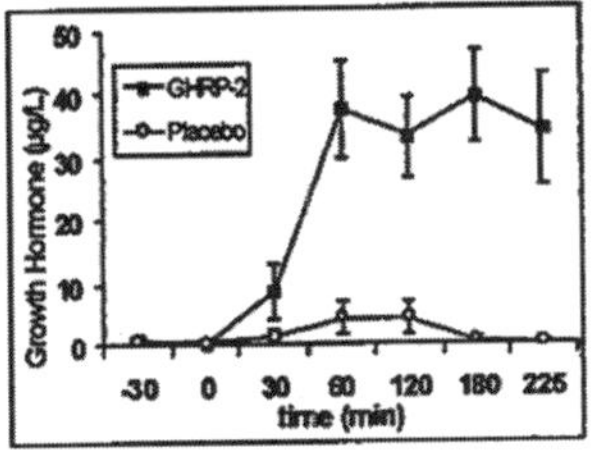

Fig. 8.12 Infusion of GHRP-2 subcutaneously for 270 min to seven lean healthy men at a dose of 1 µg kg^{-1} h^{-1} increased food intake of both individual and mean ± SEM changes in energy intake after an ad libitum buffet lunch (1 kJ = 0.239 kcal) (*left panel*) and GH levels (*right panel*). (Reproduced from Laferrere B, Abraham C, Russell CD, Bowers CY. Growth hormone releasing peptide-2 (GHRP-2), like ghrelin, increases food intake in healthy men. J Clin Endocrinol Metab 2005;90:611–614, with permission.).

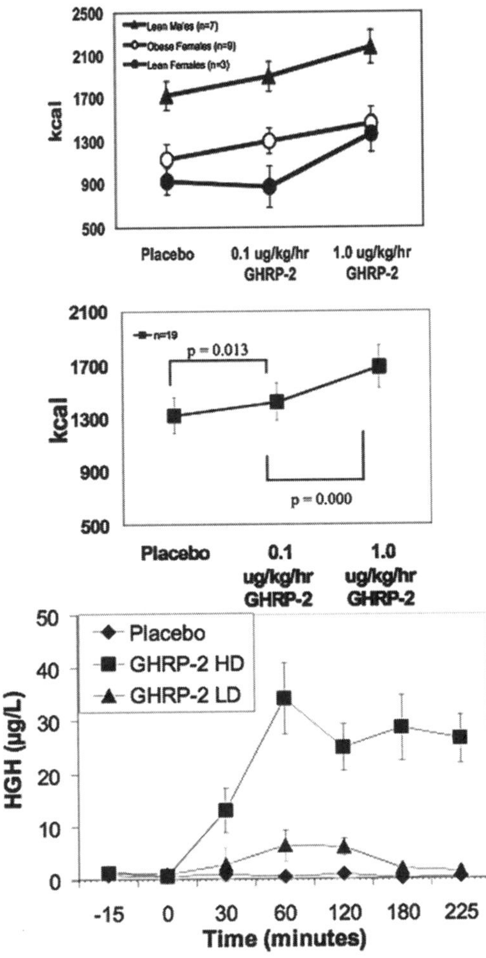

Fig. 8.13 Infusion of GHRP-2 subcutaneously for 270 min to 19 healthy subjects; 10 lean (7 men and 3 women) and 9 obese (9 women) at two dose levels (0.1 µg kg^{-1} h^{-1}, low dose [LD]; 1 µg kg^{-1} h^{-1}, high dose [HD]). Both doses increased food intake and GH levels. (Adapted from Laferrère et al., The Endocrine Society 87th Annual Meeting 2005, San Diego, p. 536, The Endocrine Society Chevy Chase, Maryland.)

GHRH, is not responsible for the impaired pituitary action of GHRH in obese subjects. Because SRIF very effectively inhibits the pituitary GH releasing action of GHRP-2 and ghrelin, low-dose GHRP-2 would not have been expected to reverse the impaired action of GHRH if SRIF had been increased.

GHRP-2 LONG-TERM CONTINUOUS DELIVERY APPROACH

In Figure 8.14 are examples of results obtained by continuous subcutaneous infusion of placebo or GHRP-2 for 30, 60, and 90 days via an ambulatory infusion pump to normal older men and women with low serum IGF-1 levels. The most important overall results were an increase of normal physiologic pulsatile GH secretion during the entire time period GHRP-2 was administered and the concomitant elevation of the IGF-1 level. These studies reveal more about the hormonal role of the feed-forward/feedback regulation of GH *(32, 33)*. The data indicate that 1) even low-pulsatile GH levels have a marked effect in increasing IGF-I levels; 2) the decreased GH levels on days 14 and 30 are not the result of desensitization of the GHRP-2 GH response; 3) the decreased GH levels on days 14 and 30 are probably due to the negative feedback effects of IGF-1 on the hypothalamic-pituitary unit rather than to desensitization of GHRH or ghrelin actions. In these studies, hepatic, renal, metabolic, and hematologic safety data obtained on placebo day 3 and GHRP-2 day 30 were normal. In women only, fasting glucose rose from 90 ± 1.2 to 103 ± 1.3 mg/dl ($p < 0.05$) but remained within the normal range (<126 mg/dl). Glucose values did not differ in men. Insulin concentrations did not change in either cohort. There were no significant clinical adverse events.

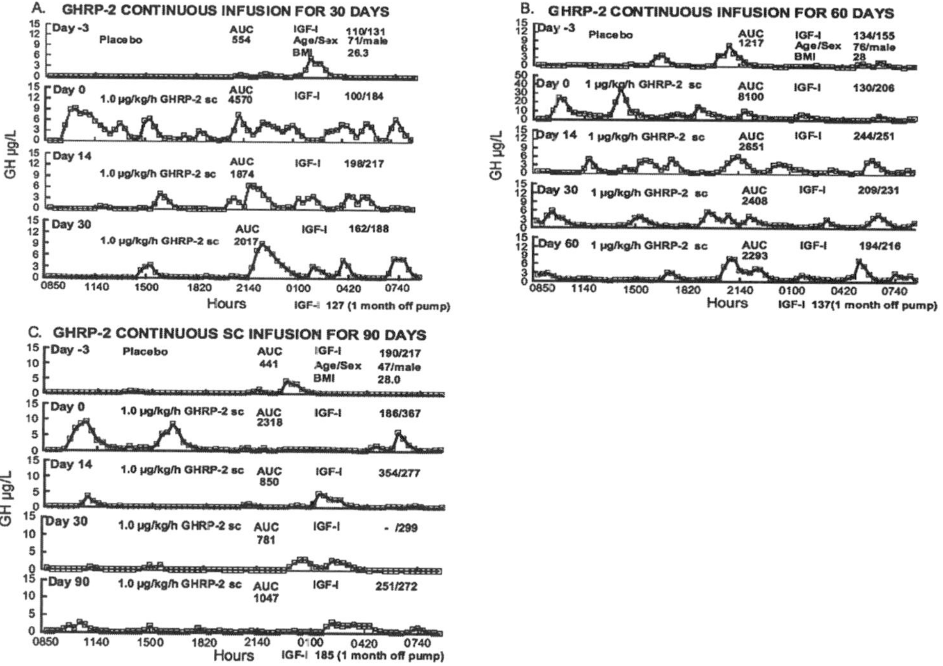

Fig. 8.14 GH and IGF-1 responses to 24-h continuous GHRP-2 infusion for 30 days (**A**); 60 days (**B**); 90 days (**C**). Even after 90 days of GHRP-2 treatment, the IGF-1 level returned to pretreatment level 1 month after the infusion was stopped.

Because the GH concentrations are lower on day 30, a negative feedback action of pulsatile GH on the hypothalamus is minimized during this equilibrated state. The persistent feed-forward action of GHRP-2 was revealed by the finding that 1 month after stopping the GHRP-2 infusion, IGF-1 returned to the low pretreatment level.

When GHRP was continuously infused subcutaneously for 30 days, n = 6 (Fig. 8.14A), 60 days, n = 5 (Fig. 8.14B), and 90 days, n = 1 (Fig. 8.14C), the same GH and IGF-1 effects were induced. Some subjects recorded an increase in appetite but this response was not evaluated.

ADDITIONAL ACTIONS OF GHRP-2 CONTINUOUS DELIVERY

Several other findings were observed in this study to support the conclusion that prolonged subcutaneous continuous GHRP-2 infusion releases GH physiologically. The release of ACTH, cortisol, and PRL, which occurs after acute intravenous bolus GHRP-2/ghrelin alone as well as with GHRH in animals and humans, did not occur during infusion of GHRP-2. In Figure 8.15 are the cortisol results, which demonstrate a normal circadian rhythm and level of cortisol on days 1 and 30. The hormonal rises of ACTH, cortisol, and PRL induced by acute intravenous bolus GHRP or ghrelin are considered to reflect pharmacologic rather than physiologic actions due to much higher blood levels of the GHRP-2. During GHRP-2 subcutaneous continuous infusion, the serum level of GHRP-2 is low and more equivalent to physiologic plasma ghrelin concentrations, which presumably, like GHRP-2 continuous subcutaneous infusion, activate the GH axis without increasing ACTH, cortisol, or PRL release. Whether the latter hormonal effects occasionally might be physiologically induced by ghrelin under select biological conditions is unknown, but it is possible because ghrelin and GHRPs definitely produce these effects in animals and humans. Other special actions in support

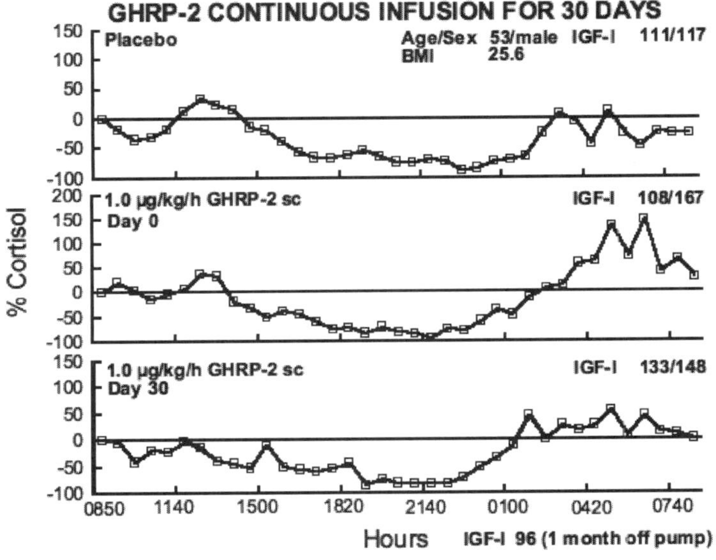

Fig. 8.15 During 30-day GHRP-2 infusion, the 24-h cortisol level and circadian rhythm remained normal.

of the physiologic actions of continuous GHRP-2 infusion include enhancement of circulating IGF-1, but not IGF-2, and increase of circulating IGFBP-3 and IGFBP-5 but not IGFBP-4 *(32)*. Leptin and adiponectin levels were unchanged. Particularly noteworthy is that the pulsatile secretion of GH is enhanced during the day and night over the entire 30-day infusion period.

TWENTY-FOUR HOUR GHRELIN CONTINUOUS DELIVERY

Acute studies with ghrelin demonstrate it effectively releases GH administered by intravenous and subcutaneous bolus injections and that these responses are essentially the same as those previously obtained with GHRPs *(48)*. When administered subcutaneously, the ghrelin GH releasing action appears to be less than with intravenous administration. Measurement of plasma desacyl + acyl ghrelin (total ghrelin) and acyl ghrelin (bioactive ghrelin) levels after subcutaneous versus intravenous administration to these patients indicates the octanoyl group is more readily cleaved after subcutaneous than intravenous administration. Revealing sites, mechanisms, and types of ghrelin degradation will be relevant to the regulation and action of ghrelin.

In our more recent studies, continuous subcutaneous infusion of ghrelin alone and together with GHRH for 24 h produced the same effects as GHRP-2 on GH and IGF-1 levels (Figs. 8.16 and 8.17). Also recorded in these figures are the plasma levels of total ghrelin (Phoenix assay) and bioactive ghrelin (Linco assay) during continuous subcutaneous infusion of ghrelin. Notable are the consistently high total ghrelin levels and the additional increase when acyl ghrelin was administered, which indicates conversion to the desacyl form of ghrelin definitely does occur. In these studies, GHRH, GH, and IGF-1 did not influence the desacyl or acyl ghrelin levels. Additionally, total ghrelin levels appeared to accumulate more than bioactive ghrelin, which needs further pharmacokinetic investigation.

In Figure 8.18 are the comparative GH and IGF-1 results of a 24-h infusion of GHRP-2 (A) and ghrelin (B) both alone and together with GHRH. In both subjects, the GH pulses were increased, and the combination of each peptide with GHRH enhanced the effect and further augmented the rise of GH and IGF-1. It is projected that in most subjects, particularly normal older subjects with low IGF-1 levels as well as idiopathic GH deficiency in short-stature children, continuous infusion of GHS alone probably would be therapeutically satisfactory to restore the function of the GH axis to normal.

During the 24-h placebo infusion even in the presence of a decreased inhibitory feedback action of IGF-1, GH concentrations were low presumably due to a lack of stimulatory feed-forward action of both endogenous GHRH and ghrelin thus indicating hypofunction of the hypothalamic-pituitary axis. Induction of normal pulsatile secretion of GH and sustained enhanced levels of IGF-1 after combined GHRP-2 + GHRH over the extended 30-day infusion period underscore the complementary physiologic action of these two peptides on GH secretion (Fig. 8.19) *(49)*. Under combined clamped administration of GHRP-2 + GHRH, the feed-forward prolonged stimulation of normal pulsatile secretion of GH is maintained and augmented and serum IGF-1 levels are raised to within normal range. This uniquely underscores SRIF in concert with GH and IGF-1 as the primary regulator of GH pulsatility.

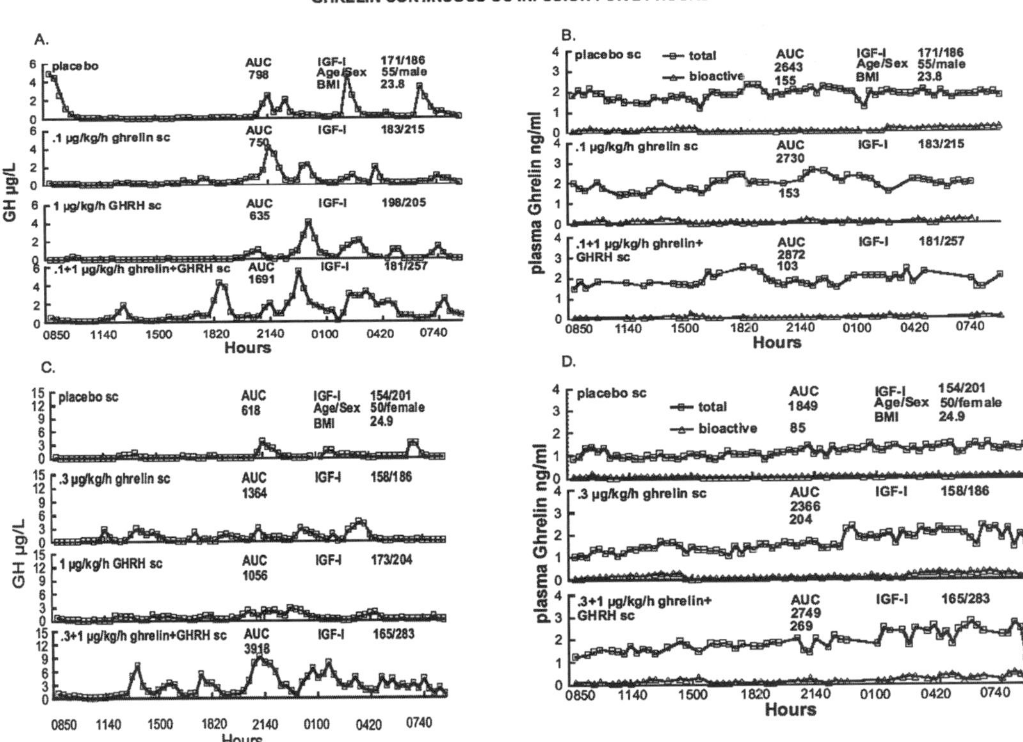

Fig. 8.16 GH responses and ghrelin levels with 24-h continuous subcutaneous infusion of 0.1 (**A** and **B**) and 0.3 $\mu g\ kg^{-1}\ h^{-1}$ ghrelin (**C** and **D**). Only a small rise in bioactive ghrelin occurred with the 0.3 $\mu g\ kg^{-1}\ h^{-1}$ dose with a greater rise in total ghrelin level; however, the IGF-1 levels rose with both the 0.1 and 0.3 $\mu g\ kg^{-1}\ h^{-1}$ doses. (Adapted from Bowers et al., The Endocrine Society 86th Annual Meeting 2004, New Orleans, p. 237, Endocrine Society Chevy Chase, Maryland.).

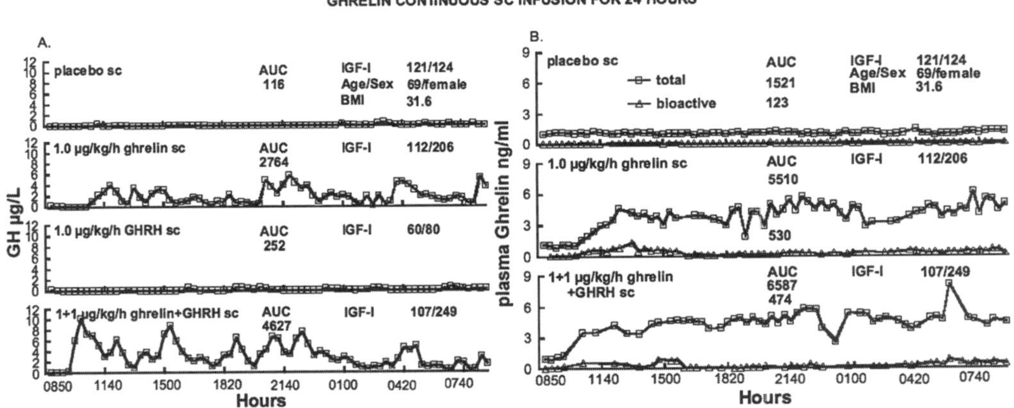

Fig. 8.17 GH responses and ghrelin levels with 24-h continuous subcutaneous infusion of 1.0 $\mu g\ kg^{-1}\ h^{-1}$ ghrelin. GH and ghrelin (both bioactive and total) levels rose considerably more with 1 $\mu g\ kg^{-1}\ h^{-1}$ ghrelin. Only the GH responses to ghrelin + GHRH rose even greater. (Adapted from Bowers et al., the Endocrine Society 86th Annual Meeting 2004, New Orleans, p. 237, The Endocrine Society Chevy Chase, Maryland.).

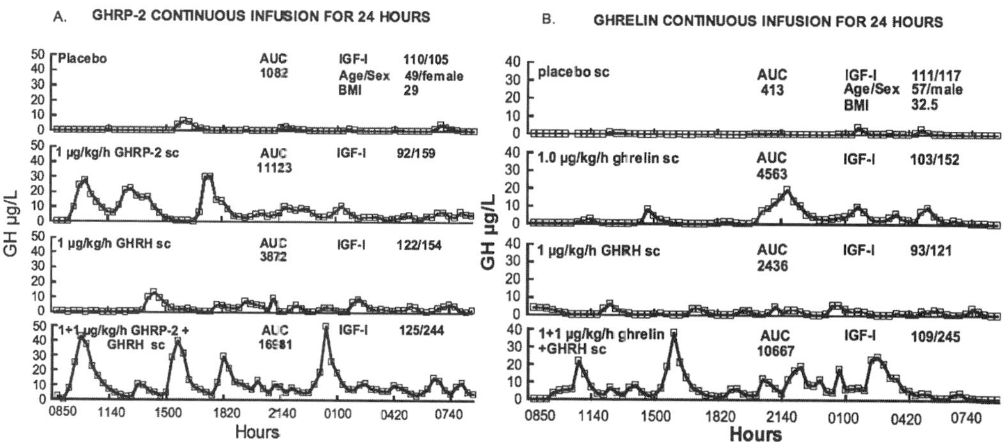

Fig. 8.18 Twenty-four hour continuous subcutaneous infusion of ghrelin produced the same effect as GHRP-2 infusion at the 1 μg kg^{-1} h^{-1} dosage, and when GHRP-2 or ghrelin was infused together with GHRH, the pulsatile GH secretion pattern was the same but the amplitude of the GH pulses was further increased. IGF-1 levels rose about the same to both peptides. (Adapted from Bowers et al., The Endocrine Society 87th Annual Meeting 2005, San Diego, p. 537, The Endocrine Society Chevy Chase, Maryland.).

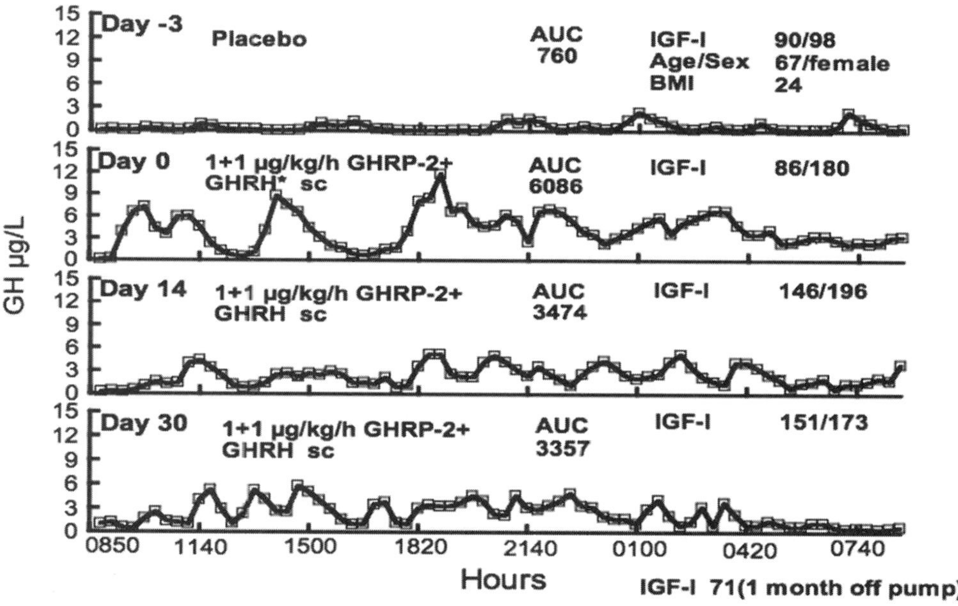

Fig. 8.19 Plasma GH profiles and IGF-1 responses over a 24-h period during 30-day subcutaneous continuous infusion of combined GHRP-2 and GHRH to 1 μg kg^{-1} h^{-1} (each peptide). Reproduced from Bowers CY. New insights into the control of growth hormone secretion. In: Kleinberg DL, Clemmons DR, eds. Central and peripheral mechanisms in pituitary disease. Bristol: UK BioScientifica Ltd.; 2002:163–175, with permission.).

Serum IGF-1 levels are low in subjects with GH resistance as well as in select normal older subjects; however, GH levels are elevated in GH-resistant subjects. Low-pulsatile GH and high IGF-1 levels indicate high efficacy of the peripheral GH action on the liver in raising serum IGF-1 levels when GH is secreted in a pulsatile pattern over the entire 24-h period.

FUTURE OUTLOOK

Even after many published studies, the pathophysiology of decreased GH secretion in obese subjects has resisted definitive explanation. Our model on the pathophysiology of decreased GH secretion in obesity is recorded in Figure 8.20. This model directly supports the conclusion that GHRH and ghrelin GH responses are both impaired in obese subjects. Physiologically, this model infers and supports the conclusion that GHRH and ghrelin are coregulators of GH secretion in normal subjects. The causes of impaired pituitary GH secretion in obesity are unknown but some possibilities include the following: a) SRIF excess, but this is improbable; b) low pituitary GH content, in part, is likely; c) low inappropriate ghrelin secretion, in part, is possible; d) GHRH receptor number and postreceptor effects are abnormal. Data on combined GHRH and GHRP-2 on GH release in obese subjects as shown in Figure 8.20 indicate GHRP-2 enhances the sensitivity and efficacy of the impaired GHRH GH response while GHRH enhances the efficacy and not the sensitivity of the impaired GHRP-2 GH response. Because GHRP-2 and ghrelin have the same actions on GH secretion, they are considered interchangeable. Also, the existence of low plasma acyl ghrelin levels has not readily been the explanation for decreased GH secretion. Nevertheless, from the above convoluted findings, the regulation of GH secretion appears to be dysfunctional in obesity because of hypofunction of the hypothalamic-pituitary axis, which involves

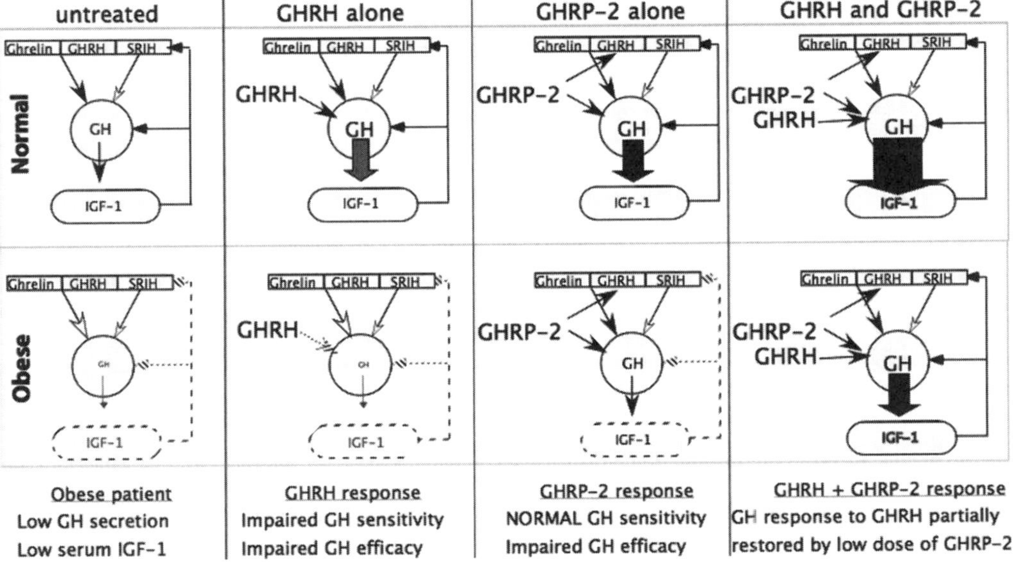

Fig. 8.20 On the pathophysiology of GH secretion in obesity.

abnormal interactions/secretion of GHRH and ghrelin. As has been emphasized by other investigators, hormonal-metabolic systems more successfully protect from weight loss and less successfully from weight gain in humans. In obese subjects, this, in part, may be due to associated decreased GH secretion, and when reversed or prevented, excess weight gain may occur less frequently and/or less easily.

Recorded in Figure 8.21 are the comparative pulsatile GH (AUC) and serum IGF-1 levels (before and after infusion) during a sustained 24-h subcutaneous infusion of placebo, GHRH 1-29NH_2, ghrelin, GHRP-2, and GHRP-3 at a dosage of 1 μg kg^{-1} h^{-1} to a normal 68-year-old obese woman with a BMI of 32.4. GHRP-3 is a newly developed, chemically and biologically stable, highly potent GHS that is 3–5 times more potent than GHRP-2. Because of the high potency and efficacy of GHRP-3 in activating the GH–IGF-1 axis, GHRP-3 is an example of a future GHS that can be readily developed for incorporation into a 3- to 6-month or longer depot formulation for clinical therapy because only a small amount would be required for formulation. Also, patient/subject drug exposure would be low.

Recorded in Figure 8.22 are mean 24-h serum GH, IGF-1, and/or immunoreactive (ir) levels of GHRP-1 in a normal woman and a normal man with low serum IGF-1 levels during continuous subcutaneous infusion of 1.5 μg kg^{-1} h^{-1} of the GHS GHRP-1 via an ambulatory pump. Blood was collected every 20 min. The values at 0 time were obtained during a 24-h infusion of placebo. The results in rats and dogs demonstrate that after a single subcutaneous injection of depot GHRP-1 Atrigel (QLT Inc vancouver, British columbia canada), the irGHRP-1 levels remained elevated in both rats and dogs over the entire 30 days. In the dogs, the mean serum IGF-1 levels were elevated and also remained so over the entire 30-day period. These results, together with our clinical data obtained with the pump approach, forecast a promising effective and efficient valuable depot approach for administration of future GHSs.

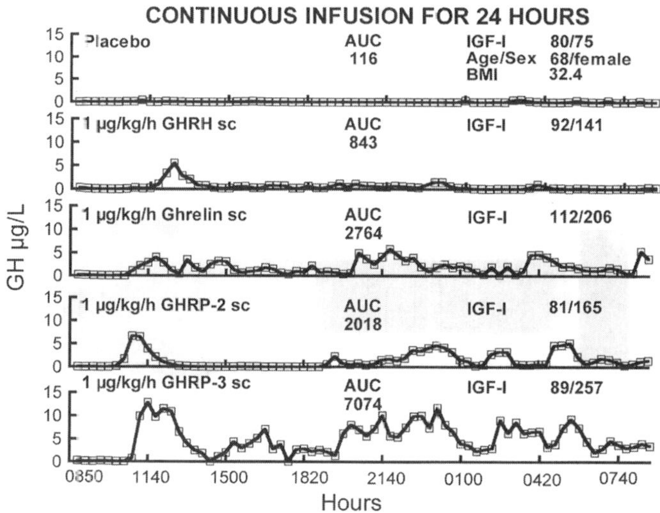

Fig. 8.21 Highly potent third-generation GHS GHRP-3.

CONTINUOUS GHRP-1

A. 30 Day sc Infusion Ambulatory Pump
Humans

Subj	Age/Sex	BMI	GH 24h•AUC µg/L Day 0	1	30	irGHRP-1 µg/L Day 0	1	30	IGF-I µg/L Day 0	1	60*
#1	60/F	24	760	2882	1622	<.2	8.3	9.5	69	131	96
#2	58/M	29	961	5754	1528	<.2	7.0	8.1	109	171	-

*1month off pump

B.Single sc injection of Depot Long Acting Atrigel* GHRP-1
Rats n=4

	Day 0	1	3	7	14	21	28
irGHRP-1 µg/L	<.1 ±0	71 ±11	50 ±8	51 ±14	35 ±6	21 ±2	8 ±1

Dogs n=6

	Hour 0	+1	+3	+6	Day 1	3	7	14	21	28
irGHRP-1 µg/L	<.1 ±0	38 ±4	50 ±9	45 ±9	17 ±3	14 ±1	8 ±1	7 ±1	7.2 ±.6	NA
IGF-I µg/L(%)	100	115 ±9	138 ±8	195 ±13	164 ±13	150 ±10	165 ±10	167 ±12	179 ±7	176 ±9

*Atrix Lab Inc.

Fig. 8.22 Once a month, long-acting formulation of GHS GHRP-1 in rats and dogs.

CONCLUSION

The essentially consistent actions on increasing GH secretion and food intake underscore these two effects are the major biological actions of the ghrelin hormone. This is supported by an infrastructure array of unique endocrine, cellular, and molecular findings. An increasing amount of data is being revealed in animals and humans about the multifunctional and expanding endocrine and also nonendocrine actions of ghrelin/GHSs. Some preliminary clinical GHSs and ghrelin results are presented that in principle forecast the potential endocrine and nonendocrine GHSs therapeutic approach. They include short-stature children, certain stages of over- and undernutrition, congestive heart failure, chronic obstructive pulmonary disease, and so forth. Some conceptual and technical points that have limited scope for the interpretation/projection of the physiologic and pathophysiologic role of ghrelin in humans concerns the following. The interesting speculation of an immediate premeal rise of plasma acyl ghrelin to initiate food intake needs more critical validation in terms of consistency, magnitude, and significance under controlled/focused clinical experimental conditions. Also, still to be elucidated is the importance of ghrelin stimulation via the circulation, afferent vagal nerve versus CNS, as well as the sensitivity of cellular and molecular CNS mediators. Furthermore, critical study of possible ghrelin receptor subtypes, direct CNS versus peripheral sites of action, and endocrine versus nonendocrine actions will be required to understand the biological role of the ghrelin system and the expanding use of ghrelin and GHSs as clinical therapeutic agents.

ACKNOWLEDGMENTS

We wish to thank the technician and fellows of the Tulane University Health Sciences Center Endocrine Section, the nurses of the General Clinical Research Center, Dr. Iranmanesh and the technicians of the Endocrine Service, Research and Development of Salem Veterans Affairs Medical Center, and Kaken Pharmaceutical Co. for supplying the GHRP-2. This work was supported in part by RR05096 (General Clinical Research Center) (GCRC).

ADDENDUM

New findings of obestatin and its proposed receptor GPR39 require continued evaluation of the fundamental aspects of the subject. Strong evidence has been obtained that GPR39 probably is not the obestatin receptor, and several groups have yet to consistently demonstrate the obestatin inhibition of food intake *(50)*. Zhang and Hsueh *(10)* reported that decreased food intake in rats was much greater after intracerebroventricular than intraperitoneal obestatin. Because most food intake studies of other investigators have been after intraperitoneal obestatin administration along with recent results indicating the instability of obestatin in serum, this may be in part the reason for the lack of reproducibility of the food intake effect *(51, 52)*. Nevertheless, some investigators have found intracerebroventricular obestatin administration to be ineffective on food intake *(53)*. In a recent publication on the processing of proghrelin to ghrelin including initial studies on the processing of obestatin, the uniqueness of this processing was revealed for it occurred by the same convertase that is known to be located within secretory vesicles, and thus this underscores a continued close interrelationship in the role of ghrelin and obestatin actions *(54)*. It is strongly implied that where and when ghrelin is synthesized so also is obestatin; however, the ghrelin octanoylation step and proghrelin processing step appear to occur independently of each other *(54)*. Selective, mainly nonparallel, obestatin-octanoyl ghrelin biosynthesis already has been reported in the perinatal rat pancreas, stomach, and plasma indicating the independence of the regulation *(55)*. Already, it has been demonstrated that obestatin increases proliferation of human retinal pigment epithelial cells in vitro, while in rats obestatin has inhibitory and ghrelin stimulatory effects on sleep, and intracerebroventricular obestatin inhibits angiotensin II–induced thirst (*56–58*). Indeed this is a convoluted story but one that is most intriguing especially as ghrelin and obestatin originate from the same gene.

REFERENCES

1. Veldhuis JD, Roemmich JN, Richmond EJ, et al. Endocrine control of body composition in infancy, childhood and puberty. Endocr Rev 2005;26:114–146.
2. Veldhuis JD, Roemmich JN, Richmond EF, Bowers CY. Somatotrophic and gonadotropic axes linkages in infancy, childhood, and the puberty-adult transition. Endocr Rev 2006;27(2):101–40.
3. Frystyk J. Free insulin-like growth factors-measurements and relationships to growth hormone secretion and glucose homeostasis. Growth Horm IGF Res 2004;14:339–375.
4. Bowers CY. Growth hormone-releasing peptide (GHRP). CMLS Cell Mol Life Sci 1998;54: 1316–1329.

5. Kojima M, Hosada H, Date Y, Nakazato M, Matsuo H, Kangawa K. Ghrelin is a growth-hormone-releasing acylated peptide from stomach. Nature 1999;402:656–660.
6. Bowers CY. Unnatural growth hormone-releasing peptide begets natural ghrelin. J Clin Endocrinol Metab 2001;86:1464–1469.
7. Ghigo E. Ghrelin. In: Ghigo E, ed. Ghrelin. Boston, MA: Kluwer Academic Publishers; 2004:1–254.
8. Van der Lely AJ, Tschop M, Heiman ML, Ghigo E. Biological, physiological, pathophysiological, and pharmacological aspects of ghrelin. Endocr Rev 2004;25:426–457.
9. Kobonits M, Goldstone AP, Gueorguiev M, Grossman AB. Ghrelin-a hormone with multiple functions. Neuroendocrinology 2004;25:27–68.
10. Zhang JV, Ren PG, Avsian-Kretchmer O, Luo CW, Rauch R, Klein C, Hsueh AJW. Obestatin, a peptide encoded by the ghrelin gene, opposes ghrelin's effects on food intake. Science 2005;370:996–999.
11. Thompson NM, Gill DAS, Davies R, Loveridge N, Houston PA, Robinson ICAF, Wells T. Ghrelin and des-octanoyl ghrelin promote adipogenesis directly in vivo by a mechanism independent of the type 1A growth hormone secretatogue receptor. Endocrinology 2004;145:234–242.
12. Toshinai K, Yamaguchi H, Sun Y, et al. Des-acyl ghrelin induces food intake by a mechanism independent of the growth hormone secretatogue receptor. Endocrinology 2006;147(5):2306–14.
13. Zigman KM, Nakano Y, Coppari R, et al. Mice lacking ghrelin receptors resist the development of diet induced obesity. J Clin Invest 2005;115:3564–3572.
14. Wortley KE, del Rincon JP, Murray JD, Garcia J, Iida K, Thorner MO, Sleeman MW. Absence of ghrelin protects against early-onset obesity. J Clin Invest 2005;115:3573–3578.
15. Gelling RW, Overduin J, Morrison CD, Morton GJ, Frayo RS, Cummings DE, Schwartz MW. Effect of uncontrolled diabetes on plasma ghrelin concentrations and ghrelin-induced feeding. Endocrinology 2004;145:4575–3582.
16. English PJ, Ghatei MA, Malik IA, Bloom SR, Wilding JP. Food fails to suppress ghrelin levels in obese humans. J Clin Endocrinol Metab 2002;87:2984–2987.
17. Barazzoni R, Bosutti A, Stebel M, et al. Ghrelin regulated mitochondrial-lipid metabolism gene expression and tissue fat distribution in liver and skeletal muscle. Am J Physio meta Endocrinol 2005;288:228–235.
18. Lall S, Tung LYC, Ohlsson C, Jansson JO, Dickson SL. Growth hormone (GH)-independent stimulation of adipostiy by GH secretagogue. Biochem Biophys Res Commun 2001;280:132–138.
19. Mesotten DD, Van den Berghe G. Changes within the GH/IGF-I/IGFBP axis in critical illness. Crit Care Clin 2006;22:17–28.
20. Chung TT, Hinds CJ. Treatment with GH and IGF-I in Critical Illness. Crit Care Clin 2006;22:29–40.
21. De Groot LJ. Non-thyroidal illness syndrome is a manifestation of hypothalamic-pituitary dysfunction, and in view of current evidence should be treated with appropriate replacement therapies. Crit Care Clin 2006;22:57–86.
22. Camina JP. Cell biology of the ghrelin receptor. J Neuroendocrinol 2006;18:65–76.
23. Ariyasu H, Takaya K, Iwakura H, et al. Transgenic mice overexpressing des-acyl ghrelin show small phenotype. Endocrinology 2005;146:355–364.
24. Bodart V, Febbraio M, Demers A, et al. CD36 mediates cardiovascular action of growth hormone-releasing peptides in the heart. Circ Res 2002;90:844–849.
25. Holst B, Cygankiewicz A, Jensen TH, Ankersen M, Schwartz TW. High constitutive signaling of the ghrelin receptor-identification of a potent inverse agonist. Mol Endocrinol 2003;17(11):2201–2210.
26. Holst B, Holliday ND, Bach A, Elling CE, Cox HM, Schwartz TW. Common structural basis for constitutive activity of the ghrelin receptor family. J Biol Chem 2004;279:53805–53817.
27. Petersen PS, Wolsbye D, Lang M, Beck-Sickinger A, Schwartz TW, Holst B. Effect of icv infusion of the ghrelin receptor selective inverse agonist [$DArg^1$,$DPhe^5$,$DTrp^{7,9}$,Leu^{11}]-Sub P on body weight Gain in rats. Keystone Symposia Silverthorne Colorado Gut Hormone and Other Regulators of Appetite, Satiety and Energy Expenditure. March 2–7, 2006:53.

28. Wang H-J, Geller F, Dempfle A, et al. Ghrelin receptor gene: Identification of several sequences variants in extremely obese children and adolescents, healthy normal-weight and underweight students, and children with short normal stature. J Clin Endocrinol Metab 2004;89:157–162.
29. Pantel J, Legendre M, Cabrol S, Hilal L, Hajaji Y, Morisset S et al. Loss of constitutive activity of the growth hormone secretatogue receptor in familial short stature. J Clin Invest 2006;116:760–768.
30. Holst B, Schwartz TW. Ghrelin receptor mutations-too little height and too much hunger. J Clin Invest 2006;116:637–641.
31. Zigman JM, Jones JE, Lee CE, Saper CB, Elmquist JK. Expression of ghrelin receptor mRNA in the rat and the mouse brain. J Comp Neurol 2006;494:528–548.
32. Bowers CY, Granda R, Mohan S, Kuipers J, Baylink D, Veldhuis JD. Sustained elevation of pulsatile growth hormone (GH) secretion and insulin-like growth factor I (IGF-I), IGF-binding protein-3 (IGFBP-3), and IGFBP-5 concentrations during 30-day continuous subcutaneous infusion of GH-releasing peptide-2 in older men and women. J Clin Endocrinol Metab 2004;89:2290–2300.
33. Veldhuis JD, Erickson D, Iranmanesh A, Miles JM, Bowers CY. Sex steroids control of the aging somatotropic axis. Endocrinol Metab Clin North Am 2005;34(4):877–893, viii.
34. Klinger B, Silbergeld A, Deghenghi R, Laron Z. Desensitization from long-term intranasal treatment with hexarelin does not interfere with the biological effects of this growth hormone-releasing peptide in short children. Eur J Endocrinol 1996;134:716–719.
35. Pihoker C, Badger TM, Reynolds GA, Bowers CY. Treatment effects of intranasal growth hormone releasing peptide-2 in children with short stature. J Endocrinol 1997;155:79–86.
36. Mericq V, Cassorla F, Salazar T, Avila A, Iniguez G, Bowers CY, Merriam GR. Effects of eight months treatment with graded doses of a growth hormone releasing peptide in GH deficient children. J Clin Endocrinol Metab 1998;83:2355–2360.
37. Mericq V, Cassorla F, Bowers CY, Avila A, Gonen B, Merriam G. Changes in appetite and body weight in response to long-term oral administration of the ghrelin agonist GHRP-2 in GH deficient children. J Clin Endocrinol Metab 2003;16:981–985.
38. Hurley DL, Smith EP, Reynolds, GA, Veldhuis JD, Bowers CY. GH releasing peptide-1 treatment for 7 days causes a dose-dependent decrease in GH mRNA but increases GH intron-containing transcripts in rats. The Endocrine Society 86th Annual Meeting 2004, New Orleans, p. 503, The Endocrine Society Chevy Chase, Maryland.
39. Murthy MG, Plunkett LM, Gertz BJ, Wittreich J, Polvino WM, Clemmons DR. MK-677, an orally active growth hormone secretagogue, reverses diet induced catabolism. J Clin Endocrinol Metab 1998;83:320–325.
40. Svensson J. Two month treatment of obese subjects with the oral growth hormone (GH) secretagogue MK-677 increases GH secretion, fat mass, and energy expenditure. J Clin Endocrinol Metab 1998;83:362–369.
41. Nagaya N, Moriya J, Yasumura Y, et al. Effects of ghrelin administration on left ventricular function, exercise capacity, and muscle wasting in patients with chronic heart failure. Circulation 2004;110:3674–3679.
42. Nagaya N, Itoh T, Murakami S, et al. Treatment of cachexia with ghrelin in patients with COPD. Chest 2005;128:1187–1193.
43. Akamizu T, Shinomiya T, Irako T, Fukunaga M, Nakai Y, Nakai Y, Kangawa K. Separate measurement of plasma levels of acylated and desacyl ghrelin in healthy subjects using a new ELISA assay. J Clin Endocrinol Metab 2005;90:6–9.
44. Wren AM, Seal LJ, Cohen MA, et al. Ghrelin enhances appetite and increases food intake in humans. J Clin Endocrinol Metab 2001;86:5992–5995.
45. Druce MR, Wren Am, Park AJ, et al. Ghrelin increases food intake in obese as well as lean subjects. Int J Obes (Lond) 2005;29(9):1130–1136.

46. Laferrere B, Abraham C, Russell CD, Bowers CY. Growth hormone releasing peptide-2 (GHRP-2), like ghrelin, increases food intake in healthy men. J Clin Endocrinol Metab 2005;90:611–614.
47. Laferrere B, Hart AB, Bowers CY. Obese subjects respond to the stimulatory effect of the ghrelin agonist growth hormone releasing peptide-2 (GHRP-2) on food intake. Obes, (Silverspring) 2006;14(6):1056–63.
48. Bowers CY, Veldhuis JD, Theuma P, et al. On the pathophysiology of GH secretion in obese humans. The Endocrine Society 86th Annual Meeting 2004, New Orleans, p. 237. The Endocrine Society Chevy Chase, Maryland.
49. Bowers CY. New insights into the control of growth hormone secretion. In: Kleinberg DL, Clemmons DR, eds. Central and peripheral mechanisms in pituitary disease. Bristol: UK BioScientifica Ltd.; 2002:163–175.
50. Holst B, Kristoffer LE, Schild E, et al. GPR39 signaling is stimulated by zinc ions but not by obestatin. Endocrinology 2006;70(3):936–46.
51. Bresciani E, Rapetti D, Dona F, et al. Obestatin inhibits feeding but does not modulate GH and corticosterone secretion in the rat. J Endocrinol Invest 2006;29(8):16–18.
52. Weihong P, Tu H, Kastin AJ. Differential BBB interactions of three ingestive peptides: Obestatin, ghrelin, and adiponectin. Peptides 2006;27:911–916.
53. Nogueiras R, Pfluger P, Tovar S, et al. Effect of obestatin on energy balance and growth hormone secretion in rodents. Endocrinology 2006;148(1):21–6.
54. Zhu X, Cao Y, Voodg K, Steiner DF. On the processing of proghrelin to ghrelin. J Biol Chem 2006;281(50):38867–70.
55. Chanoine JP, Wong A, Barrios V. Obestatin, acylated and total ghrelin concentrations in the perinatal rat pancreas. Horm Res 2006;66:81–88.
56. Camina J, Campos JF, Caminos JE, Dieguez C, Casanueva FF. Obestatin-mediated proliferation of human retinal pigment epithelial cells: regulatory mechanism. J Cell Physiol 2006;211(1):1–9.
57. Szentirmai E, Krueger JM. Obestatin alters sleep in rats. Neurosci Lett 2006;222–226.
58. Samson WK, White MM, Price C, Ferguson AV. Obestatin acts in brain to inhibit thirst. Am J Physiol Regul Integr Comp Physiol 2006;292(1):R637–43.

9 Interaction Between Physical Activity and Genetic Factors in Complex Metabolic Disease

Paul W. Franks and Stephen M. Roth

CONTENTS

Abstract

Obesity and diabetes have become increasingly prevalent during the past century. Concomitant with this rise, the consumption of *trans*-fatty acids and processed carbohydrates is likely to have increased and physical activity levels declined. However, the rates at which obesity and diabetes have increased differ across people of varying ethnicities living in the same environment, suggesting the presence of interaction between ethnic-specific factors, such as genes, and changing environments and lifestyles. Quantifying these interactions is difficult because the interaction effect is often small, and precise measurement of lifestyle factors, such as diet and habitual physical activity, is difficult. Conventional interaction studies aim to test whether the magnitude of the association between the lifestyle exposures and the disease outcome is different in those who carry the variant allele at a given locus by comparison with those who do not. Because exercising skeletal muscle is a major site for glucose and lipid metabolism, variants in the genes that are located within muscle and that are up-regulated in response to physical activity present interesting candidates for testing in studies of gene × physical activity interaction in diabetes. However, numerous methodological limitations seriously hinder attempts to test such hypotheses. This chapter describes (1) a brief review of studies that provide evidence of gene × physical activity interaction in diabetes (and related traits), (2) functional evidence for interaction between genetic factors and physical activity in metabolic dysregulation, and (3) some common methodological issues that face the study of gene × environment interaction in human populations.

From: *Contemporary Endocrinology: Energy Metabolism and Obesity: Research and Clinical Applications*
Edited by: P. A. Donohoue © Humana Press Inc., Totowa, NJ

Key Words: physical activity energy expenditure, genetics, diabetes, metabolism, gene × environment interaction.

INTRODUCTION

Until relatively recently, human evolution has been characterized by a hunter–gatherer lifestyle that involved daily bouts of physical activity energy expenditure (PAEE) followed by rest, food deprivation followed by binge eating, and, depending on the population, climatic exposure to extremes of heat and cold *(1)*. Each of these factors placed specific burdens on the physiological regulation of energy metabolism, and, through survival advantage, they have sculpted the development of *Homo sapien*. Across time, those who survived to procreate were those most suited to the environment in which they lived. Thus, human evolution has involved ongoing refinement of the species, governed by the stresses imposed by the evolutionary environment. This refinement has involved allelic purification, where genomic regions that were well suited to cope with the common environmental exposures were retained, and other regions that were incompatible with the environmental stressors were lost.

In contrast to the many millennia of human evolution, the past 50–100 years has witnessed a reduction in energy expenditure and significant adaptations in dietary composition *(2)*. Alterations in chronic energy flux, combined with an excess of energy intake over expenditure, have lead to the emergence of cardiovascular disease as the leading cause of death in the industrialized world; in 1990, the two leading causes, coronary heart disease and stroke, account for 7.0 million and 5.5 million deaths, respectively *(3)*. However, because the architecture of the human genome has evolved over a much longer time-course than have changes in the environment, genetic intolerance to a modern industrialized way of life appears to exist in specific ethnic subgroups. This may explain why the global prevalence of metabolic and cardiovascular diseases differs considerably across ethnicities, even when the environment in which these groups reside is similar *(4)*. Thus, complete prevention of diabetes in certain groups through lifestyle modification would quite likely necessitate very high levels of habitual energy expenditure and/or diets that are bereft of processed carbohydrates and saturated animal fats.

There are essentially two reasons to study the interaction between environmental and genetic factors. The first is to better understand the pathophysiology of disease, and the second is to aid in the interpretation of genetic data and guide its application to disease prevention. Because genetic association studies are often conducted using cross-sectional observations *(5)*, in the presence of gene × environment interaction (GEI), the direction and magnitude of the observed genetic effect may differ when comparing individuals with contrasting lifestyles (*6–11*), or when comparing the same individuals on separate occasions where the environment has changed *(8)*. Such interactions could partly explain why genetic associations with complex disease frequently fail to replicate *(5)*, and why the relationship between genomic variation and disease risk is sometimes inconsistent across environmentally diverse populations (*12–14*).

The aims of this chapter are (1) to briefly review studies that provide some degree of evidence that physical activity and genetic factors interact to modify the risk of diabetes and related metabolic disorders, (2) to describe selected functional biological evidence for interaction between genetic factors and physical activity in metabolic dysregulation, and thus provide a series of candidate genes to test in interaction studies, and (3) to discuss some of the methodological issues that confront testing hypotheses of GEI in humans. The environmental exposure on which we will focus is PAEE, this is known to be an important antecedent of diabetes *(15)* and other related conditions (*16–19*) and exerts many of its effects by modulating gene expression and protein formation *(20)*. To address our first aim, we present a selected review of literature reporting evidence for gene × physical activity interaction in diabetes-related traits. For our second aim, we describe the functional biology and mechanisms of interaction with PAEE for the peroxisome proliferator-activated receptor γ coactivator 1α (*PPARGC1A;* PGC-1α) gene, and several of the genes that *PPARGC1A* regulates. To engage our third aim, we discuss the numerous methodological limitations that complicate the detection of true positive GEIs and describe some of the recent methodological and technical advances that will affect future studies of GEI.

In this chapter, the term GEI refers to the interaction between a gene and other non-genetic factors, most often PAEE. It is, however, worthwhile considering that in virtually all studies of GEI, where the "environment" is behavioral (such as food intake, smoking, or physical activity level) or biological (such as level of obesity or cardiorespiratory fitness), these factors themselves are likely to be determined to an extent by genetic factors. Thus, epistasis (interaction between genes) likely underlies some of the interaction effects observed when assessing gene interactions with behavioral or biological exposures; this in essence represents a form of genetic confounding. In the case of behavioral exposures, the possibility of genetic confounding may be greatest in observational epidemiological studies, such as in cohort and case–control studies, where participants are free-living. This is because in such studies participants may maintain genetically predisposed behaviors to a greater extent than in intervention studies where behavior is prescribed and is to a lesser extent self-determined. Thus, the between-person variance in physical activity level within arms of an intervention study should, if the intervention is adhered to and is sufficiently potent to overcome a genetic predisposition for inactivity, be far less than in the free-living scenario. Therefore, the extent to which genes explain this variance will also be small. Accordingly, the extent to which gene × gene interactions will be misclassified as GEIs will also be less in a trial by comparison with a free-living study. Nonetheless, even in randomized controlled intervention studies, precise quantification of adherence will be necessary to distinguish those who are "exercise responders" or "non-responders" from those who are "exercise adherers" and "non-adherers."

The concept of GEI and disease predisposition pivots on three assumptions; the first is that common functional genetic variation results in functional variation in the protein complex, and/or substrate specificity, activity, phosphorylation, or variation in the amount of the protein transcribed by the gene, such that the phenotype is affected (this assumption is also made in the study of conventional genetic association); second, environmental factors, such as diet, physical activity, and smoking, modulate the activity of genes, which, in turn, modulate disease-related phenotypes; third, in combination, these factors result in differential regulation of the gene and expression of the phenotype, which depends simultaneously on the level of the environmental exposure and the extent of genetic variation at a given locus (Fig. 9.1).

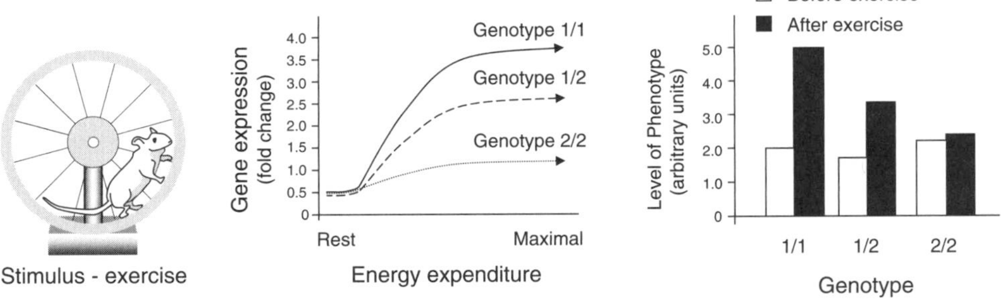

Fig. 9.1 Hypothetical example of how energy expenditure (through exercise) interacts with genotype to modify a phenotype. Before exercise (at rest), gene expression is similar between genotypes, as is the corresponding level of the phenotype. However, energy expenditure differentially regulates gene activity, depending on genotype, which affects the phenotypic expression of the gene. In this example, it is assumed that gene expression is highly correlated with the respective protein levels.

PRE-EXISTING EVIDENCE FOR GENE x PHYSICAL ACTIVITY INTERACTIONS IN TYPE 2 DIABETES

The mechanisms through which PAEE modulates metabolic homeostasis are many, but include decreased sympathetic outflow, shear stress, hyperemia, tissue proliferation, and mitochondrial biogenesis. Many of these physiological adaptations both cause and result from the regulation of genes involved in beneficial metabolic processes central to the transportation and phosphorylation of lipids and glucose. Thus, whilst habitual physical inactivity often results in chronically dysregulated metabolism, interventions designed to increase physical activity can prevent and correct these ailments (*21–24*). However, because the protective effects of physical activity are mediated by changes in gene expression and protein synthesis, it is plausible that functional genetic variation results in adaptations to physical activity interventions that differ by genotype at a given locus. This is one possible explanation for the high inter-individual variability that is frequently observed in physiological adaptation to lifestyle intervention *(25)*.

The following section describes some of the published studies that provide evidence of interaction between physical activity and genotype on phenotypes related with type 2 diabetes. These include metabolic, vascular, and anthropometric traits that have been directly linked with diabetes, either as antecedents or as sequelae.

Much of the evidence for GEI in diabetes comes from cross-sectional studies where the genetic "exposure" is characterized using single-nucleotide polymorphisms (SNPs) (see ref. *26* for a systematic review of this literature). However, most studies have tested the association between a genetic factor and phenotype at different activity levels without formally testing hypotheses of interaction, with only a few reporting statistically significant gene × physical activity interactions. Almost all observational studies have subjectively assessed physical activity through questionnaire, diary, or interview, whereas some have used direct biological measurements of energy expenditure (*6–11*). None has used the gold-standard of doubly labeled water. The most commonly studied gene is the *APOE* gene, for which outcomes include dyslipidemia, body composition, and blood pressure (*27–30*). The second most frequently studied gene is the β-adrenergic receptor (*ADRB*) isoforms 2 and 3. Outcomes include obesity

(11, 31) and dyslipidemia *(32)*. Single studies have explored the association, at different activity levels, between the *UCP3* gene and obesity in French females *(32)*, the *LPL* gene and cholesterol in Dutch males *(33)*, the *VDR* gene and fasting glucose in German males *(34)*, the *FGA* gene and plasma fibrinogen in Finnish postmenopausal females *(35)*, *NOS3* and systolic blood pressure (SBP) in Japanese *(36)*, and, in UK Caucasian adults, *PPARG* and insulin resistance *(9)*, *GPR-10* and blood pressure *(7)*, *NOS3* and glucose intolerance *(10)*, and *PPARGC1A* and VO2max *(6)*.

Only two case–control studies have been reported *(37, 38)*. Both used questionnaires to assess activity levels. Neither was nested within a pre-existing prospective cohort study, nor did they formally tested hypotheses of interaction. The first study *(37)* focused on the *ADRB2* gene in active and inactive obese women. In Gln27 allele homozygotes, the association between physical activity and BMI was significantly stronger than in that Glu27 allele homozygotes. The second study *(38)* reported putative interactions between physical activity and SNPs in the *APOE*, *APOA2*, *FABP2*, and *LIPC* genes on LDL-C and HDL-C levels in Italian adults.

Two prospective cohort studies have been reported *(39, 40)*. The first used a questionnaire to assess activity levels in 397 Hispanic and 569 Caucasian males and females and focused on the association between the C480T variant in the *LIPC* gene and incident CHD at different baseline activity levels *(39)*. The second study *(40)* in 568 obese and 717 non-obese young Danish males, which also used a questionnaire to assess physical activity, reported no evidence of interaction between physical activity and variants in the *UCP2* and *UCP3* genes on changes in BMI occurring during the subsequent 40 years.

Although data from intervention studies are often considered strong evidence of causality, the value of the evidence is partly contingent upon whether the participants are selected at random from the population and randomly assigned to either an intervention arm or a control arm. A further consideration is whether the study is large enough to be powered with reasonable probability to detect interaction and whether adjustments for multiple-hypothesis testing have been made. Very few studies of gene × exercise intervention exist where all of these criteria are met.

Although absent of a control arm, the Health, Risk Factors, Exercise Training, and Genetics (HERITAGE) study provides some of the most convincing evidence that adaptation to exercise training is dependent on genotype. HERITAGE involved a 20-week structured aerobic exercise intervention in more than 700 Canadian Blacks and Whites emanating from 99 nuclear families *(41)*. The availability of pedigrees facilitated a genome-wide scan (GWS) utilizing approximately 500 microsatellite markers, frequently spaced (~6.0 cM) across the autosome. In addition, participants were exquisitely phenotyped for a wide array of cardiovascular risk factors. Thus far, multiple publications have emanated from the HERITAGE data, many of which have included linkage approaches to describe genomic regions where genes that influence adaptation to exercise intervention may be harbored. Lakka et al. *(42, 43)*, for example, reported that a quantitative trait loci (QTL) on chromosome 7q31 influence exercise induced adaptation in fasting insulin levels, and Rankinen et al. *(44)* reported that differential adaptations in blood pressure response to exercise were associated with the *NOS3* Glu298Asp polymorphism.

The Finnish Diabetes Prevention Study (DPS) compared the 3-year risk of progressing from impaired glucose tolerance (IGT) to type 2 diabetes in two groups of adults (N = 522) assigned to either a control arm of normal health care or an intervention arm involving an intensive diet and exercise program *(45)*. The diabetes risk reduction at the end of the trial was 58% in those receiving the lifestyle intervention in comparison with those in the control group. At 1 year, weight reductions were 4.5 kg in the intervention and 1.0 kg in the control groups, and at 3 years, weight reductions were 3.5 and 0.9 kg in the intervention and control groups, respectively. Thus far, several genes have been reported to modulate adaptation to the lifestyle intervention in DPS. These include the Pro12Ala polymorphism in the *PPARG* gene *(45)*, the G308A polymorphism in the *TNF4A* gene *(46)*, and the G250A variant in the hepatic lipase gene *(47)*.

One of the most promising studies for testing hypotheses of gene × lifestyle interactions is the US Diabetes Prevention Program (DPP) *(48)*. DPP is similar in design to the Finnish DPS and achieved similar results in terms of weight reduction and diabetes prevention. However, DPP is several-fold larger than DPS and is thus well suited for the study of GEI. The primary outcomes are weight loss and diabetes incidence, although multiple sub-phenotypes were also measured. So far, reports from the DPP have examined variants in the *TCF7L2 (49)*, *KCNJ11 (50)*, and *PPARG (51, 52)* genes.

Functional Evidence for Interaction Between Genetic Factors and Physical Activity in Metabolic Dysregulation

Type 2 diabetes is related with distinct metabolic disturbances that include diminished insulin-stimulated glucose uptake, increased hepatic gluconeogenesis, and impaired insulin secretion by pancreatic β cells *(53)*. Although the liver is important in maintaining glucose homeostasis, the primary site for insulin-mediated glucose deposition and metabolism is high-oxidative skeletal muscle *(54)*. Thus, impaired insulin-stimulated glucose uptake by muscle is an important stage in the pathogenesis of diabetes *(55)*. Because aerobic and resistance exercise increases both insulin-dependent and insulin-independent glucose uptake, exercise training is a suitable intervention for the primary and secondary prevention of type 2 diabetes and several of the sub-phenotypes that precede it *(56)*.

The mechanisms through which physical activity improves muscle-specific glucose uptake are complex and are influenced by factors such as nutrition, cardiorespiratory fitness, and existing micro- and macro-vascular disease. For skeletal muscle glucose metabolism to occur, glucose must traverse from the blood through the interstitium into the intracellular space for phosphorylation to glucose-6-phosphate (*G6P*). The transportation of glucose from blood to the intracellular space is determined by several factors. These include blood flow to skeletal muscle tissue, capillary recruitment, the permeability of the endothelium to glucose, and the availability of the glucose trafficking molecule GLUT4 *(57)*. Because of the relatively small quantity of intracellular glucose and the higher affinity of glucose for phosphorylation compared with transport, insulin-stimulated glucose transportation into the muscle cell is generally considered the rate-determining factor in basal muscle glucose uptake, although evidence to this effect is largely derived from studies where extra-cellular glucose levels are very low.

PPARGC1A as a Master Regulator of Metabolism

PPARGC1A mRNA is expressed predominantly in tissues with high metabolic activity, the majority of which are rich in mitochondria. These include heart, high-oxidative (type I) skeletal muscle, brown fat, kidney, liver and brain, and other tissue such as white adipose. Through coactivation of an array of genes, *PPARGC1A* modulates the transportation, storage, and oxidation of lipids and glucose in various tissues.

During exercise, disposal of glucose and lipids occurs largely in high-oxidative skeletal muscle. The mechanisms through which *PPARGC1A* improves the capacity for lipid and glucose disposal in skeletal muscle are complex but include (1) coactivation of genes including the nuclear respiratory transcription factors (NRF-1 and NRF-2), cytochrome c oxidase 4 (*COX4*), and the mitochondrial transcription factors (mtTFA, mtTFB1, mtTFB2), which in a coordinated manner powerfully induce mitochondrial biogenesis; (2) the formation of muscle fibers characterized by a high capacity for oxidative phosphorylation following coactivation of genes such as *PPARD*; and (3) regulation in muscle of glucose transporter (GLUT4) levels (see ref. *58* for an in depth review). Inactivation of these signaling cascades may result in attenuation of oxidative capacity and disordered metabolism that manifests as an insulin-resistance-like syndrome. This is supported by observations in patients with type 2 diabetes, where the skeletal muscle expression of the *OXPHOS* genes is coordinately down-regulated *(59)*, and in morbid obesity where PGC-1α mRNA is threefold lower in subcutaneous and omental adipose tissue by comparison with tissue of lean controls *(60)*. Although the expression characteristics of PGC-1α in skeletal muscle in comparison with adipose in obese individuals is potentially more interesting, owing to this being the primary expression site, such data are yet to be reported.

Animal Studies

In rodents, over-expression of *PPARGC1A* is associated with higher oxidative capacity of skeletal muscles and prolonged time to fatigue during electronically stimulated contractions (*61–65*). Lin et al. *(63)* reported that muscle-specific transgenic over-expression of PGC-1α is associated with a higher ratio of slow- (oxidative) to fast- (glycolytic) twitch muscle fiber, and a corresponding increase in whole-body oxidative capacity. Elsewhere, Wu et al. have proposed that *PPARGC1A*-induced mitochondrial biogenesis is itself controlled by calcium-regulated signaling pathways *(65)*.

The physiological adaptations characteristic of the *PPARGC1A* transgenic mouse support the thesis that over-expression of *PPARGC1A* improves the capacity for glucose and lipid oxidation and ATP synthesis. Importantly, long-duration low-intensity aerobic exercise also increases the expression of PGC-1α mRNA in healthy wild-type rodents *(62,64,66)*. These observations suggest that the induction of *PPARGC1A* through exercise appears to facilitate beneficial health adaptations that involve changes in skeletal muscle content of oxidative enzymes and mitochondria count, which in turn improves the capacity for substrate metabolism, ATP synthesis, and exercise.

Over-expression of the Glucose Transporter 4 (*SLC2A4*; GLUT4) gene occurs in response to various physiological (e.g., muscle contraction) and pharmacological (e.g., insulin, Troglitazone, and α-lipoic acid) stimuli (*67–69*), some of which are mediated by induction of the *PPARGC1A* gene. *PPARGC1A* over-expression powerfully induces endogenous GLUT4 production in cultured myotubes (L6 cells) from *SLC2A4* null mice *(70)* through cAMP-responsive transcription factor (CREB)-dependent coactivation of the myocyte enhancer factor (*MEF*)2 *(71, 72)*. Thus, coactivation of the *SLC2A4* gene through *PPARGC1A* enables the repletion of the GLUT4 protein to levels observed in skeletal muscle of healthy animals but does not improve insulin sensitivity *(70)*. In rodents, transgenic GLUT4 over-expression increases whole-body glucose utilization, glycogen synthesis, and habitual wheel running *(73)* (for a thorough review of exercise mediated glucose transport see *(68)*).

During rest, the GLUT4 protein is sequestered by the intracellular vesicles and upon insulin or contractile stimulation is translocated to the sarcolemma and T-tubules. Knockout studies in mice indicate that GLUT4 is the primary glucose transporter in both basal and insulin-stimulated conditions *(74)*. In these studies, basal glucose transportation was reduced by approximately 80% and insulin-mediated glucose disposal was completely blunted. Over-expression of GLUT4 in genetically diabetic (*db/db*) mice ameliorates insulin resistance and improves whole-body glucose uptake in both basal and insulin-stimulated conditions *(75)*. Thus, *SLC2A4* represents an attractive molecular target for improving glucose control in human type 2 diabetes, and control of *PPARGC1A* through physiological or pharmacological processes may facilitate this objective.

Human Studies

In humans, a single 3-h bout of exhaustive exercise corresponds with an increased generation of PGC-1α mRNA, which peaks within 2 h of exercise *(76)*. Elsewhere, PGC-1α mRNA has been shown to increase markedly following 3 h of one-legged knee extensor exercise at 50% maximal work capacity; at 1 h post-exercise, PGC-1a mRNA increased 2.5-fold and rose to 8.5-fold above the pre-exercise level at 3 h. At 8 h post-exercise, PGC-1α mRNA remained elevated by sixfold but had returned to the pre-exercise level by 20 h. Furthermore, by restricting blood flow to the exercising limb, PGC-1α mRNA expression is enhanced *(77)*, demonstrating that metabolic perturbation influences PGC-1α regulation. However, the effect of long-term exercise training on PGC-1α expression is less clear. Short et al. *(78)* recently reported 1.5-fold increases in PGC-1α mRNA levels in men and women following a 16-week exercise training program consisting of stationary cycling (3–4× week at 70–80% maximum heart rate), and Russell et al. *(79)* reported chronic increases in PGC-1α mRNA expression (2.7-fold) following 6 weeks running training; importantly these changes in expression appear independent of changes in muscle fiber type ratio and quantity. However, others have been unable to detect changes in PGC-1α expression after 9 days of cycle training and following 4 weeks (5× week) of one-legged isometric resistance training *(80)*. The many possible explanations for these disparate findings included differences in total energy expenditure during the intervention, intensity and type of exercise performed, the baseline characteristics of study subjects, and biopsy protocols.

PPARGC1A may play an important role in modifying the protective effect of physical activity on risk of human diabetes. Several studies have reported an association between a common variant in the *PPARGC1A* gene (Gly482Ser) and type 2 diabetes, where the frequency of the Ser482 allele is higher in diabetics than normal glucose tolerant controls *(81)*. In healthy older Danish individuals, Ling et al. *(82)* reported that carriers of the Ser482 allele had lower levels of *PPARCG1A* and *PPARGC1B* mRNA by comparison with Gly482 homozygotes. Ling et al. also reported a lower mean VO_2max in the Ser482 allele carriers. In a recent study, we compared the allele frequencies at the Gly482Ser locus of the *PPARGC1A* gene in Olympic-class endurance athletes and unfit controls *(83)*. In athletes, the Gly482 allele was significantly more common than in controls. When the three groups were combined, VO_2max was significantly lower in carriers of the Ser482 allele than in Gly482 carriers. Thus, these data indicate that the presence of the Ser482 allele may be associated with low cardiorespiratory fitness. Notably, the frequency of the Ser482 allele in unfit population controls (40%) is similar to that reported previously in cohorts with diabetes (~37%) *(81)*. By contrast, fit controls in our study had a lower Ser482 allele frequency (33%), and Olympic-class athletes had the lowest allele frequency (29%) of all groups. Thus, given that a low level of cardiorespiratory fitness is a strong risk factor for diabetes, it is possible that the previously reported relationship between Gly482Ser and diabetes is partly mediated by VO_2max.

Although several studies have explored the effects of exercise on *PPARGC1A* expression in humans, it remains unclear how modulation of energy balance through the simultaneous manipulation of energy intake and energy expenditure affects the expression of *PPARGC1A* and other *OXPHOS* genes. Understanding how energy-balance modulation affects *OXPHOS* gene expression is likely to provide insight into the molecular disturbances that, following physical inactivity, promote metabolic dyshomeostasis, as observed in type 2 diabetes. Thus, quantifying these complex mechanisms may ultimately facilitate targeted prevention of disease. To test the hypothesis that sequence variation at *PPARGC1A* affects the response of VO_2max and glucose and lipid oxidation to exercise in humans, a well-controlled etiological trial, involving precise measurement of energy balance, is likely to be necessary.

The reason precise measures of energy balance, and not simply records of attendance at exercise sessions, are necessary is that participants in exercise intervention trials may compensate for their increased energy expenditure during the intervention by decreasing habitual activity and altering diet at other times during the trial *(84, 85)*. Moreover, because the effects of single genes are often small, the adequate investigation of gene–physical activity interaction probably requires the precise characterization of energy balance, or at least energy expenditure, which is yet to be achieved in an intervention trial. The following section outlines some of the important methodological limitations that complicate the identification of true-positive GEIs in complex metabolic disease.

METHODOLOGICAL ISSUES IN THE STUDY OF GEI IN HUMAN POPULATIONS

Preserving Statistical Power in Studies of Interaction

The ubiquitous limitation of studies that have sought to assess whether the effects of physical activity on metabolic traits differ by genotype, is insufficient statistical power. Increasing the sample size is usually the simplest way to improve power, but is often infeasible owing to the associated financial and logistical burdens. The other principal factors that limit statistical power are measurement error in the exposures (genetic and environmental) and the outcome (phenotype), the frequency of the minor allele at the specified locus, and the magnitude of the interaction term (i.e., the between-genotype difference in the slope of the effect at a given locus) *(86)*.

The majority of studies that have sought to assess gene × physical activity interaction have measured the environmental exposure (physical activity) and the phenotypes with relatively low precision. Where PAEE is quantified using questionnaire, the correlation between observed PAEE and true PAEE approximates 0.30 or less *(87)*. If the outcome of interest is insulin sensitivity, and this is assessed using corrected insulin response to OGTT, the correlation between the observed and true level of insulin sensitivity would be around 0.40 *(88)*. Measurement error decreases considerably if PAEE is assessed, for example, using the combination of doubly labeled water and respiratory gas exchange *(87)*, and insulin sensitivity is measured using the hyperinsulinemic euglycemic clamp technique *(88, 89)*. In this example of improved measurement, the sample size required to detect interaction for a given allele frequency and effect size would dramatically diminish.

Because the allele frequency is an important determinant of statistical power in studies of genetic association and interaction, existing exercise studies, which are often small in sample size and/or have poorly characterized exposures and phenotypes, are unlikely to be sufficiently powered for the meaningful examination of low frequency risk alleles. However, unless rare alleles are highly penetrant, that is, the proportion of those who carry the variant allele and who develop the disease is high, the relevance of such issues in the context of public health will be limited. Furthermore, although protein-coding regions of the genome generally have lower mean allele frequencies (MAFs) than non-coding regions, this is primarily true for genetic variants that have always been detrimental for survival and have interfered with reproduction, thus causing their progressive deselection, or purification, from the species. This is true for most diseases that show a Mendelian pattern of inheritance. However, the genes associated with disease phenotypes that were once preferential for survival, which happen to include many of those of interest in studies of GEI, are likely to be relatively common. Thus, the genetic variants associated with the ability to lay down fat reserves, an attribute that may have conferred a survival advantage throughout much of human evolution, particularly in traditionally nomadic populations such Native Americans *(90)*, are likely to be relatively frequent in these populations today.

Characterizing the Architecture of "Interaction" Genes

An emerging approach for the assessment of genetic association is the so-called genome-wide association (GWA) study, made possible by SNP microarrays that allow the large-scale characterization of variation across the human genome *(91)*. Currently available technology allows for the genotyping of approximately 1,000,000 SNPs *(92)*, with copy number variation arrays also available. GWA studies have been shown to be successful in the identification of a number of possible causal variants across multiple diseases, including age-related macular degeneration (AMD) *(93)*, coronary heart disease *(94, 95)*, type 2 diabetes *(96–98)*, and others *(99, 100)*. In the AMD study, an SNP was strongly associated with AMD in the initial GWA analysis, and, using the HapMap database and additional genotyping in the regions that neighbored the initial SNP to define the allelic structure of the region, the causal variant was subsequently identified. An important note is that AMD, CHD, and type 2 diabetes are considered complex multi-factorial traits, much like many of the phenotypes of interest in studies of gene × physical activity interaction *(101)*, indirectly arguing that GWA studies may be equally useful for these phenotypes.

It has long been argued that association studies are more powerful than linkage studies for the identification of disease-causing loci where the effect on the phenotype is modest *(102)*. However, as Wang et al. *(103)* highlight, this may be because most linkage studies are relatively small, with less than 500 affected sib-pairs studied on average, whereas association studies of unrelated individuals are frequently several-fold larger. Thus, to conclude that linkage studies have failed as a means through which disease-causing genes can be identified may be premature. Nonetheless, the majority of irrefutable disease-causing genes, of which around 50 have been found to date *(103)*, have emerged from association studies.

Because strong patterns of LD (i.e., where the correlation between alleles within a region is higher than would be expected by chance) exist across approximately 80% of the human genome *(104)*, for association studies to be efficient, the LD patterns within the region of interest must be determined, and genetic variation characterized in the form of haplotypes. Haplotypes are combinations of alleles at multiple loci located within a single chromosomal region that are in high LD. These regions, known as "haplotype blocks," can be tagged using polymorphisms, known as "haplotype tagging SNPs" or "tSNPs," that explain the majority of the variation explained by the remaining SNPs within the block *(104)*. Because a haplotype by comparison with a single genetic locus contains sequence variability from a number of linked loci, it improves the estimate of the effect of the true, but unobserved, functional variant. An awareness of the need to characterize genomic variation and patterns of LD provided the impetus for the formation of the International HapMap Consortium *(104)*. The objective of the consortium was to characterize patterns of DNA variation across the human genome and to compare the genetic sequences of different individuals to identify chromosomal regions where genetic variants are shared. Nearly seven million SNPs were eventually genotyped in 269 samples from four populations of African, Asian, and European descent *(105)*. By providing open access to the haplotype structure of the genome, the hope was that this information would aid the discovery of disease-causing genes using genome-wide association methods *(106)*, and this expectation has already been fulfilled as evidenced by the GWA studies discussed above, all of which relied to some extent on HapMap data.

One of the potential limitations of the haplotype approach is that the number of haplotype combinations can be vast where extensive recombination exists within a region. Therefore, methods have been developed to reduce the quantity of haplotypic information to a manageable level. For example, could construct haplotypes from only tSNPs and subsequently combine the haplotypes that confer a similar direction and magnitude of effect *(10)*. However, alleles within exons are generally in lower LD than alleles outside exons. Thus, adequate characterization of these sectors may be unachievable using haplotypes or tSNPs, and dense genotyping will be required *(107)*.

The fact that advances in statistical tools have not kept pace with technological advances in the area of genetics is well recognized *(108)*. While the capacity to genotype DNA and array RNA from large populations has expanding to a million datapoints per subject, the availability of adequate statistical methods lags behind.

One fundamental problem is how to manage the data. As discussed above, genotyping technology allows the assessment of around a million markers per individual, and the new generation of gene expression tools similarly permit the characterization of over a million putative transcripts per tissue sample. Thus, the sheer volume of data prohibits the use of many conventional analytical approaches *(108)*. This reality is reinforced when considering that a conventional multipoint two-way interaction model on data from a 1,000,000 SNP chip would take many years of processing time, even if the fastest available processing facilities were used. Therefore, statistical approaches that begin with data reduction strategies will be necessary. These will likely involve algorithms that reduce the dimensionality of the data by pooling genotypes from multiple loci into a smaller number of functional classes (e.g., high-risk vs. low-risk groups) *(109)*. Such algorithms include the combinatorial-partition method (CPM), the multifactor dimensionality reduction (MDR) technique, and the related generalized MDR (GMDR), all of which attempt to address this issue data dimensionality *(110–113)*. These approaches have been successful in identifying gene × gene interactions for a number of complex traits, including breast cancer *(111)*, elevated plasma triglyceride levels *(110)*, and type 2 diabetes *(114)*. Cho et al. *(114)* used the MDR technique to study interactions among 23 loci in 15 genes and successfully identified a two-locus interaction between variants in the *UCP2* and *PPARG* genes, which was significantly related with type 2 diabetes risk. These approaches are also suitable for use with GEI models, although the higher degree of measurement error associated with environmental exposure data may decrease the relative success of these methods by comparison with the gene x gene scenario.

Functional Studies

Functional investigation of a genetic association is considered the gold standard for evidence of causality (i.e., providing molecular evidence in support of an interaction identified in an epidemiological setting). Indeed some have proposed that variants that are not supported by functional evidence should not be considered in association studies, unless the study hypothesis and design focus specifically on LD-structure approaches for identifying a potentially causal allele *(115)*.

The objectives of functional studies include identifying allelic influences on transcriptional regulation, RNA stability and posttranscriptional process, and protein expression, posttranslational processing, and function. How functional evidence is sought will depend on the characteristics and expression sites of the target genes, a full discussion of which is beyond the scope of this review. That said, functional studies of metabolic hypotheses often demand access to human tissues such as hypothalamus, liver, kidney, and pancreas, which are difficult to obtain. However, the study of molecular genetic hypotheses involving physical activity may be less constrained, because the genes through which physical activity exerts its effects are frequently expressed in adipose and skeletal muscle tissues, which are generally more accessible. A purpose of conducting such studies could be to provide information on gene expression and translation that would help qualify an association between genotype and the more distal clinical phenotypes such as insulin sensitivity and adiposity. Animal models and in vitro techniques may also be required to complement studies of human tissue.

CONCLUSION

While it is widely believed that most complex diseases are likely to involve GEI, the effect of interactions at a single genetic locus may be small. Thus, the detection of interaction is inherently difficult, and the clinical relevance of such interactions may be limited. The testing of biological candidate genes (i.e., those that have sound a priori evidence supporting their role in modifying the effects of physical activity on metabolism) improves the probability that an observed effect is true. Ascertainment of appropriate candidate genes is likely to require that the answer to the following questions is "yes": (1) Does physical activity modify the expression/transcription of the gene? (2) Have functional variants at this locus been identified? (3) Does the protein complex encoded by the gene influence the phenotype of interest? Studies utilizing screening strategies, where large batteries of genes are tested for interaction, are likely to reveal novel pathways that are unlikely to be discovered using the approach described above. However, where a screening approach is used to derive data, which is likely to become increasingly popular as access to whole-genome technologies improves, very large cohorts and/or replication studies will be necessary to confirm or refute whether the initial observations are true or simply due to chance.

Although observations of interaction made in epidemiological studies are likely to help refine the search, they do not provide firm evidence that interaction exists. This is partly attributable to the limitations described in this chapter, but also because the majority of interaction studies are conducted in cross-sectional data, and thus inference of causal direction is difficult. To demonstrate convincingly that genetic variation at a specific locus modifies the effect of PAEE on a metabolic trait is likely to require a combination of in vivo functional studies, where expression levels are manipulated through intervention in genetic wild-type and knockout animals and through human etiological trials where metabolic adaptation to PAEE intervention is shown to differ by genotype. Other human experiments that involve the modulation of energy balance may also be necessary to observe effect modification by genotype. Importantly, these approaches should aim to demonstrate that by intervening on PAEE, expression and translation of candidate genes differ depending on genotype at the respective locus, and that more distal clinical phenotypes, such as insulin sensitivity and lipid oxidation rates, relate in the hypothesized direction with the functional allele. The success of such studies is likely to pivot on the ability to construct sound a priori hypotheses, the measurement precision of the exposures/treatments and phenotypes, the manner in which data are analyzed, and the size of the study. Depending on the expression site(s) of a given candidate gene, access to appropriate tissue will also limit the ability to demonstrate the functional basis of GEI in humans.

ACKNOWLEDGMENTS

PWF was funded in part by an NIH Visiting Scientist Research Fellowship. SMR was supported by grant AG-022791. We thank Dr. William C. Knowler for his helpful comments on this paper.

REFERENCES

1. Wendorf M. Diabetes, the ice free corridor, and the Paleoindian settlement of North America. Am J Phys Anthropol 1989;79(4):503–20.
2. Prentice AM, Jebb SA. Obesity in Britain: gluttony or sloth? BMJ 1995;311(7002):437–9.
3. Murray CJ, Lopez AD. Mortality by cause for eight regions of the world: Global Burden of Disease Study. Lancet 1997;349(9061):1269–76.
4. King H, Rewers M. Global estimates for prevalence of diabetes mellitus and impaired glucose tolerance in adults. WHO Ad Hoc Diabetes Reporting Group. Diabetes Care 1993;16(1):157–77.
5. Hirschhorn JN, Lohmueller K, Byrne E, Hirschhorn K. A comprehensive review of genetic association studies. Genet Med 2002;4(2):45–61.
6. Franks PW, Barroso I, Luan JA, et al. PGC-1alpha genotype modifies the association of volitional energy expenditure with VO_2max. Med Sci Sports Exerc 2003;35(12):1998–2004.
7. Franks PW, Bhattacharyya S, Luan J, et al. Association between physical activity and blood pressure is modified by variants in the G-protein coupled receptor 10. Hypertension. 2004;43(2):224–8.
8. Franks PW, Knowler WC, Nair S, et al. Interaction between an 11betaHSD1 gene variant and birth era modifies the risk of hypertension in Pima Indians. Hypertension 2004;44(5):681–8.
9. Franks PW, Luan J, Browne PO, et al. Does peroxisome proliferator-activated receptor gamma genotype (Pro12ala) modify the association of physical activity and dietary fat with fasting insulin level? Metabolism 2004;53(1):11–6.
10. Franks PW, Luan Ja, Barroso I, et al. Variation in the eNOS gene modifies the association between total energy expenditure and glucose intolerance. Diabetes 2005;54(9):2795–801.
11. Meirhaeghe A, Helbecque N, Cottel D, Amouyel P. Beta2-adrenoceptor gene polymorphism, body weight, and physical activity. Lancet 1999;353(9156):896.
12. Li T, Stefansson H, Gudfinnsson E, et al. Identification of a novel neuregulin 1 at-risk haplotype in Han schizophrenia Chinese patients, but no association with the Icelandic/Scottish risk haplotype. Mol Psychiatr 2004;9(7):698–704.
13. Stefansson H, Sarginson J, Kong A, et al. Association of neuregulin 1 with schizophrenia confirmed in a Scottish population. Am J Hum Genet 2003;72(1):83–7.
14. Stefansson H, Sigurdsson E, Steinthorsdottir V, et al. Neuregulin 1 and susceptibility to schizophrenia. Am J Hum Genet 2002;71(4):877–92.
15. Burchfiel CM, Sharp DS, Curb JD, et al. Physical activity and incidence of diabetes: the Honolulu Heart Program. Am J Epidemiol 1995;141(4):360–8.
16. Boule NG, Haddad E, Kenny GP, Wells GA, Sigal RJ. Effects of exercise on glycemic control and body mass in type 2 diabetes mellitus: a meta-analysis of controlled clinical trials. JAMA 2001;286(10):1218–27.
17. Kujala UM, Kaprio J, Sarna S, Koskenvuo M. Relationship of leisure-time physical activity and mortality: the Finnish twin cohort. JAMA 1998;279(6):440–4.
18. U.S. Department of Health and Human Services, Health Resources and Services Administration, Maternal and Child Health Bureau. Child Health USA 2004. Rockville, Maryland: U.S. Department of Health and Human Services; 2004.
19. Pols MA, Peeters PH, Twisk JW, Kemper HC, Grobbee DE. Physical activity and cardiovascular disease risk profile in women. Am J Epidemiol 1997;146(4):322–8.
20. Teran-Garcia M, Rankinen T, Koza RA, Rao DC, Bouchard C. Endurance training-induced changes in insulin sensitivity and gene expression. Am J Physiol Endocrinol Metab 2005;288(6):E1168–78.
21. Pan XR, Li GW, Hu YH, et al. Effects of diet and exercise in preventing NIDDM in people with impaired glucose tolerance. The Da Qing IGT and Diabetes Study. Diabetes Care 1997;20(4):537–44.
22. Tuomilehto J, Lindstrom J, Eriksson JG, et al. Prevention of type 2 diabetes mellitus by changes in lifestyle among subjects with impaired glucose tolerance. N Engl J Med 2001;344(18):1343–50.

23. Knowler WC, Barrett-Connor E, Fowler SE, et al. Reduction in the incidence of type 2 diabetes with lifestyle intervention or metformin. N Engl J Med 2002;346(6):393–403.
24. Ramachandran A, Snehalatha C, Mary S, Mukesh B, Bhaskar AD, Vijay V. The Indian Diabetes Prevention Programme shows that lifestyle modification and metformin prevent type 2 diabetes in Asian Indian subjects with impaired glucose tolerance (IDPP-1). Diabetologia 2006;49(2):289–97.
25. Bouchard C, Rankinen T. Individual differences in response to regular physical activity. Med Sci Sports Exerc 2001;33(Suppl 6):S446–51.
26. Franks PW, Mesa JL, Harding AH, Wareham NJ. Gene-lifestyle interaction on risk of type 2 diabetes. Nutr Metab Cardiovasc Dis2007;17(2):104–24.
27. Bernstein MS, Costanza MC, James RW, et al. Physical activity may modulate effects of ApoE genotype on lipid profile. Arterioscler Thromb Vasc Biol 2002;22(1):133–40.
28. Corella D, Guillen M, Saiz C, et al. Environmental factors modulate the effect of the APOE genetic polymorphism on plasma lipid concentrations: ecogenetic studies in a Mediterranean Spanish population. Metabolism 2001;50(8):936–44.
29. Senti M, Elosua R, Tomas M, et al. Physical activity modulates the combined effect of a common variant of the lipoprotein lipase gene and smoking on serum triglyceride levels and high-density lipoprotein cholesterol in men. Hum Genet 2001;109(4):385–92.
30. Taimela S, Lehtimaki T, Porkka KV, Rasanen L, Viikari JS. The effect of physical activity on serum total and low-density lipoprotein cholesterol concentrations varies with apolipoprotein E phenotype in male children and young adults: The Cardiovascular Risk in Young Finns Study. Metabolism 1996;45(7):797–803.
31. McCole SD, Shuldiner AR, Brown MD, et al. Beta2- and beta3-adrenergic receptor polymorphisms and exercise hemodynamics in postmenopausal women. J Appl Physiol 2004;96(2):526–30.
32. Otabe S, Clement K, Dina C, et al. A genetic variation in the 5' flanking region of the UCP3 gene is associated with body mass index in humans in interaction with physical activity. Diabetologia 2000;43(2):245–9.
33. Boer JM, Kuivenhoven JA, Feskens EJ, et al. Physical activity modulates the effect of a lipoprotein lipase mutation (D9N) on plasma lipids and lipoproteins. Clin Genet 1999;56(2):158–63.
34. Ortlepp JR, Metrikat J, Albrecht M, von Korff A, Hanrath P, Hoffmann R. The vitamin D receptor gene variant and physical activity predicts fasting glucose levels in healthy young men. Diabet Med 2003;20(6):451–4.
35. Rauramaa R, Vaisanen S, Nissinen A, et al. Physical activity, fibrinogen plasma level and gene polymorphisms in postmenopausal women. Thromb Haemost 1997;78(2):840–4.
36. Kimura T, Yokoyama T, Matsumura Y, et al. NOS3 genotype-dependent correlation between blood pressure and physical activity. Hypertension 2003;41(2):355–60.
37. Corbalan MS, Marti A, Forga L, Martinez-Gonzalez MA, Martinez JA. The 27Glu polymorphism of the beta2-adrenergic receptor gene interacts with physical activity influencing obesity risk among female subjects. Clin Genet 2002;61(4):305–7.
38. Pisciotta L, Cantafora A, Piana A, et al. Physical activity modulates effects of some genetic polymorphisms affecting cardiovascular risk in men aged over 40 years. Nutr Metab Cardiovasc Dis 2003;13(4):202–10.
39. Hokanson JE, Kamboh MI, Scarboro S, Eckel RH, Hamman RF. Effects of the hepatic lipase gene and physical activity on coronary heart disease risk. Am J Epidemiol 2003;158(9):836–43.
40. Berentzen T, Dalgaard LT, Petersen L, Pedersen O, Sorensen TI. Interactions between physical activity and variants of the genes encoding uncoupling proteins -2 and -3 in relation to body weight changes during a 10-y follow-up. Int J Obes (Lond) 2005;29(1):93–9.
41. Bouchard C, Leon AS, Rao DC, Skinner JS, Wilmore JH, Gagnon J. The HERITAGE family study. Aims, design, and measurement protocol. Med Sci Sports Exerc 1995 May;27(5):721–9.

42. Lakka TA, Rankinen T, Weisnagel SJ, et al. Leptin and leptin receptor gene polymorphisms and changes in glucose homeostasis in response to regular exercise in nondiabetic individuals: the HERITAGE family study. Diabetes 2004;53(6):1603–8.
43. Lakka TA, Rankinen T, Weisnagel SJ, et al. A quantitative trait locus on 7q31 for the changes in plasma insulin in response to exercise training: the HERITAGE Family Study. Diabetes 2003;52(6):1583–7.
44. Rankinen T, Rice T, Perusse L, et al. NOS3 Glu298Asp genotype and blood pressure response to endurance training: the HERITAGE family study. Hypertension 2000;36(5):885–9.
45. Lindi VI, Uusitupa MI, Lindstrom J, et al. Association of the Pro12Ala polymorphism in the PPAR-gamma2 gene with 3-year incidence of type 2 diabetes and body weight change in the Finnish Diabetes Prevention Study. Diabetes 2002;51(8):2581–6.
46. Kubaszek A, Pihlajamaki J, Komarovski V, et al. Promoter polymorphisms of the TNF-alpha (G-308A) and IL-6 (C-174G) genes predict the conversion from impaired glucose tolerance to type 2 diabetes: the Finnish Diabetes Prevention Study. Diabetes 2003;52(7):1872–6.
47. Todorova B, Kubaszek A, Pihlajamaki J, et al. The G-250A promoter polymorphism of the hepatic lipase gene predicts the conversion from impaired glucose tolerance to type 2 diabetes mellitus: the Finnish Diabetes Prevention Study. J Clin Endocrinol Metab 2004;89(5):2019–23.
48. The Diabetes Prevention Program Research Group. The Diabetes Prevention Program: recruitment methods and results. Control Clin Trials 2002;23(2):157–71.
49. Florez JC, Jablonski KA, Bayley N, et al. TCF7L2 polymorphisms and progression to diabetes in the Diabetes Prevention Program. N Engl J Med 2006;355(3):241–50.
50. Florez JC, Jablonski KA, Kahn SE, et al. Type 2 diabetes-associated missense polymorphisms KCNJ11 E23K and ABCC8 A1369S influence progression to diabetes and response to interventions in the Diabetes Prevention Program. Diabetes 2007;56(2):531–6.
51. Florez JC, Jablonski KA, Sun MW, et al. Effects of the type 2 diabetes-associated PPARG P12A polymorphism on progression to diabetes and response to troglitazone. J Clin Endocrinol Metab 2007;92(4):1502–9.
52. Franks PW, Jablonski KA, Florez JC, et al. The Pro12Ala variant at the PPARG gene and change in obesity-related traits in the Diabetes Prevention Program. Diabetologia (in press).
53. DeFronzo RA. Insulin resistance: a multifaceted syndrome responsible for NIDDM, obesity, hypertension, dyslipidaemia and atherosclerosis. Neth J Med 1997;50(5):191–7.
54. Wasserman D. An overview of muscle glucose uptake during exercise: sites of regulation. London: Plenum; 1998.
55. Shulman GI. Cellular mechanisms of insulin resistance in humans. Am J Cardiol 1999;84(1A):3J–10J.
56. World Health Organisation WHO Expert Committee on Diabetes. Second Report. Geneva: World Health Organisation; 1980.
57. Richter EA, Nielsen JN, Jorgensen SB, Frosig C, Wojtaszewski JF. Signalling to glucose transport in skeletal muscle during exercise. Acta Physiol Scand 2003;178(4):329–35.
58. Soyal S, Krempler F, Oberkofler H, Patsch W. PGC-1alpha: a potent transcriptional cofactor involved in the pathogenesis of type 2 diabetes. Diabetologia 2006;49(7):1477–88.
59. Mootha VK, Lindgren CM, Eriksson KF, et al. PGC-1alpha-responsive genes involved in oxidative phosphorylation are coordinately downregulated in human diabetes. Nat Genet 2003;34(3):267–73.
60. Semple RK, Crowley VC, Sewter CP, et al. Expression of the thermogenic nuclear hormone receptor coactivator PGC-1alpha is reduced in the adipose tissue of morbidly obese subjects. Int J Obes Relat Metab Disord 2004;28(1):176–9.
61. Baar K, Wende A, Jones TE, et al. Adaptations of skeletal muscle to exercise: rapid increase in the transcriptional coactivator PGC-1. FASEB J 2002;16(14):1879–86.
62. Goto M, Terada S, Kato M, et al. cDNA Cloning and mRNA analysis of PGC-1 in epitrochlearis muscle in swimming-exercised rats. Biochem Biophys Res Commun 2000;274(2):350–4.

63. Lin J, Wu H, Tarr PT, et al. Transcriptional co-activator PGC-1 alpha drives the formation of slow-twitch muscle fibres. Nature 2002;418(6899):797–801.
64. Terada S, Goto M, Kato M, Kawanaka K, Shimokawa T, Tabata I. Effects of low-intensity prolonged exercise on PGC-1 mRNA expression in rat epitrochlearis muscle. Biochem Biophys Res Commun 2002;296(2):350–4.
65. Wu H, Kanatous SB, Thurmond FA, et al. Regulation of mitochondrial biogenesis in skeletal muscle by CaMK. Science 2002;296(5566):349–52.
66. Terada S, Tabata I. Effects of acute bouts of running and swimming exercise on PGC-1alpha protein expression in rat epitrochlearis and soleus muscle. Am J Physiol Endocrinol Metab 2004;286(2): E208–16.
67. Konrad D, Somwar R, Sweeney G, et al. The antihyperglycemic drug alpha-lipoic acid stimulates glucose uptake via both GLUT4 translocation and GLUT4 activation: potential role of p38 mitogen-activated protein kinase in GLUT4 activation. Diabetes 2001;50(6):1464–71.
68. Richter EA, Nielsen JN, Jorgensen SB, Frosig C, Birk JB, Wojtaszewski JF. Exercise signalling to glucose transport in skeletal muscle. Proc Nutr Soc 2004;63(2):211–6.
69. Yonemitsu S, Nishimura H, Shintani M, et al. Troglitazone induces GLUT4 translocation in L6 myotubes. Diabetes 2001;50(5):1093–101.
70. Michael LF, Wu Z, Cheatham RB, et al. Restoration of insulin-sensitive glucose transporter (GLUT4) gene expression in muscle cells by the transcriptional coactivator PGC-1. Proc Natl Acad Sci USA 2001;98(7):3820–5.
71. Handschin C, Rhee J, Lin J, Tarr PT, Spiegelman BM. An autoregulatory loop controls peroxisome proliferator-activated receptor gamma coactivator 1alpha expression in muscle. Proc Natl Acad Sci USA 2003;100(12):7111–6.
72. Herzig S, Hedrick S, Morantte I, Koo SH, Galimi F, Montminy M. CREB controls hepatic lipid metabolism through nuclear hormone receptor PPAR-gamma. Nature 2003;426(6963):190–3.
73. Tsao TS, Li J, Chang KS, et al. Metabolic adaptations in skeletal muscle overexpressing GLUT4: effects on muscle and physical activity. FASEB J 2001;15(6):958–69.
74. Zisman A, Peroni OD, Abel ED, et al. Targeted disruption of the glucose transporter 4 selectively in muscle causes insulin resistance and glucose intolerance. Nat Med 2000;6(8):924–8.
75. Gibbs EM, Stock JL, McCoid SC, et al. Glycemic improvement in diabetic db/db mice by overexpression of the human insulin-regulatable glucose transporter (GLUT4). J Clin Invest 1995;95(4):1512–8.
76. Pilegaard H, Saltin B, Neufer PD. Exercise induces transient transcriptional activation of the PGC-1alpha gene in human skeletal muscle. J Physiol 2003;546(Pt 3):851–8.
77. Norrbom J, Sundberg CJ, Ameln H, Kraus WE, Jansson E, Gustafsson T. PGC-1alpha mRNA expression is influenced by metabolic perturbation in exercising human skeletal muscle. J Appl Physiol 2004;96(1):189–94.
78. Short KR, Vittone JL, Bigelow ML, et al. Impact of aerobic exercise training on age-related changes in insulin sensitivity and muscle oxidative capacity. Diabetes 2003;52(8):1888–96.
79. Russell AP, Feilchenfeldt J, Schreiber S, et al. Endurance training in humans leads to fiber type-specific increases in levels of peroxisome proliferator-activated receptor-gamma coactivator-1 and peroxisome proliferator-activated receptor-alpha in skeletal muscle. Diabetes 2003;52(12):2874–81.
80. Tunstall RJ, Mehan KA, Wadley GD, et al. Exercise training increases lipid metabolism gene expression in human skeletal muscle. Am J Physiol Endocrinol Metab 2002;283(1):E66–72.
81. Barroso I, Luan J, Sandhu M, Franks PW, Crowley V, Schafer A, et al. Meta-analysis of the Gly482Ser variant in PPARGC1A in type 2 diabetes and related phenotypes. Diabetologia 2006;49(3):501–5.
82. Ling C, Poulsen P, Carlsson E, et al. Multiple environmental and genetic factors influence skeletal muscle PGC-1alpha and PGC-1beta gene expression in twins. J Clin Invest 2004;114(10):1518–26.

83. Lucia A, Gomez-Gallego F, Barroso I, et al. PPARGC1A genotype (Gly482Ser) predicts exceptional endurance capacity in European men. J Appl Physiol 2005;99(1):344–8.
84. Kempen KP, Saris WH, Westerterp KR. Energy balance during an 8-wk energy-restricted diet with and without exercise in obese women. Am J Clin Nutr 1995;62(4):722–9.
85. Van Etten LM, Westerterp KR, Verstappen FT, Boon BJ, Saris WH. Effect of an 18-wk weight-training program on energy expenditure and physical activity. J Appl Physiol 1997;82(1):298–304.
86. Wong MY, Day NE, Luan JA, Chan KP, Wareham NJ. The detection of gene-environment interaction for continuous traits: should we deal with measurement error by bigger studies or better measurement? Int J Epidemiol 2003;32(1):51–7.
87. Montoye H, Kemper H, Saris WHS, Washburn R. Measuring Phsyical Activity and Energy Expenditure. Champaign, IL: Human Kinetics; 1996.
88. Hanson RL, Pratley RE, Bogardus C, et al. Evaluation of simple indices of insulin sensitivity and insulin secretion for use in epidemiologic studies. Am J Epidemiol 2000;151(2):190–8.
89. Matsuda M, DeFronzo RA. Insulin sensitivity indices obtained from oral glucose tolerance testing: comparison with the euglycemic insulin clamp. Diabetes Care 1999;22(9):1462–70.
90. Neel JV. Diabetes mellitus: a "thrifty" genotype rendered detrimental by "progress"? Am J Hum Genet 1962;14:353–62.
91. Musani SK, Shriner D, Liu N, et al. Detection of gene x gene interactions in genome-wide association studies of human population data. Hum Hered 2007;63(2):67–84.
92. Steemers FJ, Gunderson KL. Whole genome genotyping technologies on the BeadArray platform. Biotechnol J 2007;2(1):41–9.
93. Klein RJ, Zeiss C, Chew EY, et al. Complement factor H polymorphism in age-related macular degeneration. Science 2005;308(5720):385–9.
94. Helgadottir A, Thorleifsson G, Manolescu A, et al. A common variant on chromosome 9p21 affects the risk of myocardial infarction. Science 2007;316(5830):1491–3.
95. McPherson R, Pertsemlidis A, Kavaslar N, et al. A common allele on chromosome 9 associated with coronary heart disease. Science 2007;316(5830):1488–91.
96. Saxena R, Voight BF, Lyssenko V, et al. Genome-wide association analysis identifies loci for type 2 diabetes and triglyceride levels. Science 2007;316(5829):1331–6.
97. Scott LJ, Mohlke KL, Bonnycastle LL, et al. A genome-wide association study of type 2 diabetes in Finns detects multiple susceptibility variants. Science 2007;316(5829):1341–5.
98. Zeggini E, Weedon MN, Lindgren CM, et al. Replication of genome-wide association signals in UK samples reveals risk loci for type 2 diabetes. Science 2007;316(5829):1336–41.
99. Genome-wide association study of 14,000 cases of seven common diseases and 3,000 shared controls. Nature 2007;447(7145):661–78.
100. Chanock SJ, Manolio T, Boehnke M, et al. Replicating genotype-phenotype associations. Nature 2007;447(7145):655–60.
101. Heck AL, Barroso CS, Callie ME, Bray MS. Gene-nutrition interaction in human performance and exercise response. Nutrition 2004;20(7–8):598–602.
102. Risch N, Merikangas K. The future of genetic studies of complex human diseases. Science 1996;273(5281):1516–7.
103. Wang WY, Barratt BJ, Clayton DG, Todd JA. Genome-wide association studies: theoretical and practical concerns. Nat Rev Genet 2005;6(2):109–18.
104. The International HapMap Project. Nature 2003;426(6968):789–96.
105. A haplotype map of the human genome. Nature 2005;437(7063):1299–320.
106. Crawford DC, Nickerson DA. Definition and clinical importance of haplotypes. Annu Rev Med 2005;56:303–20.
107. Neale BM, Sham PC. The future of association studies: gene-based analysis and replication. Am J Hum Genet 2004;75(3):353–62.

108. Elston RC, Anne Spence M. Advances in statistical human genetics over the last 25 years. Stat Med 2006;25(18):3049–80.
109. Heidema AG, Boer JM, Nagelkerke N, Mariman EC, van der AD, Feskens EJ. The challenge for genetic epidemiologists: how to analyze large numbers of SNPs in relation to complex diseases. BMC Genet 2006;7:23.
110. Nelson MR, Kardia SL, Ferrell RE, Sing CF. A combinatorial partitioning method to identify multilocus genotypic partitions that predict quantitative trait variation. Genome Res 2001;11(3): 458–70.
111. Ritchie MD, Hahn LW, Roodi N, et al. Multifactor-dimensionality reduction reveals high-order interactions among estrogen-metabolism genes in sporadic breast cancer. Am J Hum Genet 2001;69(1): 138–47.
112. Thornton-Wells TA, Moore JH, Haines JL. Genetics, statistics and human disease: analytical retooling for complexity. Trends Genet 2004;20(12):640–7.
113. Lou XY, Chen GB, Yan L, et al. A generalized combinatorial approach for detecting gene-by-gene and gene-by-environment interactions with application to nicotine dependence. Am J Hum Genet 2007;80(6):1125–37.
114. Cho YM, Ritchie MD, Moore JH, et al. Multifactor-dimensionality reduction shows a two-locus interaction associated with Type 2 diabetes mellitus. Diabetologia 2004;47(3):549–54.
115. Rebbeck TR, Spitz M, Wu X. Assessing the function of genetic variants in candidate gene association studies. Nat Rev Genet 2004;5(8):589–97.

10 11β-Hydroxysteroid Dehydrogenase Type 1 and Obesity

Roland H. Stimson and Brian R. Walker

CONTENTS

Abstract

Individuals with central obesity and the metabolic syndrome appear phenotypically similar to those with Cushing syndrome, a disease of primary glucocorticoid excess. Although morning plasma cortisol concentrations are low or normal in obesity, it is possible that tissue cortisol levels are increased. The enzyme 11β-hydroxysteroid dehydrogenase type 1 (11β-HSD1) catalyzes the conversion of inactive cortisone to active cortisol and is present in many tissues including liver and adipose tissue. Transgenic mice overexpressing 11β-HSD1 selectively in adipose tissue develop central obesity with all the features of the metabolic syndrome. In humans, tissue-specific dysregulation of glucocorticoids occurs in simple obesity, with increased 11β-HSD1 activity in subcutaneous adipose tissue and decreased activity in the liver. 11β-HSD1 is highly regulated, and altered plasticity may predispose to metabolic disease. Genetic studies have shown associations between polymorphisms in the *HSD11B1* gene and components of the metabolic syndrome. Nonspecific inhibition of this enzyme leads to improved hepatic insulin sensitivity, while more selective compounds are being developed to potentially treat central obesity and the associated metabolic complications.

From: *Contemporary Endocrinology: Energy Metabolism and Obesity: Research and Clinical Applications*
Edited by: P. A. Donohoue © Humana Press Inc., Totowa, NJ

Key Words: adipose tissue, glucocorticoids, 11β-hydroxysteroid dehydrogenases, metabolic syndrome, obesity.

INTRODUCTION

With the increasing obesity epidemic, a relatively new metabolic disorder has emerged. An increased body mass index (BMI), especially in those with a central fat distribution, is associated with type 2 diabetes mellitus (T2DM), hypertension, hypertriglyceridemia, and decreased high density lipoprotein cholesterol (HDL-C). This cluster has been termed the *metabolic syndrome*, or *Reaven's syndrome X (1)*. People with the metabolic syndrome have an increased risk of developing cardiovascular disease. Central obesity, for example, as measured by a high ratio of waist-to-hip circumference (WHR), has been shown to be associated with increased cardiovascular disease and mortality *(2)*. It has long been observed that those with central obesity or the metabolic syndrome are phenotypically similar to those with Cushing's syndrome, and it has been postulated that dysregulation of cortisol production or metabolism could be a common feature in both of these entities *(3)*.

PRIMARY GLUCOCORTICOID EXCESS

Cushing's syndrome is a disease characterized by high circulating levels of cortisol, often caused by tumors in the pituitary or the adrenal cortex secreting excessive amounts of adrenocorticotropin hormone (ACTH) or cortisol respectively. Patients with Cushing's syndrome are often obese, while a higher proportion of their total body fat is deposited centrally compared with those with simple obesity *(4)*, especially in the visceral adipose tissue *(5, 6)*. The steroid excess also causes hypertension, insulin resistance, and dyslipidemia. After surgical resection and plasma cortisol levels have decreased to normal, total fat mass decreases *(7)* with the visceral compartment declining disproportionately compared with the subcutaneous adipose tissue and other sites *(8)*. The glucocorticoid receptor antagonist RU38486 also decreases plasma glucose levels, triglycerides, and improves hypertension and mood disturbance in Cushing's syndrome *(9, 10)*. This indicates that primary glucocorticoid excess can cause all the features of the metabolic syndrome.

The mechanisms by which glucocorticoids induce features of the metabolic syndrome are complex and are mediated in several tissues, including liver and adipose tissue. During fasting, gluconeogenesis occurs in the liver to convert pyruvate to glucose in order to meet the body's metabolic demands. The cytosolic form of the enzyme phosphoenolpyruvate kinase (PEPCK-C) catalyzes a key rate-limiting step in this pathway, converting oxaloacetate to phosphoenolpyruvate, and is regulated by several factors including glucocorticoids. Glucocorticoids increase PEPCK-C messenger RNA (mRNA) expression in rat liver in vivo *(11)* and in vitro *(12, 13)*. By this and other pathways, glucocorticoid excess leads to increased hepatic gluconeogenesis, which also occurs in type 2 diabetes mellitus. PEPCK-C is also a key enzyme in the glyceroneogenesis pathway, which generates the glycerol-3-phosphate needed for re-esterification of fatty acids released by intra-adipose lipolysis. Increased PEPCK-C expression in the liver would potentially increase triglyceride synthesis in the liver with resultant efflux into the circulation.

PEPCK-C is also present in adipose tissue, which is the other major organ of glyceroneogenesis. Glucocorticoids appear to regulate this enzyme in a tissue-specific manner, with dexamethasone leading to decreased PEPCK-C expression *(14)* and activity *(15, 16)* in white adipose tissue (WAT) in rats. Increased PEPCK-C activity in white adipose tissue has also been seen in adrenalectomized rats, which is suppressible with dexamethasone *(17)*. Thus, glucocorticoid excess could decrease glyceroneogenesis and increase the proportion of free fatty acids (FFAs) released into the circulation by adipose tissue. Increased plasma FFAs are also seen in people with type 2 diabetes mellitus *(18)*. Glucocorticoids have also been inconsistently shown in rat adipocytes to increase the expression of hormone sensitive lipase (HSL) *(19)*, which catalyzes the hydrolysis of intra-adipose triglycerides into glycerol and FFAs. This would lead to increased lipolysis and higher plasma FFA concentrations.

However, in Cushing's syndrome, there are lipogenic as well as lipolytic effects, with increased fat mass being deposited centrally. Adipose tissue contains adipose precursor cells (preadipocytes) in addition to mature adipocytes, although these precursors are far fewer in number. In vitro, cortisol dramatically increases the rate of differentiation of these cells into adipocytes *(20, 21)*, potentially increasing adipose mass in states of chronic glucocorticoid excess. The hormone lipoprotein lipase (LpL), which catalyzes the hydrolysis of circulating triglycerides prior to the uptake of FFAs and re-esterification by adipose tissue, is also regulated by glucocorticoids. Dexamethasone increases LpL expression and activity in human adipose tissue *(22)*, which could potentially lead to increased fat deposition. Interestingly, one study found increased LpL activity in central subcutaneous adipose tissue in Cushing's syndrome patients compared with healthy controls but found no difference in femoral adipose tissue *(23)*. This could partly account for the increased lipogenesis seen centrally compared with peripheral sites in chronic glucocorticoid excess.

GLUCOCORTICOIDS IN OBESITY AND THE METABOLIC SYNDROME

It has been observed that there is increased activity of the hypothalamic-pituitary-adrenal (HPA) axis in those with hypertension and hypertriglyceridemia, components of the metabolic syndrome *(24)*. Mildly elevated morning plasma cortisol levels are associated with hypertension (*25–28*), insulin resistance *(26, 27, 29)*, and hypertriglyceridemia *(26, 27)*. Increased cortisol secretion and enhanced tissue cortisol sensitivity are also noted in those with insulin resistance *(30, 31)*. However, in simple obesity, morning plasma cortisol levels are often low (*27,32–38*) or normal (*39–42*), but with increased HPA axis activity *(34, 39)*. The combination of low plasma cortisol with elevated cortisol production rate can be explained by the finding of elevated levels of urinary cortisol metabolites *(36, 38, 43, 44)*, which indicate an increased metabolic clearance rate of endogenous glucocorticoids in obesity. This appears, at least in part, to be due to increased 5α- and 5β-reductase activity in the liver *(44, 45)*, while increased 5β-reductase activity has also been shown in people with type 2 diabetes mellitus *(31)* and with the insulin resistance associated with nonalcoholic fatty liver disease *(44)*. These findings indicate that glucocorticoid secretion and metabolism are altered in obesity but do not explain the phenotypic similarities with Cushing's syndrome.

THE 11β-HYDROXYSTEROID DEHYDROGENASES

In Cushing's syndrome, plasma cortisol is elevated, and although those with components of the metabolic syndrome have mildly elevated levels, in simple obesity morning concentrations are low/normal. If these two phenotypically similar disorders are both due to cortisol excess, there must be increased local concentrations or action of glucocorticoids in obesity. The 11β-hydroxysteroid dehydrogenase (11β-HSD) enzymes provide a mechanism for such tissue-specific changes in cortisol concentrations. There are two isozymes, 11β-HSD type 1 and type 2, which vary in their site and action (Fig. 10.1). 11β-HSD2 is an exclusive dehydrogenase that is nicotinamide adenine dinucleotide (NAD) dependent and is found primarily in the kidney, colon, placenta, sweat glands, and the salivary glands *(46, 47)*. This enzyme functions to catalyze the conversion of active cortisol to the inactive cortisone in humans (corticosterone to 11-deoxycorticosterone in rodents), thus protecting mineralocorticoid receptors in target tissues from being activated by glucocorticoids *(48, 49)*. Inactivation of this enzyme by gene mutations leads to the syndrome of apparent mineralocorticoid excess (SAME), which is characterized by hypertension and hypokalemia *(50)*.

In contrast, 11β-HSD type 1 is a bidirectional enzyme that is present in many tissues, with high expression in the liver, adipose tissue, and the brain. This enzyme is nicotinamide adenine dinucleotide phosphate (NADPH) (NAD dependent and catalyzes the interconversion of the inactive glucocorticoid cortisone to the physiologically active cortisol and vice versa *(51)*. Initially, it was thought that this enzyme was only involved in the metabolism of cortisol, as in vitro it acts mainly as a dehydrogenase converting cortisol to cortisone. However, in intact cells, 11β-HSD1 acts primarily as a reductase, converting cortisone to cortisol and thereby increasing local concentrations of active cortisol in the tissues where it is expressed *(52–54)*. It has been noted that the active catalytic site 11β-HSD1 resides in the lumen of the endoplasmic reticulum (ER) *(55)*. Hexose-6-phosphate dehydrogenase, which is also present in the ER, has been shown to influence the directionality of 11β-HSD1 by generating the NADPH needed for it to act as an oxoreductase *(56)*. This may explain the respective reaction directions observed in vivo and in tissue homogenates. Inhibition of 11β-HSD1 in the liver was found to increase hepatic insulin sensitivity in healthy men, indicating that increased

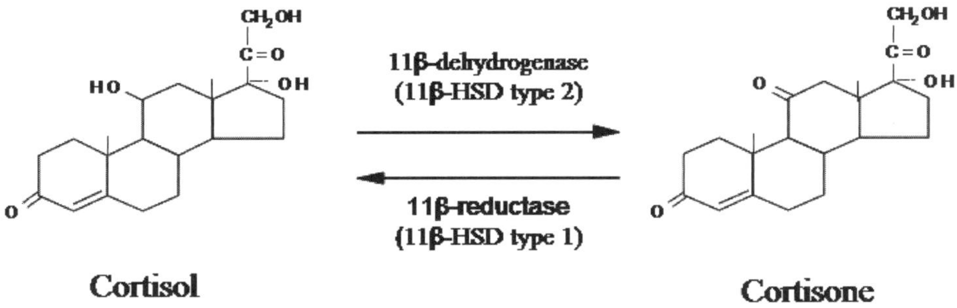

Fig. 10.1 The 11β-hydroxysteroid dehydrogenases. 11β-HSD2 is solely a dehydrogenase, converting cortisol to cortisone. 11β-HSD1 is bidirectional, able to act as a dehydrogenase or reductase. The reductase direction predominates in intact cells, thereby increasing tissue cortisol concentrations where it is expressed.

hepatic 11β-HSD1 activity could potentially cause insulin resistance *(57)*. Significant 11β-HSD1 reductase activity was also observed in omental fat, leading to the idea that central obesity could be caused by "Cushing's disease of the omentum" *(58)*, without necessarily affecting plasma cortisol levels.

TRANSGENIC MANIPULATION OF 11β-HSD1 IN MICE

In order to test this hypothesis, transgenic mice were created that overexpressed the 11β-HSD1 enzyme specifically in certain tissues. When expression is increased selectively in adipose tissue, utilizing the fatty acid binding protein (AP2) promoter, these mice become centrally obese with an increase in mesenteric fat mass out of proportion to other sites. These mice also develop dyslipidemia, hypertension, insulin resistance, and glucose intolerance *(59,60)*. Of note, corticosterone levels are low/normal in plasma, as a result of a compensatory adjustment of corticosterone production, but are raised two- to three-fold in the adipose tissue. Utilizing the apolipoprotein E (ApoE) promoter, transgenic mice overexpressing 11β-HSD1 selectively in the liver have also been created to examine the potential contribution of hepatic cortisol generation to the metabolic syndrome *(61)*. These mice again have normal plasma corticosterone levels despite having a substantial increase in hepatic 11β-HSD1 activity. They develop mild insulin resistance, dyslipidemia, fatty liver, and hypertension but do not become hyperglycemic or obese.

Conversely, 11β-HSD1 knockout mice appear healthy and have a normal life span. They resist hyperglycemia and weight gain on a high-fat diet and deposit fat in physiologically "safer" sites (away from the abdominal depots) *(62,63)*. The 11β-HSD1 knockout mice also have decreased plasma triglycerides due to improved lipid oxidation, and increased HDL-C *(64)*. 11β-HSD1 knockout mice on a MF1 and 129/Ola background have higher morning plasma corticosterone levels *(62)*, although they have lower corticosterone concentrations in tissues that normally express 11β-HSD1 *(65)*. However, morning plasma corticosterone concentrations are not elevated in young 11β-HSD1 knockout mice on the C57Bl6 background (unpublished data).

11β-HSD1 IN HUMAN IDIOPATHIC OBESITY

The transgenic mice have shown that tissue-specific dysregulation of cortisol generation could potentially be critical in the pathogenesis of obesity and the metabolic syndrome. Consequently, much recent work has focused on whether these results translate to human obesity. Examination of urinary cortisol metabolites was formerly regarded as the gold standard method of examining global 11β-HSD1 activity. Cortisol is metabolized predominately in the liver by the A-ring reductases 5α- and 5β-reductase and the 3α-hydroxysteroid dehydrogenases before excretion in the urine largely as its tetrahydrometabolites 5β-THF (THF), 5α-THF (α-THF), and 5β-THE (THE) (Fig. 10.2). Examination of the ratio of urinary concentration of cortisol:cortisone metabolites [(THF + α-THF)/THE] has been used as a marker for 11β-HSD1 activity, whereas 11β-HSD2 activity is generally measured by the ratio of free urinary cortisol/cortisone (UFF/UFE) *(66)*.

However, studies of the (THF + α-THF)/THE ratio in human obesity have found it to be increased *(38,45,67)*, normal *(24,44,68,69)* or even decreased *(43,70)*. The

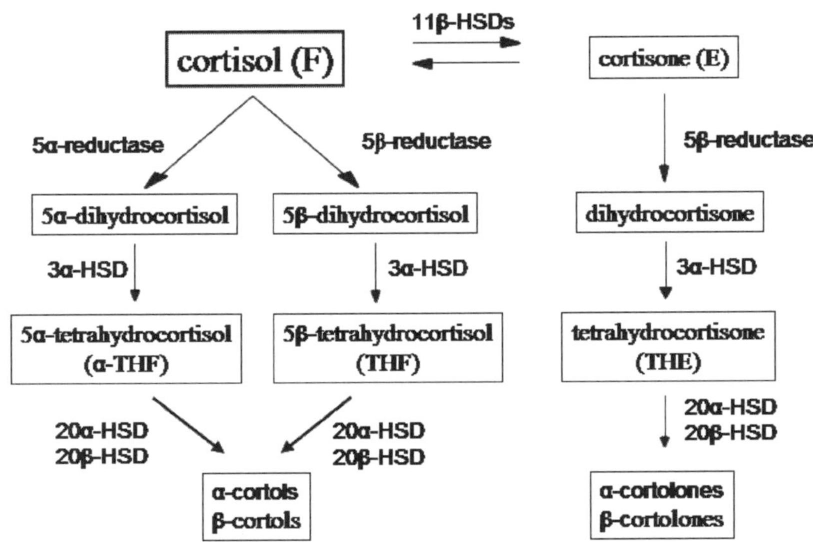

Fig. 10.2 Cortisol metabolism. Cortisol (F) and cortisone (E) are partly excreted by the kidneys in their unbound form. However, the majority of F and E are excreted as their tetrahydrometabolites, after metabolism by the A-ring reductases and 3α-HSD. These can be further metabolized by the 20α-HSDs to form the cortols and cortolones.

(THF + α-THF)/THE ratio has also been examined in patients with type 2 diabetes, who have no change in 11β-HSD1 activity when compared with healthy controls *(31, 71, 72)*. Some of the inconsistency between studies may be accounted for by gender differences in 11β-HSD1 activity, as the ratio has been found to be decreased in females *(73, 74)*. Altered activity of the A-ring reductases could also be a contributory factor in women *(74, 75)* while liver fat content can also alter 5β-reductase activity *(44)*. These potential confounding factors are not accounted for in most of the above studies.

Recently, infusions of deuterated 9,11,12,12-$^{2}H_4$-cortisol (d4F) have been performed in humans. The deuterium on the 11th carbon atom is removed when the cortisol is converted to cortisone (d3E) by 11β-HSD2 and is replaced by an unlabeled hydrogen atom when converted by 11β-HSD1 to cortisol again (d3F) (Fig. 10.3). Differences in enrichment between d4F and d3F can be used to calculate 11β-HSD1 activity *(76)*. One study has examined whole body cortisol generation in obese and lean individuals using deuterated cortisol and found no change in 11β-HSD1 activity between the two groups *(77)*. However, the above studies only look at total body 11β-HSD1 activity so of course cannot take into account differences in tissue-specific regulation. Consequently, other methods have to be used in order to measure 11β-HSD1 activity within individual tissues.

11β-HSD1 in Liver

Tissue-specific abnormalities in 11β-HSD1 have been observed in obese Zucker rats, which are leptin resistant due to a mutation in the leptin receptor gene. Hepatic 11β-HSD1 mRNA and activity are decreased in the obese, whereas omental adipose tissue activity is increased *(78)*. In humans, measuring the conversion of orally administered cortisone to cortisol has been used to assess the activity of hepatic 11β-HSD1.

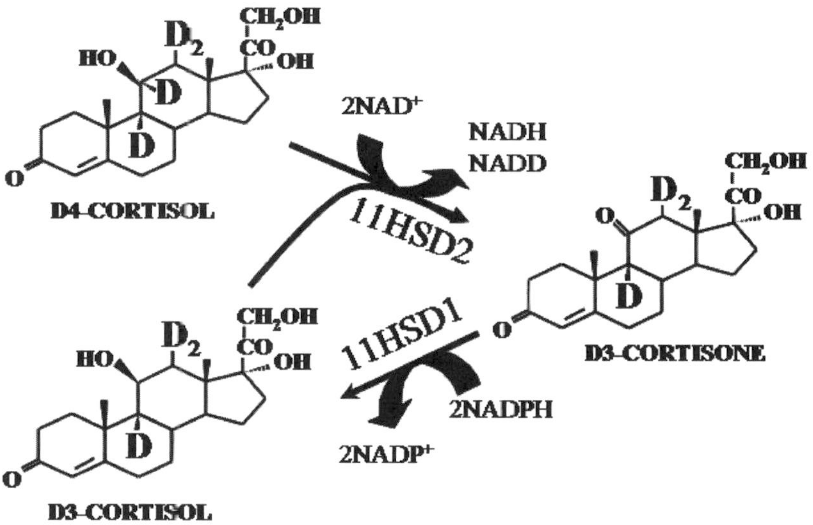

Fig. 10.3 Quantifying cortisol production using deuterated cortisol. Deuterated cortisol can be used to measure global 11β-HSD1 activity. 9,11,12,12-$^2H_4$-Cortisol (d4-cortisol) is converted mainly in the kidney to d3-cortisone, with the loss of the deuterium on C_{11}. The d3-cortisone is then reduced by 11β-HSD1, predominately in the liver and adipose tissue, with the addition of an unlabeled hydrogen to form d3-cortisol. Differences between d3-cortisol and d4-cortisol metabolism therefore reflect 11βHSD1 reductase activity.

A consistent finding is a decrease in activity in obese humans compared with normal-weight individuals *(38, 43, 70)*. Decreased hepatic 11β-HSD1 activity has also been observed in association with glucose intolerance *(31)*, which of course is a component of the metabolic syndrome, although the magnitude of this difference is substantially less than the effect of obesity per se.

11β-HSD1 in Subcutaneous Adipose Tissue

Adipose tissue has been examined extensively for variations in steroid metabolism. Subcutaneous adipose tissue has been studied most frequently as biopsies can be obtained easily. Messenger RNA levels of 11β-HSD1 were increased in obese subjects compared with lean individuals in most studies *(79–84)*, although no difference was detected in one article *(85)*. Increased 11β-HSD1 activity is also observed in obesity *(38, 43, 79, 80)*, while 11β-HSD1 mRNA has been shown to correlate with enzyme activity *(79, 80)*. This work has been criticized because 11β-HSD1 activity was measured in the dehydrogenase direction, by incubation with cortisol, rather than in the reductase direction by incubation with cortisone *(86)*. However, the dehydrogenase is the more stable activity in homogenized tissue in vitro and is linearly related to the total 11β-HSD1 protein present, so that we have argued that it gives a reliable estimate of 11β-HSD1 protein. It is true, however, that no measurement in vitro can necessarily predict the reaction direction or activity of 11β-HSD1 in vivo. To address this, arteriovenous differences in cortisol and cortisone have been measured across subcutaneous adipose tissue in vivo and showed a correlation between fat mass and cortisone clearance rates, which is a marker of 11β-HSD1 activity *(87)*. More recently, microdialysis has been used to infuse tritiated cortisone into subcutaneous adipose tissue, demonstrating more robustly that local conversion to cortisol is increased in obese individuals *(77)*.

Insulin resistance also positively correlates with either 11β-HSD1 mRNA or activity in many of these studies (*79–82,84*), again indicating the potential importance of glucocorticoid regeneration in the pathogenesis of the metabolic syndrome. Interestingly, intra-adipose cortisol concentrations do not appear to correlate with 11β-HSD1 mRNA or activity *(79, 80)*, which may indicate that analysis techniques are insufficiently sensitive to detect any changes that exist, or that the rate of cortisol generation by 11β-HSD1 in subcutaneous adipose tissue is small by comparison with the influx of cortisol from plasma, so that the adipose tissue is not exposed to substantially higher concentrations in obese individuals, despite two- to threefold differences in enzyme expression and activity.

11β-HSD1 in Visceral Adipose Tissue

It has been argued that increased glucocorticoid regeneration in the visceral adipose depot may be more important than subcutaneous tissue in central obesity and its associated metabolic phenotype *(58)*. 11β-HSD1 mRNA and activity are reported to be higher in cultured visceral adipose stromal cells (ASCs) compared with subcutaneous ASCs *(58, 88)*. Moreover, in the only study published to date comparing 11β-HSD1 in visceral adipose biopsies of lean and obese subjects, mRNA did not differ in freshly isolated tissue, but enzyme activity in cultured omental preadipocytes was lower in obese subjects *(85)*. In vivo work is needed to quantify visceral adipose cortisol production in obesity.

Portal and peripheral concentrations of cortisol have been analyzed in a small number of morbidly obese patients, and no differences were noted between the two sites *(89)*. However, only six patients were studied, and changes in concentration could be difficult to detect during the stress of intra-abdominal surgery. Two groups have utilized deuterated cortisol infusions with hepatic venous sampling to measure splanchnic (visceral) cortisol production. One group found that cortisol was produced by the splanchnic tissues at 15.6 nmol/min, although this included hepatic and intra-adipose 11β-HSD1, so is impossible to determine what proportion visceral fat contributed *(90)*. In contrast, under the conditions we used, we found that the splanchnic tissues generated 45 nmol of cortisol per min. In addition we measured first-pass metabolism of cortisone to cortisol and calculated that only 15 nmol/min cortisol production was due to hepatic 11β-HSD1 in steady state *(91)*. The remainder of splanchnic production (~30 nmol/min) is largely due to visceral fat, although other tissues with 11β-HSD1 activity, such as the pancreas, may also contribute.

11β-HSD1 in Skeletal Muscle

Skeletal muscle has been investigated and found to contain 11β-HSD1 mRNA in humans *(92)*, but most groups have found low enzyme activity in most species. In cultured human myoblasts, in the presence of glucocorticoids, there are positive correlations between 11β-HSD1 mRNA expression with BMI, insulin resistance, and systolic blood pressure *(93)*. The only other study in this area was performed in Pima Indians, which found no correlation between 11β-HSD1 mRNA levels and body composition in homogenized skeletal muscle tissue *(82)*. More work is needed to clarify the importance of enzyme expression in human skeletal muscle.

11β-HSD1 IN OTHER FORMS OF OBESITY

Polycystic Ovarian Syndrome

Polycystic ovarian syndrome (PCOS) is a disorder characterized by infertility, hyperandrogenism, and hirsutism. This is often accompanied by obesity, and it has been suggested that this disorder could be partly due to activation of the HPA axis secondary to alterations in glucocorticoid metabolism *(94)*. The urinary 11-hydroxy/11-keto cortisol metabolite ratio has been inconsistently reported to be decreased in PCOS women compared with healthy controls, suggesting decreased total body 11β-HSD1 activity *(95, 96)*. However, no correlation was seen between 11β-HSD1 activity and androgen production. This decreased activity has been further examined and found not to be due to endogenous inhibitors of this enzyme *(97)*. Further studies are needed into this disorder to examine tissue specific differences in glucocorticoid regeneration in these patients.

HIV Treatment–Associated Lipodystrophy

Highly active antiretroviral therapy (HAART) is used very successfully in the treatment of human immunodeficiency virus (HIV). However, these patients can develop a lipodystrophy on this therapy that leads to redistribution of fat to the abdomen, nape of neck, and face accompanied by insulin resistance and dyslipidemia; this looks remarkably like Cushing's syndrome. These people have normal plasma cortisol levels *(98)* but may have tissue-specific dysregulation of cortisol regeneration. Only one study has examined 11β-HSD1 in these patients, but it has found increased mRNA levels in subcutaneous abdominal adipose tissue, and increased cortisol: cortisone metabolite ratios compared with controls *(99)*. This does not appear to be a direct effect of protease inhibitors, which decrease rather than increase 11β-HSD1 activity in preadipocytes in vitro *(100)* and were prescribed to both the lipodystrophic and nonlipodystrophic group in the in vivo study *(99)*. It may be that reduction of intra-adipose cortisol regeneration will be a useful strategy to reduce metabolic complications in HIV lipodystrophy.

Growth Hormone Deficiency and Hypothalamic Obesity

Growth hormone (GH) deficiency is generally seen in patients who have hypothalamic or pituitary disease, either before or after surgical resection. These patients often become obese in a central distribution *(101)*, again leading to parallels with Cushing's syndrome. Moreover, GH decreases 11β-HSD1 expression, probably indirectly through insulin-like growth factor 1 (IGF-1), in vivo and in vitro *(102, 103)*.

There is circumstantial evidence in support of the hypothesis that increased 11β-HSD1 is important in mediating the obesity of GH deficiency. Increased (α-THF + THF)/THE ratios have been observed in hypothalamic obesity, suggesting increased total body 11β-HSD1 activity, although no correlation with BMI was confirmed *(104)*. Several studies have shown that 11-OH/11-keto cortisol metabolite ratios decrease when GH therapy is given to combined ACTH- and GH-deficient patients (*105–108*), although this is not universal *(109)*. These studies did not show any association between the 11-OH/11-keto cortisol metabolite ratio and body composition, although another study found a correlation between a decreased ratio and increased BMI and fat mass *(110)*. Conversely, in the treatment of acromegaly, a decrease in GH action leads to an increase in the 11-OH/11-keto ratio, but is not associated with changes in body fat *(111)*. Interpretation of these studies is complicated because these patients are often dependent on exogenous glucocorticoids due to associated ACTH deficiency and potential confounding effects of obesity and gender influencing urinary steroid ratios.

GH therapy leads to a reduction in fat mass in GH-deficient patients *(101, 106)*, and it has been postulated that use of GH in simple obesity could lead to similar results, possibly through inhibition of 11β-HSD1. One study used prolonged (8 months) GH treatment of simple obesity, which led to a decreased plasma cortisol/cortisone ratio but no change in fat mass *(112)*. It is difficult to know whether 11β-HSD1 dysregulation contributes to hypothalamic obesity, and there has been no research examining tissue specific activity or 11β-HSD1 inhibition in these subjects.

PLASTICITY OF 11β-HSD1

The studies described above illustrate that static observation of 11β-HSD1 suggests tissue-specific changes in obesity. In parallel, investigations in cells and in animals have illustrated that 11β-HSD1 is highly regulated. Further consideration of regulation of enzyme expression and function is crucial to understand the physiologic role of 11β -HSD1 and the basis for its dysregulation in obesity.

Effects of Diet and Weight Loss

Although most studies show increased 11β-HSD1 in subcutaneous adipose tissue in association with increasing BMI, it is unclear whether this is a primary cause or a secondary effect. The effect of weight loss on adipose tissue has been investigated to address the reversibility of increased 11β-HSD1, but the two published studies show conflicting results. One used primary cultures of abdominal subcutaneous adipocytes before and after 5% weight loss and found no change in 11β-HSD1 mRNA levels *(84)*. The other study used gluteal biopsies and found no change in mRNA expression in whole adipose tissue after 14% weight loss *(113)*; however, an increase in 11β-HSD1 mRNA expression was seen in isolated adipocytes. The discrepancies between these studies may be explained by using different sites to biopsy adipose tissue or by different diets. In the first study, volunteers were on ad libitum diets for several days both before and after weight loss. In the second study, volunteers were studied on ad libitum diet before weight loss and while continuing a very-low-calorie diet (VLCD) after weight loss. In rodents, high-fat feeding has been found to decrease adipose tissue 11β-HSD1 mRNA and activity over just a few days *(114, 115)*, and it is possible that dietary variations in humans can also alter 11β-HSD1 expression more acutely than any effect of weight loss or gain. Only one study has looked in more detail at human dietary modulation of 11β-HSD1 thus far and found no change in activity in people eating a VLCD *(116)*; however, this was assessed by urinary metabolites and reflects total body activity so does not allow for tissue specific regulation.

Hormonal Regulation

GH and IGF-1 (see above) are not the only factors known to regulate 11β-HSD1 activity. A good deal of conflicting data exists on regulatory factors of 11β-HSD1, and some of this is due to differences between in vitro and in vivo measurements. 11β-HSD1 is also regulated in a tissue-specific manner, so certain factors may have effects in some tissues but not in others. Only the work examining hepatic and adipose tissue is discussed here. In vitro, in human preadipocytes and adipocytes cortisol increases expression and activity of 11β-HSD1, potentially leading to positive feedback in these cells *(84, 88, 113)*. Inflammatory cytokines like TNF-α and IL-1β have also been shown to upregulate 11β-HSD1 in preadipocytes and adipocytes *(100, 117, 118)*. Interestingly, no effect was seen in hepatocytes *(100)*, indicating that regulation probably occurs in a tissue-specific manner. Despite inhibiting 11β-HSD1 in hepatocytes *(54)*, insulin has not been shown to have a direct effect on 11β-HSD1 in adipose tissue in vitro *(88, 118)*, although interestingly it did prevent the increase induced by TNF-α. In vivo, however, insulin decreased 11β-HSD1 activity acutely in healthy men but not in those with obesity *(77)*. PPARγ agonists downregulate 11β-HSD1 expression in vitro in mouse-derived 3T3-L1 adipocytes *(119)*. However, the only human in vivo trial published found no effect on 11β-HSD1 expression in adipose tissue in healthy controls or type 2 diabetic patients *(120)*. It is likely that many factors interact to regulate 11β-HSD1 expression and activity in specific tissues, and much more work is needed to unravel this complex field.

11β-HSD1 POLYMORPHISMS AND OBESITY

It has been postulated that mutations in the gene encoding the 11β-HSD1 enzyme could lead to altered activity and be pathogenically linked to obesity and the metabolic syndrome. Consequently, studies have been performed searching for correlations between metabolic parameters and certain single nucleotide polymorphisms (SNPs) and microsatellite repeat markers in the *HSD11B1* gene. This gene is situated on chromosome 1 and contains six exons *(121)*, while it is approximately 30 kb in size *(122)*. SNPs in the 5′ region of *HSD11B1* can lead to reduced transcription rates *(123)*, but most studies have not shown a link between genetic polymorphisms and body composition (*82,124–126*). There are two studies that have reported a correlation between polymorphisms and anthropometric measurements. One was performed in children, where homozygosity for an insertion in intron 3 was associated with an increased BMI and insulin resistance *(127)*. However, there were only 11 homozygotes in the study, and there was no trend seen in heterozygotes. The other study showed that shorter microsatellite repeat markers in intron 4 correlated with increased waist:hip ratios in women in one population, but found no significance in men or in a second study population *(122)*.

However, other components of the metabolic syndrome have been correlated with polymorphisms of the *HSD11B1* gene. A SNP in the 5' region has been shown to be associated with insulin resistance *(82)* and hypertension *(126)*, although no correlation was noted with 11β-HSD1 mRNA expression in adipose tissue or muscle. However, these studies have not examined 11β-HSD1 enzyme activity in relation to variations in the *HSD11B1* gene, and it is difficult in humans ethically to examine mRNA levels in other metabolically important sites like the liver.

Cortisone Reductase Deficiency

In 1984, a rare disorder was characterized called *cortisone reductase deficiency (CRD) (128)*. These patients are mostly women and present with hyperandrogenism, hirsutism, and infertility (*129–132*). Males can present with precocious puberty *(133)*. Some of these patients are lean but some are obese. These people have all been found to have a markedly decreased ability to reduce inactive cortisone to cortisol, and a very low urinary (α-THF + THF)/THE ratio. The most likely biochemical explanation is generalized 11β-HSD1 deficiency, the closest human equivalent to the 11β-HSD1 knockout mouse. However, unlike the mouse (which lacks the capacity to secrete adrenal androgens), the compensatory increase in HPA axis drive—to maintain plasma cortisol levels in the absence of peripheral regeneration of cortisol from cortisone—leads to adrenal androgen excess in affected humans.

Genetic studies have been performed in many of these patients, looking for a functional defect in the *HSD11B1* gene. However, no coding mutations were seen in any affected individuals *(130, 132, 134)*. However, as described above, hexose-6-phosphate dehydrogenase influences the reaction direction of 11β-HSD1. One group examined three patients with CRD and found that all had mutations in intron 3 of the *HSD11B1* gene and in exon 5 of the H6PD gene *(135)*. It was hypothesized that mutations in both genes are needed to produce this rare genetic disorder. This proposal needs to be revisited, however, because a more recent study in PCOS patients and healthy controls has found as many as nine patients with the combined mutations in the *HSD11B1* and *H6PD* genes, none of whom had the biochemical features of cortisone reductase deficiency *(136)*. Further work is needed to clarify the precise genetic abnormality that causes this disorder.

INHIBITION OF 11β-HSD1

With the epidemic rise of obesity and the concurrent metabolic syndrome, new treatments are urgently needed. Whether 11β-HSD1 is a primary cause or a secondary mechanism in the pathogenesis of obesity, inhibition of this enzyme remains an exciting prospect for therapy. Most of the human work in this field has been performed using carbenoxolone, the hemisuccinate derivative of glycyrrhetinic acid. This compound nonselectively inhibits both 11β-HSD1 and 11β-HSD2 activity *(137)*. Carbenoxolone has been shown to improve hepatic insulin sensitivity and decrease hepatic glucose production in healthy men and in men with type 2 diabetes *(57, 138)*. However, its effects appear to be limited to the liver *(77)*, are insufficient to impact upon glycemic control in type 2 diabetes *(139)*, and are attenuated in obese patients in whom hepatic 11β -HSD1 is already impaired *(77)*. Unfortunately, this drug also causes hypertension and hypokalemia secondary to concurrent 11-βHSD2 inhibition so would not be appropriate for general use, but it shows the potential benefit of specific 11β-HSD1 inhibitors. Inhibition of adipose tissue 11β-HSD1 would seem to offer greater potential, although carbenoxolone does not seem to accumulate in adipose tissue. Two studies, one in humans and one in Zucker rats, found that carbenoxolone had no effect on adipose 11β-HSD1 activity despite significant inhibition of hepatic 11β-HSD1 *(77, 140)* (Fig. 10.4).

At present, the pharmaceutical industry is hard at work attempting to create specific 11β-HSD type 1 inhibitors. A new class of drugs termed *arylsulfonamidothiazoles* specifically inhibit 11-βHSD1 but not 11-βHSD2 *(141)*, but to date only hepatic insulin

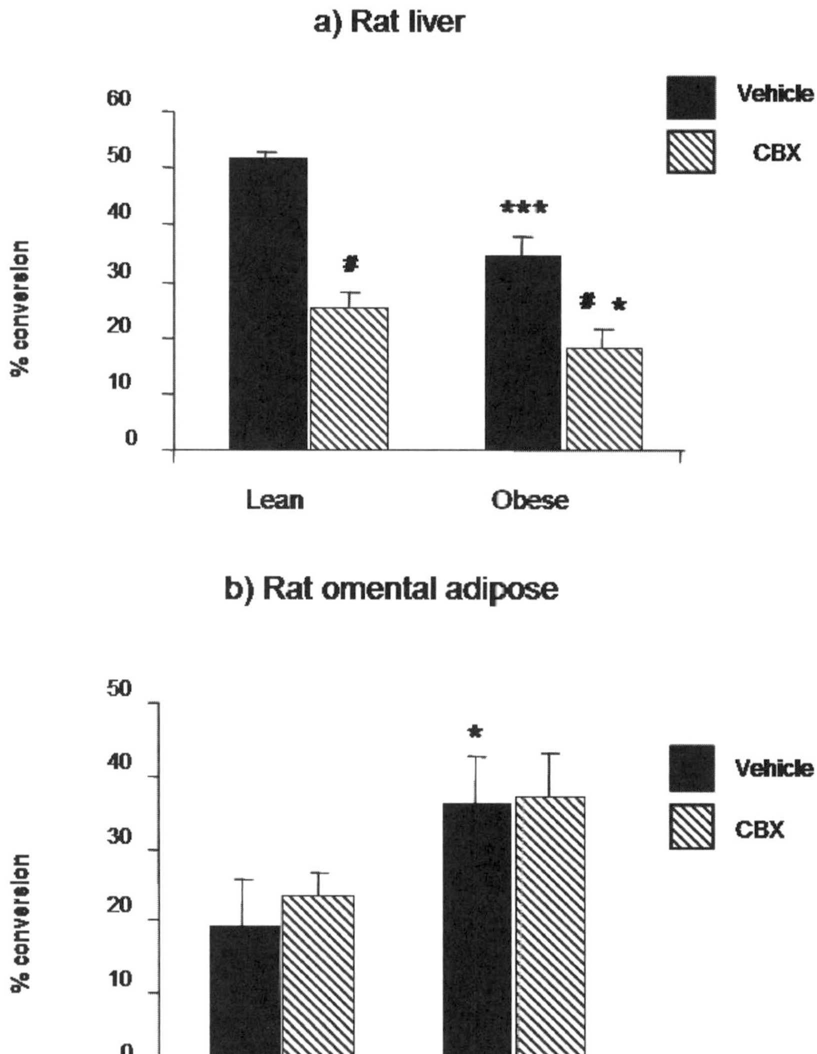

Fig. 10.4 Carbenoxolone inhibits 11β-HSD1 in the liver but not adipose tissue. (**a**) Carbenoxolone significantly inhibits hepatic 11β-HSD1 in both lean and obese Zucker rats. #, $p < 0.001$ compared with vehicle-treated group of the same phenotype. Obese Zucker rats have decreased hepatic 11β-HSD1 activity compared with lean Zucker rats. *, $p < 0.05$; ***, $p < 0.001$ compared with leans in the same treatment group. (**b**) Carbenoxolone does not inhibit 11β-HSD1 in omental adipose tissue in Zucker rats. Obese Zucker rats have increased 11β-HSD1 activity compared with lean Zucker rats. (**c**) Carbenoxolone inhibits conversion of cortisone to cortisol by hepatic 11β-HSD1 in humans. (**d**) Carbenoxolone does not inhibit cortisol generation by 11β-HSD1 in subcutaneous adipose tissue in obese humans, measured by tritiated cortisone infusion. *, $p < 0.05$ compared with carbenoxolone. CBX, carbenoxolone. (Adapted from Sandeep TC, et al. Increased in vivo regeneration of cortisol in adipose tissue in human obesity and effects of the 11beta-hydroxysteroid dehydrogenase type 1 inhibitor carbenoxolone. Diabetes 2005;54:872–879; and Livingstone DE, Walker BR. Is 11beta-hydroxysteroid dehydrogenase type 1 a therapeutic target? Effects of carbenoxolone in lean and obese Zucker rats. J Pharmacol Exp Ther 2003;305:167–172.).

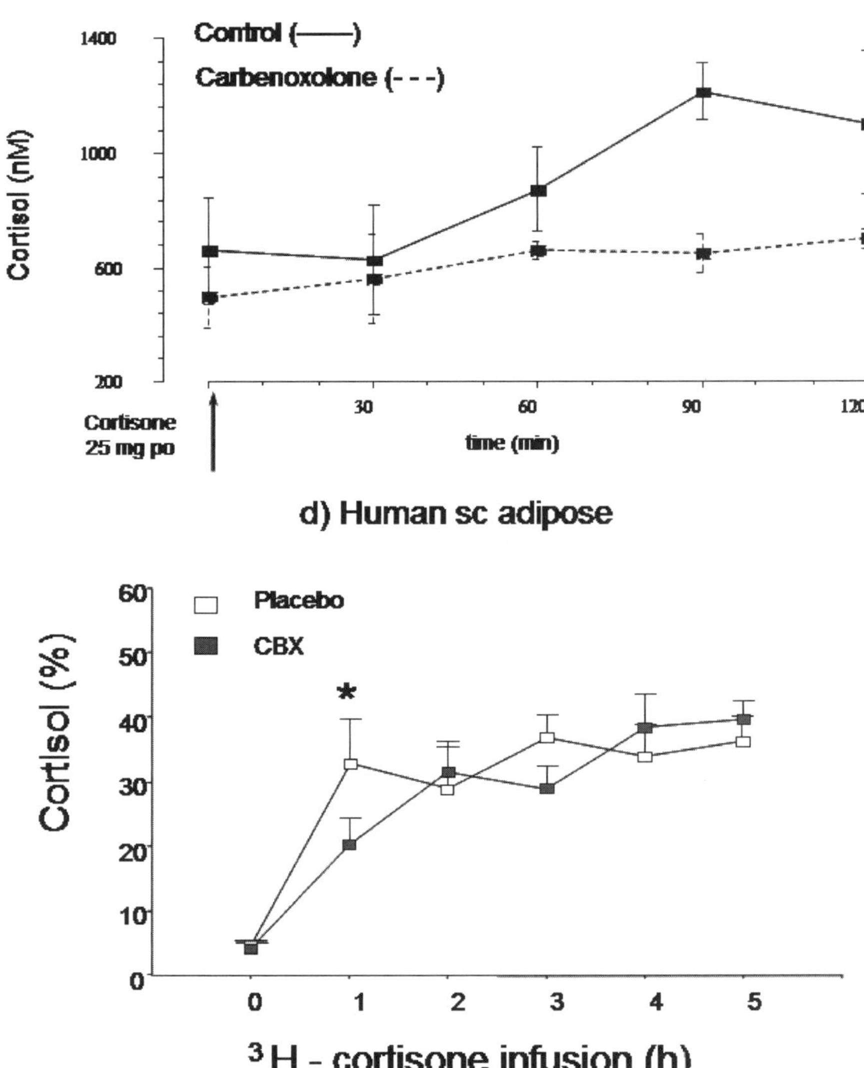

Fig. 10.4 Continued.

sensitivity has been shown to be improved by these drugs in rodents *(142)*. A number of other chemical classes of 11β-HSD1 inhibitors have been patented. The key test of the importance of altered 11β-HSD1 in human obesity will be the success or otherwise of these agents in limiting metabolic complications of obesity. Results of human studies are keenly awaited.

CONCLUSION

The 11β-HSD1 enzyme has been a focus of interest, especially since the transgenic model indicated that increased activity in adipose tissue can cause obesity and the metabolic syndrome. Human studies have discovered decreased and increased activity of 11β-HSD1 in the liver and subcutaneous adipose tissue, respectively, in obese individuals. 11β-HSD1 is known to be highly regulated by many factors, including diet. Theoretically, an individual's inability to downregulate this enzyme in our calorie-rich environment may be a key mechanism predisposing to obesity and the metabolic syndrome. In vivo work examining the plasticity of 11β-HSD1 will lead to better understanding of the important physiologic regulators of this enzyme and whether inhibition of 11β-HSD1 can protect against obesity. The introduction of specific 11β-HSD1 inhibitors in the near future will also test the metabolic benefits of decreasing tissue glucocorticoids, which could pave the way for new drug treatments of diabetes, heart disease, and obesity.

ACKNOWLEDGMENTS

This work was supported by grants from the British Heart Foundation and Wellcome Trust.

REFERENCES

1. Reaven G. Metabolic syndrome: pathophysiology and implications for management of cardiovascular disease. Circulation 2002; 106(3):286–288.
2. Welborn TA, Dhaliwal SS, Bennett SA. Waist-hip ratio is the dominant risk factor predicting cardiovascular death in Australia. Med J Aust 2003; 179(11–12):580–585.
3. Bjorntorp P. Visceral fat accumulation: the missing link between psychosocial factors and cardiovascular disease? J Intern Med 1991; 230:195–201.
4. Garrapa GG, Pantanetti P, Arnaldi G, Mantero F, Faloia E. Body composition and metabolic features in women with adrenal incidentaloma or Cushing's syndrome. J Clin Endocrinol Metab 2001; 86(11):5301–5306.
5. Wajchenberg BL, Bosco A, Marone MM et al. Estimation of body fat and lean tissue distribution by dual energy X-ray absorptiometry and abdominal body fat evaluation by computed tomography in Cushing's disease. J Clin Endocrinol Metab 1995; 80(9):2791–2794.
6. Rockall AG, Sohaib SA, Evans D et al. Computed tomography assessment of fat distribution in male and female patients with Cushing's syndrome. Eur J Endocrinol 2003; 149(6):561–567.
7. Pirlich M, Biering H, Gerl H et al. Loss of body cell mass in Cushing's syndrome: effect of treatment. J Clin Endocrinol Metab 2002; 87(3):1078–1084.
8. Lonn L, Kvist H, Ernest I, Sjostrom L. Changes in body composition and adipose tissue distribution after treatment of women with Cushing's syndrome. Metabolism 1994; 43(12):1517–1522.
9. Nieman LK, Chrousos GP, Kellwar C et al. Successful treatment of Cushing's syndrome with the glucocorticoid antagonist RU486. J Clin Endocrinol Metab 1985; 61:536–540.
10. Chu JW, Matthias DF, Belanoff J, Schatzberg A, Hoffman AR, Feldman D. Successful long-term treatment of refractory Cushing's disease with high-dose mifepristone (RU 486). J Clin Endocrinol Metab 2001; 86(8):3568–3573.
11. Lamers WH, Hanson RW, Meisner HM. cAMP stimulates transcription of the gene for cytosolic phosphoenolpyruvate carboxykinase in rat liver nuclei. Proc Natl Acad Sci U S A 1982; 79(17): 5137–5141.

12. Wang XL, Herzog B, Waltner-Law M, Hall RK, Shiota M, Granner DK. The synergistic effect of dexamethasone and all-trans-retinoic acid on hepatic phosphoenolpyruvate carboxykinase gene expression involves the coactivator p300. J Biol Chem 2004; 279(33):34191–34200.
13. Sasaki K, Cripe TP, Koch SR et al. Multihormonal regulation of phosphoenolpyruvate carboxykinase gene transcription. The dominant role of insulin. J Biol Chem 1984; 259(24):15242–15251.
14. Nechushtan H, Benvenisty N, Brandeis R, Reshef L. Glucocorticoids control phosphoenolpyruvate carboxykinase gene expression in a tissue specific manner. Nucleic Acids Res 1987; 15(16):6405–6417.
15. Meyuhas O, Reshef L, Ballard FJ, Hanson RW. Effect of Insulin and Glucocorticoids on Synthesis and Degradation of Phosphoenolpyruvate Carboxykinase (Gtp) in Rat Adipose-Tissue Cultured In Vitro. Biochem J 1976; 158(1):9–16.
16. Meyuhas O, Reshef L, Gunn JM, Hanson RW, Ballard FJ. Regulation of Phosphoenolpyruvate Carboxykinase (Gtp) in Adipose-Tissue In Vivo by Glucocorticoids and Insulin. Biochem J 1976; 158(1):1–7.
17. Reshef L, Ballard FJ, Hanson RW. The role of the adrenals in the regulation of phosphoenolpyruvate carboxykinase of rat adipose tissue. J Biol Chem 1969; 244(20):5577–5581.
18. Reaven GM, Hollenbeck C, Jeng CY, Wu MS, Chen YD. Measurement of plasma glucose, free fatty acid, lactate, and insulin for 24 h in patients with NIDDM. Diabetes 1988; 37(8):1020-1024.
19. Slavin BG, Ong JM, Kern PA. Hormonal regulation of hormone-sensitive lipase activity and mRNA levels in isolated rat adipocytes. J Lipid Res 1994; 35(9):1535–1541.
20. Hauner H, Schmid P, Pfeiffer EF. Glucocorticoids and insulin promote the differentiation of human adipocyte precursor cells into fat cells. J Clin Endocrinol Metab 1987; 64(4):832–835.
21. Hauner H, Entenmann G, Wabitsch M et al. Promoting effect of glucocorticoids on the differentiation of human adipocyte precursor cells cultured in a chemically defined medium. J Clin Invest 1989; 84(5):1663–1670.
22. Fried SK, Russell CD, Grauso NL, Brolin RE. Lipoprotein lipase regulation by insulin and glucocorticoid in subcutaneous and omental adipose tissues of obese women and men. J Clin Invest 1993; 92(5):2191-2198.
23. Rebuffe-Scrive M, Krotkiewski M, Elfverson J, Bjorntorp P. Muscle and adipose tissue morphology and metabolism in Cushing's syndrome. J Clin Endocrinol Metab 1988; 67(6):1122–1128.
24. Reynolds RM, Walker BR, Phillips DIW et al. Altered control of cortisol secretion in adult men with low birthweight and cardiovascular risk factors. J Clin Endocrinol Metab 2001; 86:245-250.
25. Filipovsky J, Ducimetiere P, Eschwege E, Richard JL, Rosselin G, Claude JR. The relationship of blood pressure with glucose, insulin, heart rate, free fatty acids and plasma cortisol levels according to degree of obesity in middle-aged men. J Hypertens 1996; 14:229–235.
26. Phillips DI, Barker DJ, Fall CH et al. Elevated plasma cortisol concentrations: a link between low birth weight and the insulin resistance syndrome? J Clin Endocrinol Metab 1998; 83(3):757-760.
27. Walker BR, Soderberg S, Lindahl B, Olsson T. Independent effects of obesity and cortisol in predicting cardiovascular risk factors in men and women. J Intern Med 2000; 247:198–204.
28. Phillips DIW, Walker BR, Reynolds RM et al. Low birthweight and elevated plasma cortisol concentrations in adults from three populations. Hypertension 2000; 35:1301–1306.
29. Stolk RP, Lamberts SWJ, de Jong FH, Pols HAP, Grobbee DE. Gender differences in the associations between cortisol and insulin sensitivity in healthy subjects. J Endocrinol 1996; 149:313–318.
30. Walker BR, Phillips DIW, Noon JP et al. Increased glucocorticoid activity in men with cardiovascular risk factors. Hypertension 1998; 31:891–895.
31. Andrews RC, Herlihy O, Livingstone DE, Andrew R, Walker BR. Abnormal cortisol metabolism and tissue sensitivity to cortisol in patients with glucose intolerance. J Clin Endocrinol Metab 2002; 87(12):5587–5593.
32. Reynolds RM, Syddall HE, Walker BR, Wood PJ, Phillips DI. Predicting cardiovascular risk factors from plasma cortisol measured during oral glucose tolerance tests. Metabolism 2003; 52(5):524–527.

33. Jessop DS, Dallman MF, Fleming D, Lightman SL. Resistance to glucocorticoid feedback in obesity. J Clin Endocrinol Metab 2001; 86(9):4109–4114.
34. Solano MP, Kumar M, Fernandez B, Jones L, Goldberg RB. The pituitary response to ovine corticotropin-releasing hormone is enhanced in obese men and correlates with insulin resistance. Horm Metab Res 2001; 33(1):39–43.
35. Hautanen A, Raikkonen K, Adlercreutz H. Associations between pituitary-adrenocortical function and abdominal obesity, hyperinsulinaemia and dyslipidaemia in normotensive males. J Intern Med 1997; 241(6):451–461.
36. Strain GW, Zumoff B, Kream J, Strain JJ, Levin J, Fukushima D. Sex difference in the influence of obesity on the 24 hr mean plasma concentration of cortisol. Metabolism 1982; 31:209–212.
37. Phillips DI, Walker BR, Reynolds RM et al. Low birth weight predicts elevated plasma cortisol concentrations in adults from 3 populations. Hypertension 2000; 35(6):1301–1306.
38. Rask E, Walker BR, Soderberg S et al. Tissue-specific changes in peripheral cortisol metabolism in obese women: increased adipose 11beta-hydroxysteroid dehydrogenase type 1 activity. J Clin Endocrinol Metab 2002; 87(7):3330–3336.
39. Pasquali R, Cantobelli S, Casimirri F et al. The hypothalamic-pituitary-adrenal axis in obese women with different patterns of body fat distribution. J Clin Endocrinol Metab 1993; 77:341–346.
40. Weaver JU, Kopelman PG, McLoughlin L, Forsling ML, Grossman A. Hyperactivity of the hypothalamo-pituitary-adrenal axis in obesity: a study of ACTH, AVP, -lipotrophin and cortisol responses to insulin-induced hypoglycaemia. Clin Endocrinol 1993; 39:345–350.
41. Yanovski JA, Yanovski SZ, Gold PW, Chrousos GP. Differences in corticotropin-releasing hormone-stimulated adrenocorticotropin and cortisol before and after weight loss. J Clin Endocrinol Metab 1997; 82(6):1874–1878.
42. Kopelman PG, Grossman A, Lavender P, Besser GM, Rees LH, Coy D. The cortisol response to corticotrophin-releasing factor is blunted in obesity. Clin Endocrinol (Oxf) 1988; 28(1):15–18.
43. Rask E, Olsson T, Soderberg S et al. Tissue-specific dysregulation of cortisol metabolism in human obesity. J Clin Endocrinol Metab 2001; 86(3):1418–1421.
44. Westerbacka J, Yki-Jarvinen H, Vehkavaara S et al. Body fat distribution and cortisol metabolism in healthy men: enhanced 5beta-reductase and lower cortisol/cortisone metabolite ratios in men with fatty liver. J Clin Endocrinol Metab 2003; 88(10):4924–4931.
45. Andrew R, Phillips DIW, Walker BR. Obesity and gender influence cortisol secretion and metabolism in man. J Clin Endocrinol Metab 1998; 83:1806–1809.
46. Rusvai E, Naray-Fejes-Toth A. A new isoform of 11β-hydroxysteroid dehydrogenase in aldosterone target cells. J Biol Chem 1993; 268:10717–10720.
47. Brown RW, Chapman KE, Edwards CRW, Seckl JR. Human placental 11β-hydroxysteroid dehydrogenase: evidence for and partial purification of a distinct NAD-dependent isoform. Endocrinology 1993; 132:2614–2621.
48. Edwards CRW, Stewart PM, Burt D et al. Localisation of 11β-hydroxysteroid dehydrogenase- tissue specific protector of the mineralocorticoid receptor. Lancet 1988; ii:986–989.
49. Funder JW, Pearce PT, Smith R, Smith AI. Mineralocorticoid action: target tissue specificity is enzyme, not receptor mediated. Science 1988; 242:583–585.
50. Ulick S, Levine LS, Gunczler P et al. A syndrome of apparent mineralocorticoid excess associated with defects in the peripheral metabolism of cortisol. J Clin Endocrinol Metab 1979; 49:757–764.
51. Lakshmi V, Monder C. Purification and characterization of the corticosteroid 11β-dehydrogenase component of the rat liver 11β-hydroxysteroid dehydrogenase complex. Endocrinology 1988; 123:2390–2398.
52. Hundertmark S, Buhler H, Ragosch V et al. Correlation of surfactant phosphatidylcholine synthesis and 11beta- hydroxysteroid dehydrogenase in the fetal lung. Endocrinology 1995; 136(6):2573–2578.

53. Low SC, Chapman KE, Edwards CRW, Seckl JR. 'Liver-type' 11β-hydroxysteroid dehydrogenase cDNA encodes reductase but not dehydrogenase activity in intact mammalian COS-7 cells. J Mol Endocrinol 1994; 13:167–174.
54. Jamieson PM, Chapman KE, Edwards CRW, Seckl JR. 11β-Hydroxysteroid dehydrogenase is an exclusive 11β-reductase in primary cultures of rat hepatocytes: effect of physicochemical and hormonal manipulations. Endocrinology 1995; 136:4754–4761.
55. Ozols J. Lumenal orientation and post-translational modifications of the liver microsomal 11beta-hydroxysteroid dehydrogenase. J Biol Chem 1995; 270(5):2305–2312.
56. Atanasov AG, Nashev LG, Schweizer RA, Frick C, Odermatt A. Hexose-6-phosphate dehydrogenase determines the reaction direction of 11beta-hydroxysteroid dehydrogenase type 1 as an oxoreductase. FEBS Lett 2004; 571(1-3):129–133.
57. Walker BR, Connacher AA, Lindsay RM, Webb DJ, Edwards CRW. Carbenoxolone increases hepatic insulin sensitivity in man: a novel role for 11-oxosteroid reductase in enhancing glucocorticoid receptor activation. J Clin Endocrinol Metab 1995; 80:3155–3159.
58. Bujalska IJ, Kumar S, Stewart PM. Does central obesity reflect 'Cushing's disease of the omentum'? Lancet 1997; 349:1210–1213.
59. Masuzaki H, Paterson J, Shinyama H et al. A transgenic model of visceral obesity and the metabolic syndrome. Science 2001; 294:2166–2170.
60. Masuzaki H, Yamamoto H, Kenyon CJ et al. Transgenic amplification of glucocorticoid action in adipose tissue causes high blood pressure in mice. J Clin Invest 2003; 112(1):83–90.
61. Paterson JM, Morton NM, Fievet C et al. Metabolic syndrome without obesity: Hepatic overexpression of 11beta-hydroxysteroid dehydrogenase type 1 in transgenic mice. Proc Natl Acad Sci U S A 2004; 101(18):7088–7093.
62. Kotelevtsev YV, Holmes MC, Burchell A et al. 11β-Hydroxysteroid dehydrogenase type 1 knockout mice show attenuated glucocorticoid inducible responses and resist hyperglycaemia on obesity and stress. Proc Natnl Acad Sci USA 1997; 94:14924–14929.
63. Morton NM, Paterson JM, Masuzaki H et al. Novel adipose tissue-mediated resistance to diet-induced visceral obesity in 11β-hydroxysteroid dehydrogenase type 1-deficient mice. Diabetes 2004; 53(4):931-938.
64. Morton NM, Holmes MC, Fievet C et al. Improved lipid and lipoprotein profile, hepatic insulin sensitivity, and glucose tolerance in 11β-hydroxysteroid dehydrogenase type 1 null mice. J Biol Chem 2001; 276:41293–41300.
65. Yau JLW, Noble JM, Kenyon CJ et al. Lack of tissue glucocorticoid reactivation in 11β-hydroxysteroid dehydrogenase type 1 knockout mice ameliorates age-related learning impairments. Proc Natnl Acad Sci USA 2001; 98:4716–4721.
66. Palermo M, Shackleton CHL, Mantero F, Stewart PM. Urinary free cortisone and the assessment of 11beta- hydroxysteroid dehydrogenase activity in man. Clin Endocrinol (Oxf) 1996; 45:605–611.
67. Fraser R, Ingram MC, Anderson NH, Morrison C, Davies E, Connell JMC. Cortisol effects on body mass, blood pressure, and cholesterol in the general population. Hypertension 1999; 33:1364–1368.
68. Andrew R, Gale CR, Walker BR, Seckl JR, Martyn CN. Glucocorticoid metabolism and the Metabolic Syndrome: associations in an elderly cohort. Exp Clin Endocrinol Diabetes 2002; 110(6):284–290.
69. Dimitriou T, Maser-Gluth C, Remer T. Adrenocortical activity in healthy children is associated with fat mass. Am J Clin Nutr 2003; 77(3):731–736.
70. Stewart PM, Boulton A, Kumar S, Clark PMS, Shackleton CHL. Cortisol metabolism in human obesity: impaired cortisone - cortisol conversion in subjects with central adiposity. J Clin Endocrinol Metab 1999; 84:1022–1027.
71. Valsamakis G, Anwar A, Tomlinson JW et al. 11beta-hydroxysteroid dehydrogenase type 1 activity in lean and obese males with type 2 diabetes mellitus. J Clin Endocrinol Metab 2004; 89(9):4755–4761.

72. Kerstens MN, Riemens SC, Sluiter WJ, Pratt JJ, Wolthers BG, Dullaart RP. Lack of relationship between 11beta-hydroxysteroid dehydrogenase setpoint and insulin sensitivity in the basal state and after 24h of insulin infusion in healthy subjects and type 2 diabetic patients. Clin Endocrinol (Oxf) 2000; 52(4):403–411.
73. Raven PW, Taylor NF. Sex differences in the human metabolism of cortisol. Endocrine Research 1996; 22:751–755.
74. Toogood AA, Taylor NF, Shalet SM, Monson JP. Sexual dimorphism of cortisol metabolism is maintained in elderly subjects and is not oestrogen dependent. Clin Endocrinol (Oxf) 2000; 52(1):61–66.
75. Finken MJJ, Andrews RC, Andrew R, Walker BR. Cortisol metabolism in healthy young adults: sexual dimorphism in activities of A-ring reductase but not 11β-hydroxysteroid dehydrogenases. J Clin Endocrinol Metab 1999; 84:3316–3321.
76. Andrew R, Smith K, Jones GC, Walker BR. Distinguishing the activities of 11beta-hydroxysteroid dehydrogenases in vivo using isotopically labeled cortisol. J Clin Endocrinol Metab 2002; 87(1): 277–285.
77. Sandeep TC, Andrew R, Homer NZ, Andrews RC, Smith K, Walker BR. Increased in vivo regeneration of cortisol in adipose tissue in human obesity and effects of the 11beta-hydroxysteroid dehydrogenase type 1 inhibitor carbenoxolone. Diabetes 2005; 54(3):872–879.
78. Livingstone DEW, Jones GC, Smith K, Andrew R, Kenyon CJ, Walker BR. Understanding the role of glucocorticoids in obesity: tissue-specific alterations of corticosterone metabolism in obese Zucker rats. Endocrinology 2000; 141:560–563.
79. Lindsay RS, Wake DJ, Nair S et al. Subcutaneous adipose 11 beta-hydroxysteroid dehydrogenase type 1 activity and messenger ribonucleic acid levels are associated with adiposity and insulinemia in Pima Indians and Caucasians. J Clin Endocrinol Metab 2003; 88(6):2738–2744.
80. Wake DJ, Rask E, Livingstone DE, Soderberg S, Olsson T, Walker BR. Local and systemic impact of transcriptional up-regulation of 11beta-hydroxysteroid dehydrogenase type 1 in adipose tissue in human obesity. J Clin Endocrinol Metab 2003; 88(8):3983–3988.
81. Kannisto K, Pietilainen KH, Ehrenborg E et al. Overexpression of 11beta-hydroxysteroid dehydrogenase-1 in adipose tissue is associated with acquired obesity and features of insulin resistance: studies in young adult monozygotic twins. J Clin Endocrinol Metab 2004; 89(9):4414–4421.
82. Nair S, Lee YH, Lindsay RS et al. 11beta-Hydroxysteroid dehydrogenase Type 1: genetic polymorphisms are associated with Type 2 diabetes in Pima Indians independently of obesity and expression in adipocyte and muscle. Diabetologia 2004; 47(6):1088–1095.
83. Paulmyer-Lacroix O, Boullu S, Oliver C, Alessi MC, Grino M. Expression of the mRNA coding for 11beta-hydroxysteroid dehydrogenase type 1 in adipose tissue from obese patients: an in situ hybridization study. J Clin Endocrinol Metab 2002; 87(6):2701–2705.
84. Engeli S, Bohnke J, Feldpausch M et al. Regulation of 11beta-HSD genes in human adipose tissue: influence of central obesity and weight loss. Obes Res 2004; 12(1):9–17.
85. Tomlinson JW, Sinha B, Bujalska I, Hewison M, Stewart PM. Expression of 11beta-hydroxysteroid dehydrogenase type 1 in adipose tissue is not increased in human obesity. J Clin Endocrinol Metab 2002; 87(12):5630–5635.
86. Tomlinson JW, Walker EA, Bujalska IJ et al. 11beta-hydroxysteroid dehydrogenase type 1: a tissue-specific regulator of glucocorticoid response. Endocr Rev 2004; 25(5):831–866.
87. Katz JR, Mohamed-Ali V, Wood PJ, Yudkin JS, Coppack SW. An in vivo study of the cortisol-cortisone shuttle in subcutaneous abdominal adipose tissue. Clin Endocrinol 1999; 50:63–68.
88. Bujalska IJ, Kumar S, Hewison M, Stewart PM. Differentiation of adipose stromal cells: The roles of glucocorticoids and 11beta-hydroxysteroid dehydrogenase. Endocrinology 1999; 140(7):3188–3196.
89. Aldhahi W, Mun E, Goldfine AB. Portal and peripheral cortisol levels in obese humans. Diabetologia 2004; 47(5):833–836.

90. Basu R, Singh RJ, Basu A et al. Splanchnic cortisol production occurs in humans: evidence for conversion of cortisone to cortisol via the 11-beta hydroxysteroid dehydrogenase (11beta-hsd) type 1 pathway. Diabetes 2004; 53(8):2051–2059.
91. Andrew R, Westerbacka J, Wahren J, Yki-Jarvinen H, Walker BR. The contribution of visceral adipose tissue to splanchnic cortisol production in healthy humans. Diabetes 2005; 54(5):1364–1370.
92. Whorwood CB, Donovan SJ, Wood PJ, Phillips DI. Regulation of glucocorticoid receptor alpha and beta isoforms and type I 11beta-hydroxysteroid dehydrogenase expression in human skeletal muscle cells: a key role in the pathogenesis of insulin resistance? J Clin Endocrinol Metab 2001; 86(5):2296–2308.
93. Whorwood CB, Donovan SJ, Flanagan D, Phillips DI, Byrne CD. Increased glucocorticoid receptor expression in human skeletal muscle cells may contribute to the pathogenesis of the metabolic syndrome. Diabetes 2002; 51(4):1066–1075.
94. Stewart PM, Shackleton CHL, Beastall GH, Edwards CRW. 5alpha-reductase activity in polycystic ovarian syndrome. Lancet 1990; 335:431–433.
95. Rodin A, Thakkar H, Taylor N, Clayton R. Hyperandrogenism in polycystic ovary syndrome: evidence of dysregulation of 11beta-hydroxysteroid dehydrogenase. N Engl J Med 1994; 330:460–465.
96. Tsilchorozidou T, Honour JW, Conway GS. Altered cortisol metabolism in polycystic ovary syndrome: insulin enhances 5alpha-reduction but not the elevated adrenal steroid production rates. J Clin Endocrinol Metab 2003; 88(12):5907–5913.
97. Walker BR, Rodin A, Taylor NF, Clayton RN. Endogenous inhibitors of 11β-hydroxysteroid dehyrogenase type 1 do not explain abnormal cortisol metabolism in polycystic ovarian syndrome. Clin Endocrinol 2000; 52:77–80.
98. Miller KK, Daly PA, Sentochnik D et al. Pseudo-Cushing's syndrome in human immunodeficiency virus-infected patients. Clin Infect Dis 1998; 27(1):68–72.
99. Sutinen J, Kannisto K, Korsheninnikova E et al. In the lipodystrophy associated with highly active antiretroviral therapy, pseudo-Cushing's syndrome is associated with increased regeneration of cortisol by 11beta-hydroxysteroid dehydrogenase type 1 in adipose tissue. Diabetologia 2004; 47(10):1668–1671.
100. Tomlinson JW, Moore J, Cooper MS et al. Regulation of expression of 11β-hydroxysteroid dehydrogenase type 1 in adipose tissue: tissue-specific induction by cytokines. Endocrinology 2001; 142:1982–1989.
101. Weaver JU, Monson JP, Noonan K et al. The effect of low dose recombinant human growth hormone replacement on regional fat distribution, insulin sensitivity, and cardiovascular risk factors in hypopituitary adults. J Clin Endocrinol Metab 1995; 80:153–159.
102. Moore JS, Monson JP, Kaltsas G et al. Modulation of 11β-hydroxysteroid dehydrogenase isozymes by growth hormone and insulin-like growth factor: in vivo and in vitro studies. J Clin Endocrinol Metab 1999; 84:4172–4177.
103. Trainer PJ, Drake WM, Perry LA, Taylor NF, Besser GM, Monson JP. Modulation of cortisol metabolism by the growth hormone receptor antagonist pegvisomant in patients with acromegaly. J Clin Endocrinol Metab 2001; 86(7):2989–2992.
104. Tiosano D, Eisentein I, Militianu D, Chrousos GP, Hochberg Z. 11 beta-Hydroxysteroid dehydrogenase activity in hypothalamic obesity. J Clin Endocrinol Metab 2003; 88(1):379–384.
105. Weaver JU, Thaventhiran L, Noonan K et al. The effect of growth hormone replacement on cortisol metabolism and glucocorticoid sensitivity in hypopituitary adults. Clin Endocrinol (Oxf) 1994; 41:639–648.
106. Toogood AA, Taylor NF, Shalet SM, Monson JP. Modulation of cortisol metabolism by low-dose growth hormone replacement in elderly hypopituitary patients. Journal of Clinical Endocrinology & Metabolism 2000; 85(4):1727–1730.

107. Gelding SV, Taylor NF, Wood PJ et al. The effect of growth hormone replacement therapy on cortisol-cortisone interconversion in hypopituitary adults: Evidence for growth hormone modulation of extrarenal 11beta-hydroxysteroid dehydrogenase activity. Clin Endocrinol (Oxf) 1998; 48(2):153–162.
108. Swords FM, Carroll PV, Kisalu J, Wood PJ, Taylor NF, Monson JP. The effects of growth hormone deficiency and replacement on glucocorticoid exposure in hypopituitary patients on cortisone acetate and hydrocortisone replacement. Clin Endocrinol (Oxf) 2003; 59(5):613–620.
109. Walker BR, Andrew R, MacLeod KM, Padfield PL. Growth hormone replacement inhibits renal and hepatic 11β-hydroxysteroid dehydrogenases in ACTH-deficient patients. Clin Endocrinol 1998; 49:257–263.
110. Weaver JU, Taylor NF, Monson JP, Wood PJ, Kelly WF. Sexual dimorphism in 11 beta hydroxysteroid dehydrogenase activity and its relation to fat distribution and insulin sensitivity; a study in hypopituitary subjects. Clin Endocrinol (Oxf) 1998; 49(1):13–20.
111. Frajese GV, Taylor NF, Jenkins PJ, Besser GM, Monson JP. Modulation of cortisol metabolism during treatment of acromegaly is independent of body composition and insulin sensitivity. Horm Res 2004; 61(5):246–251.
112. Tomlinson JW, Crabtree N, Clark PM et al. Low-dose growth hormone inhibits 11 beta-hydroxysteroid dehydrogenase type 1 but has no effect upon fat mass in patients with simple obesity. J Clin Endocrinol Metab 2003; 88(5):2113–2118.
113. Tomlinson JW, Moore JS, Clark PM, Holder G, Shakespeare L, Stewart PM. Weight loss increases 11beta-hydroxysteroid dehydrogenase type 1 expression in human adipose tissue. J Clin Endocrinol Metab 2004; 89(6):2711–2716.
114. Morton NM, Ramage L, Seckl JR. Down-regulation of adipose 11beta-hydroxysteroid dehydrogenase type 1 by high-fat feeding in mice: a potential adaptive mechanism counteracting metabolic disease. Endocrinology 2004; 145(6):2707–2712.
115. Drake AJ, Livingstone DE, Andrew R, Seckl JR, Morton NM, Walker BR. Reduced adipose glucocorticoid reactivation and increased hepatic glucocorticoid clearance as an early adaptation to high-fat feeding in Wistar rats. Endocrinology 2005; 146(2):913–919.
116. Johnstone AM, Faber P, Andrew R et al. Influence of short-term dietary weight loss on cortisol secretion and metabolism in obese men. Eur J Endocrinol 2004; 150(2):185–194.
117. Friedberg M, Zoumakis E, Hiroi N, Bader T, Chrousos GP, Hochberg Z. Modulation of 11 beta-hydroxysteroid dehydrogenase type 1 in mature human subcutaneous adipocytes by hypothalamic messengers. J Clin Endocrinol Metab 2003; 88(1):385–393.
118. Handoko K, Yang K, Strutt B, Khalil W, Killinger D. Insulin attenuates the stimulatory effects of tumor necrosis factor alpha on 11beta-hydroxysteroid dehydrogenase 1 in human adipose stromal cells. Journal of Steroid Biochemistry & Molecular Biology 2000; 72(3-4):163–168.
119. Berger J, Tanen M, Elbrecht A et al. Peroxisome proliferator-activated receptor-γ ligands inhibit adipocyte 11β-hydroxysteroid dehydrogenase type 1 expression and activity. J Biol Chem 2001; 276:12629–12635.
120. Bogacka I, Xie H, Bray GA, Smith SR. The effect of pioglitazone on peroxisome proliferator-activated receptor-gamma target genes related to lipid storage in vivo. Diabetes Care 2004; 27(7):1660–1667.
121. Tannin GM, Agarwal AK, Monder C, New MI, White PC. The human gene for 11β-hydroxysteroid dehydrogenase. J Biol Chem 1991; 266:16653–16658.
122. Draper N, Echwald SM, Lavery GG et al. Association studies between microsatellite markers within the gene encoding human 11beta-hydroxysteroid dehydrogenase type 1 and body mass index, waist to hip ratio, and glucocorticoid metabolism. J Clin Endocrinol Metab 2002; 87(11):4984–4990.
123. de Quervain DJ, Poirier R, Wollmer MA et al. Glucocorticoid-related genetic susceptibility for Alzheimer's disease. Hum Mol Genet 2004; 13(1):47–52.
124. Caramelli E, Strippoli P, Di Giacomi T, Tietz C, Carinci P, Pasquali R. Lack of mutations of type 1 11beta-hydroxysteroid dehydrogenase gene in patients with abdominal obesity. Endocr Res 2001; 27(1–2):47–61.

125. Robitaille J, Brouillette C, Houde A, Despres JP, Tchernof A, Vohl MC. Molecular screening of the 11beta-HSD1 gene in men characterized by the metabolic syndrome. Obes Res 2004; 12(10):1570–1575.
126. Franks PW, Knowler WC, Nair S et al. Interaction between an 11betaHSD1 gene variant and birth era modifies the risk of hypertension in Pima Indians. Hypertension 2004; 44(5):681–688.
127. Gelernter-Yaniv L, Feng N, Sebring NG, Hochberg Z, Yanovski JA. Associations between a polymorphism in the 11 beta hydroxysteroid dehydrogenase type I gene and body composition. Int J Obes Relat Metab Disord 2003; 27(8):983–986.
128. Taylor NF, Bartlett WA, Dawson DJ, Enoch BA. Cortisone reductase deficiency: evidence for a new inborn error in metabolism of adrenal steroids. J Endocrinol 1984; 102 (Suppl):90.
129. Phillipov G, Palermo M, Shackleton CH. Apparent cortisone reductase deficiency: a unique form of hypercortisolism. J Clin Endocrinol Metab 1996;81:3855—3860.
130. Jamieson A, Wallace AM, Walker BR et al. Apparent cortisone reductase deficiency: a functional defect in 11β-hydroxysteroid dehydrogenase type 1. J Clin Endocrinol Metab 1999; 84:3570–3574.
131. Biason-Lauber A, Suter SL, Shackleton CH, Zachmann M. Apparent cortisone reductase deficiency: a rare cause of hyperandrogenemia and hypercortisolism. Horm Res 2000; 53(5):260–266.
132. Nikkila H, Tannin GM, New MI et al. Defects in the HSD11 gene encoding 11β-hydroxysteroid dehydrogenase are not found in patients with apparent mineralocorticoid excess or 11-oxoreductase deficiency. J Clin Endocrinol Metab 1993; 77:687–691.
133. Malunowicz EM, Romer TE, Urban M, Bossowski A. 11beta-hydroxysteroid dehydrogenase type 1 deficiency ('apparent cortisone reductase deficiency') in a 6-year-old boy. Horm Res 2003; 59(4):205–210.
134. Nordenstrom A, Marcus C, Axelson M, Wedell A, Ritzen EM. Failure of cortisone acetate treatment in congenital adrenal hyperplasia because of defective 11beta-hydroxysteroid dehydrogenase reductase activity. J Clin Endocrinol Metab 1999; 84(4):1210–1213.
135. Draper N, Walker EA, Bujalska IJ et al. Mutations in the genes encoding 11beta-hydroxysteroid dehydrogenase type 1 and hexose-6-phosphate dehydrogenase interact to cause cortisone reductase deficiency. Nat Genet 2003; 34(4):434–439.
136. Millan JL, Botella-Carretero JI, Alvarez-Blasco F et al. A study of the Hexose-6-Phosphate Dehydrogenase Gene R453Q and 11{beta}-Hydroxysteroid Dehydrogenase Type 1 Gene 83557insA Polymorphisms in the Polycystic Ovary Syndrome. J Clin Endocrinol Metab 2005.
137. Stewart PM, Wallace AM, Atherden SM, Shearing CH, Edwards CRW. Mineralocorticoid activity of carbenoxolone: contrasting effects of carbenoxolone and liquorice on 11β-hydroxysteroid dehydrogenase activity in man. Clin Sci 1990; 78:49–54.
138. Andrews RC, Rooyackers O, Walker BR. Effects of the 11 beta-hydroxysteroid dehydrogenase inhibitor carbenoxolone on insulin sensitivity in men with type 2 diabetes. J Clin Endocrinol Metab 2003; 88(1):285–291.
139. Sandeep TC, Yau JL, MacLullich AM et al. 11Beta-hydroxysteroid dehydrogenase inhibition improves cognitive function in healthy elderly men and type 2 diabetics. Proc Natl Acad Sci U S A 2004; 101(17):6734–6739.
140. Livingstone DE, Walker BR. Is 11beta-hydroxysteroid dehydrogenase type 1 a therapeutic target? Effects of carbenoxolone in lean and obese Zucker rats. J Pharmacol Exp Ther 2003; 305(1):167–172.
141. Barf T, Vallgarda J, Emond R et al. Arylsulfonamidothiazoles as a new class of potential antidiabetic drugs. Discovery of potent and selective inhibitors of the 11beta-hydroxysteroid dehydrogenase type 1. J Med Chem 2002; 45(18):3813–3815.
142. Alberts P, Nilsson C, Selen G et al. Selective inhibition of 11 beta-hydroxysteroid dehydrogenase type 1 improves hepatic insulin sensitivity in hyperglycemic mice strains. Endocrinology 2003; 144(11):4755–4762.

11 Prader-Willi Syndrome: A Model of Disordered Energy Homeostasis

Andrea Haqq

CONTENTS

Key Words: energy homeostasis, etiology, growth hormone deficiency, Prader-Willi syndrome, sleep and respiratory abnormalities.

INTRODUCTION

Prader-Willi syndrome (PWS) was originally described by Andrea Prader, Alexis Labhart, and Heinrich Willi in 1956 *(1)*. It is a genetic disorder that occurs in both sexes and all races and occurs with a frequency of approximately 1 in 10,000 to 1 in 15, 000 live births *(2)*. It is one of the most commonly recognized genetic obesity syndromes. Hypothalamic dysfunction is proposed to be the basis for many of the characteristic features of this disorder, including deficient growth hormone (GH) secretion, short stature, insatiable hunger, morbid obesity, hypogonadism, aberrant body temperature control, and sleep disturbances *(3)*. Autonomic nervous system dysfunction is thought to be responsible for these individuals' thick, viscous saliva, high pain threshold, skin picking, and high threshold for vomiting *(4)*. In the newborn period, PWS individuals suffer from significant hypotonia, poor suck, decreased arousal, and failure to thrive and often require tube feedings for several weeks to months. This is followed in childhood by progressive obesity by 1 to 6 years of age, insatiable appetite, short stature, further delayed motor and cognitive development, behavioral difficulties, and

From: *Contemporary Endocrinology: Energy Metabolism and Obesity: Research and Clinical Applications*
Edited by: P. A. Donohoue © Humana Press Inc., Totowa, NJ

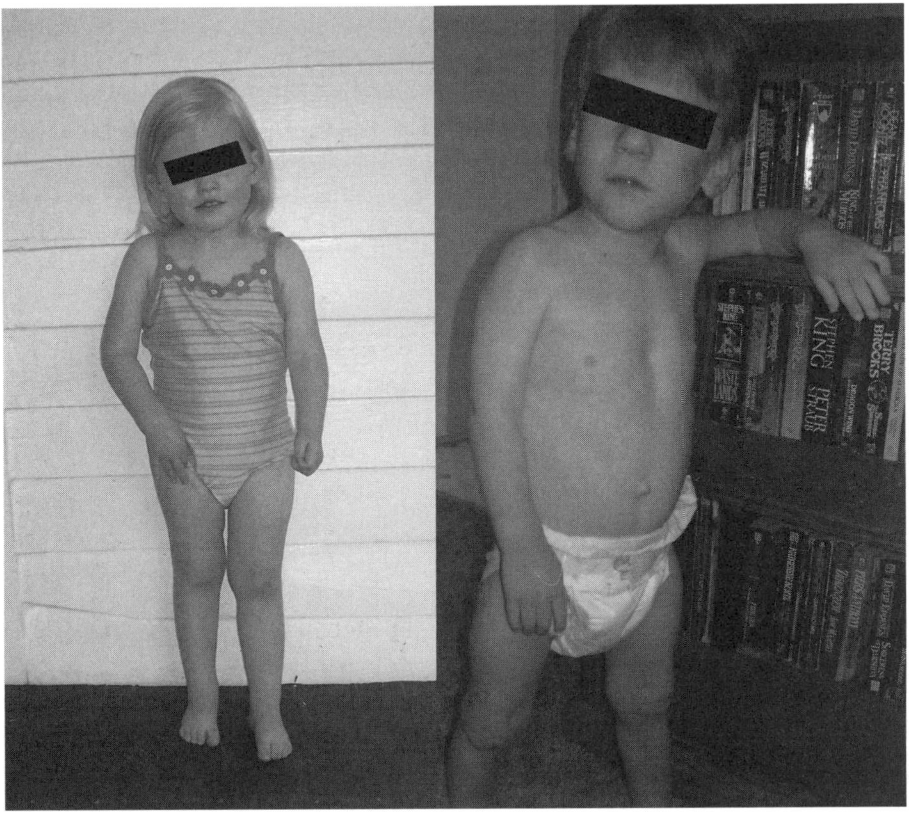

Fig. 11.1 Typical physical features of PWS appearing in a $2\frac{1}{2}$-year-old girl and a 2-year-old boy with PWS. (*see* Color Plate 4)

sleep disturbances. A photograph illustrating the typical physical features of this disorder in infancy and childhood is shown in Figure 11.1. A characteristic facial appearance may be noted including narrow bifrontal diameter, almond-shaped palpebral fissures, and down-turned mouth with a thin upper lip. Small, narrow hands with a straight ulnar border and tapering fingers, and short, broad feet are typical in Caucasians with this disorder. African-American individuals often have normal hand and foot size *(5)*. A characteristic body habitus is also present from toddlerhood, including sloping shoulders, heavy midsection, and genu valgus. One third of PWS individuals are also fairer compared with their family of origin; they have lighter skin, hair, and eye color. Additional common features include strabismus, scoliosis, and/or kyphosis.

ETIOLOGY: GENETICS OF PRADER-WILLI SYNDROME

PWS is due to lack of expression of paternally derived genes on chromosome 15q11-q13 *(6)*. The genes within this area of the chromosome are imprinted. Imprinted genes are modified in different ways depending on the gender of the parent from whom they were inherited. Therefore, the expression of the genes is dependent on the parent-of-origin. The majority of PWS cases (~70%) are due to deletions spanning 4 to 4.5 Mb of the paternal 15q11-q13. The next most common cause of PWS is maternal uniparental disomy (UPD) (20–30%), which is due to maternal meiotic nondisjunction, followed by mitotic loss of a single paternal chromosome 15 postzygotically. PWS caused by deletions or UPD does not recur. Finally, two types of imprinting defects occur in ~5% of cases: in one case there is a submicroscopic deletion of a genetic element called the imprinting center (IC), and in the other case, there is an abnormal imprint but no detectable mutation *(7, 8)*. All of the families studied in which there has been a recurrence of PWS have demonstrated a mutation in the imprinting center. There is an up-to-50% risk of recurrence in these cases, and prenatal diagnosis may be possible *(9)*. Balanced translocations are a rare cause of PWS (0.1%); most of these translocations disrupt the *SNURF-SNRPN* gene. In general, those individuals with UPD or IC defects have a milder phenotype than those with deletions *(2)*. See Figure 11.2 for an illustration of the human chromosome 15q11-13 region.

The exact gene(s) responsible for PWS is not known. However, the *SNURF-SNRPN* gene is one major candidate gene that may play a role in causing PWS. This gene locus is very complex, spanning ~465 kb and consisting of >148 exons, which can undergo alternative splicing *(10)*. This locus encodes a minimum of four functions, including elements of the *cis*-acting regulatory region called the imprinting center (IC), two independent proteins (SmN, a core spliceosomal protein; and SNURF protein, which may regulate SmN or the imprinting process), and a small nucleolar RNA (snoRNA). Several additional paternally expressed imprinted genes have been identified in 15q11-13 including NDN (encoding NECDIN protein) and MAGEL2 (MAGE-like2) and MKRN3 (Makorin 3). Recently, additional genes and transcripts have been identified in this region, but their involvement in the etiology of PWS is unknown. Detailed neuroanatomic mapping of these RNA and proteins has not been completed with the exception of NDN and MAGEL2 *(11–13)*. Except for the function of NDN in neural differentiation and survival, the functions of these genes are poorly understood *(14)*. One recent report describes gene expression studies of a novel translocation t(4;15)(q27;q11.2) associated with PWS and concludes that the

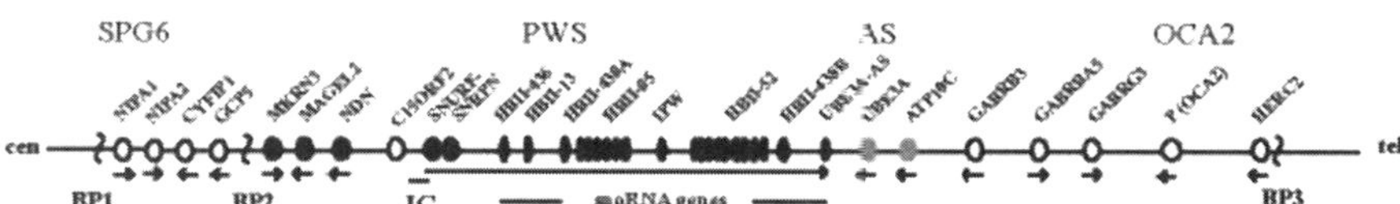

Fig. 11.2 Genetic structure of human chromosome 15q11-q13. The human ~5 Mb 15q11-q13 region flanked by PWS/AS common deletion breakpoints (BP, zig-zag lines) is shown. Symbols: *circles*, protein-coding genes; *ovals*, RNA-coding genes; *black*, paternally expressed; *gray*, maternally expressed; *white*, biparentally expressed; *line arrows*, transcriptional orientation of genes. IC, imprinting center; OCA2, oculocutaneous albinism type II; SPG6, spastic paraplegia type 6; cen, centromere; tel, telomere. The *HBII-85* and *HBII-52* snoRNAs are repeated 24 and 47 times, respectively *(181)*. (Modified from Stefan M, Portis T, Longnecker R, Nicholls RD. A nonimprinted Prader-Willi syndrome (PWS)-region gene regulates a different chromosomal domain in trans but the imprinted pws loci do not alter genome-wide mRNA levels. Genomics 2005;85:630–6340, and generously provided by Dr. Robert Nicholls.)

snoRNA, PWCR1/HBII-85, may be the cause of PWS in this individual *(15, 16)*. The function of known snoRNAs is to guide 2′-O-ribose methylation of mainly ribosomal RNA; however, this novel imprinted snoRNA has no known target. It is postulated that snoRNAs might be involved in the posttranscriptional regulation of a gene responsible for PWS. Further study in mouse models and patients may reveal more definitive evidence for the involvement of snoRNAs in the etiology of PWS.

Several mouse models of PWS exist with a consistent phenotype of neonatal lethality, hypotonia, failure to thrive, and growth retardation. However, none of these models demonstrate obesity or infertility. These models include a) maternal duplication of chromosome 7 (UPD); b) PWS deletion in which a transgene is inserted into the whole PWS syngenic region in the paternal chromosome 7C; c) deletion of the IC and Snurf-Snrpn exons 1–6; and d) specific deletion between exon 2 of Snurf-Snrpn and Ube3a not involving the IC *(6,17–19,6,20)*. Much study has been done on necdin-deficient mice, which demonstrate neonatal lethality secondary to respiratory distress with partial penetrance. The survivors show increased skin scraping activity and improved spatial learning and memory, paralleling the skin picking and propensity for jigsaw puzzles seen in humans with PWS. Finally, reductions in oxytocin and Lateinizing hormone-releasing hormone (LHRH)-producing neurons of the hypothalamus have been demonstrated in these mice *(12, 21, 22)*. Further study of such mouse strains and other specific gene-targeted knockouts is likely to aid in the understanding of the complex genetics of PWS.

CLINICAL MANAGEMENT

Diagnosis

Clinical Major and Minor Diagnostic Criteria

The original major and minor diagnostic criteria for diagnosis of PWS were proposed in 1993 by Dr. Holm *(23)* (see Table 11.1). Hallmark features of PWS include neonatal hypotonia and failure to thrive, developmental delay and mild cognitive impairment, characteristic facial appearance, early childhood onset obesity, hypogonadism with genital hypoplasia, mild short stature, and a characteristic behavior disorder. Since the publication of the original diagnostic criteria, others have suggested revised clinical criteria. One study examined the sensitivity for each criterion in a retrospective case review of 90 patients *(24)*. Based on the new sensitivity analyses, these authors proposed revised diagnostic criteria to ensure that all appropriate people are tested and that unnecessary testing of people is avoided. These revised criteria are organized into age groupings that follow the natural history of PWS (see Table 11.2).

Laboratory Diagnosis

PWS is caused by a lack of expression of the paternally active genes in the long arm of chromosome 15 (q11-13). Approximately 70% of cases result from a deletion of this region of paternal chromosome 15; 28% of cases result from UPD (two copies of the chromosome from mother and no copies from father); and less than 2% of cases are caused by an imprinting center mutation *(25–30)*. All three forms of PWS are detected by methylation analysis. If the methylation pattern is abnormal (signifying one parent of origin), then fluorescence in situ hybridization (FISH) can be used to confirm a deletion and/or microsatellite probes may be used to verify maternal UPD. Note that

Table 11.1
Diagnostic criteria for Prader-Willi syndrome

Major criteria

1. Neonatal and infantile central hypotonia with poor suck, gradually improving with age.
2. Feeding problems in infancy with need for special feeding techniques and poor weight gain/failure to thrive.
3. Excessive or rapid weight gain on weight-for-length chart (excessive is defined as crossing two centile channels) after 12 months but before 6 years of age; central obesity in the absence of intervention.
4. Characteristic facial features with dolichocephaly in infancy, narrow face or bifrontal diameter, almond-shaped eyes, small-appearing mouth with thin upper lip, down-turned corners of the mouth (three or more required).
5. Hypogonadism—with any of the following, depending on age:
   (a) Genital hypoplasia (male: scrotal hypoplasia, cryptorchidism, small penis and/or testes for age [<5th percentile]; female: absence or severe hypoplasia of labia minora and/or clitoris.
   (b) Delayed or incomplete gonadal maturation with delayed pubertal signs in the absence of intervention after 16 years of age (male: small gonads, decreased facial and body hair, lack of voice change; female: amenorrhea/oligomenorrhea after age 16).
6. Global developmental delay in a child younger than 6 years of age; mild to moderate mental retardation or learning problems in older children.
7. Hyperphagia/food foraging/obsession with food.
8. Deletion 15q11-13 on high resolution (>650 bands) or other cytogenetic/molecular abnormality of the Prader-Willi chromosome region, including maternal disomy.

Minor criteria

1. Decreased fetal movement or infantile lethargy or weak cry in infancy, improving with age.
2. Characteristic behavior problems— temper tantrums, violent outbursts, and obsessive/compulsive behavior; tendency to be argumentative, oppositional, rigid, manipulative, possessive, and stubborn; perseverating, stealing and lying (five or more of these symptoms required).
3. Sleep disturbance or sleep apnea.
4. Short stature for genetic background by age 15 (in the absence of growth hormone intervention).
5. Hypopigmentation—fair skin and hair compared to family.
6. Small hands (<25th percentile) and/or feet (<10th percentile) for height age.
7. Narrow hands with straight ulnar border.
8. Eye abnormalities (esotropia, myopia).
9. Thick viscous saliva with crusting at corners of the mouth.
10. Speech articulation defects.
11. Skin picking.

(Continued)

Table 11.1
Continued

Supportive findings (increase the certainty of diagnosis but are not scored)

1. High pain threshold.
2. Decreased vomiting.
3. Temperature instability in infancy or altered temperature sensitivity in older children and adults.
4. Scoliosis and/or kyphosis.
5. Early adrenarche.
6. Osteoporosis.
7. Unusual skill with jigsaw puzzles.
8. Normal neuromuscular studies.

Source: From Holm VA, Cassidy SB, Butler MG, Hanchett JM, Greenswag LR, Whitman BY, Greenberg F. Prader-Willi syndrome: consensus diagnostic criteria. Pediatrics 1993;91:398–340.

Table 11.2
Suggested new revised criteria to prompt DNA testing for Prader-Willi syndrome

Age at assessment	*Features sufficient to prompt DNA testing*
Birth to 2 years	1. Hypotonia with poor suck.
2–6 years	1. Hypotonia with history of poor suck. 2. Global developmental delay.
6–12 years	1. History of hypotonia with poor suck (hypotonia often persists) 2. Global developmental delay. 3. Excessive eating (hyperphagia; obsession with food) with central obesity if uncontrolled.
13 years through adult	1. Cognitive impairment; usual mild mental retardation. 2. Excessive eating (hyperphagia; obsession with food) with central obesity if uncontrolled. 3. Hypothalamic hypogonadism and/or typical behavior problems (including temper tantrums and obsessive-compulsive features).

Source: From Gunay-Aygun M, Schwartz S, Heeger S, O'Riordan MA, Cassidy SB. The changing purpose of Prader-Willi syndrome clinical diagnostic criteria and proposed revised criteria. Pediatrics 2001;108:1–5.

high-resolution chromosome analysis alone is insufficient because false positives and false negatives have occurred with this method without FISH. Finally, an abnormal methylation pattern in the presence of normal FISH and uniparental disomy studies suggests an imprinting center mutation. Analysis for mutations in the imprinting center can be done in a few select research laboratories on a research basis only.

Medical

Growth Hormone Deficiency

Mild prenatal growth retardation occurs commonly in PWS; 41% of infants have a birth weight <2.5 kg; birth length is either normal or slightly below normal. Short stature is almost always present by 1 year of age and continues throughout childhood. PWS-specific growth charts are available and should be used in clinical management of these children *(31)*. The cause of the short stature is both growth hormone deficiency and the lack of a sufficient pubertal growth spurt *(31, 32)*. The average height of PWS males is 155 cm and of PWS females is 145 cm *(33)*. The GH deficiency seen in PWS is independent of obesity and manifests in low spontaneous and pharmacologically stimulated GH secretion and low serum concentrations of insulin-like growth factor 1 (IGF-1) in both children and adults (34–45). This is unlike overnutrition in common obesity, which is associated with normal or increased IGF-1 levels. Finally, body composition studies in PWS individuals resemble that of classic GH deficiency including decreased lean mass and increased adipose tissue mass compared with age-matched controls *(46)*.

Data in Infants/Toddlers. Body fat content is increased and lean body mass is reduced in young infants and toddlers with PWS, even before progressive weight gain ensues *(47, 48)*. This finding provides a rationale for institution of GH therapy at a young age. In a randomized, blinded, controlled study, 29 infants with PWS (4–37 months of age) were randomized to GH treatment (1 mg/m^2/day) or observation for 12 months *(49)*. The GH-treated cohort demonstrated decreased percent body fat ($p < 0.001$), increased lean body mass ($p < 0.001$), increased height velocity z-scores ($p < 0.001$), and higher mobility skill acquisition when compared with controls of similar ages. No adverse effects were seen. In another 30-month study, 11 PWS children started on GH treatment before 2 years of age were compared with six infants treated only with coenzyme Q10 (a supplement postulated to enhance motor function in PWS) *(50)*. The GH-treated infants showed increases in lean mass adjusted for height ($p = 0.02$) and stabilization of percentage of fat adjusted for age. Follow-up from these studies will be important to discern whether this very early institution of therapy in infants with PWS may lead to improvements in attainment of developmental motor skills and further normalization of body composition and physical function. No adverse events were seen in these studies. However, controversy continues about whether growth hormone treatment causes an excess of mortality beyond that expected from PWS alone. These sudden deaths have been concentrated in young children, early in the course of GH therapy in individuals with a history of respiratory obstruction/infection or severe obesity (*51–59*). The exact cause of these sudden deaths has not been determined. Possibilities include impaired ventilatory responsiveness to hypercapnia and hypoxia, increased lymphoid tissue or tonsillar hyperplasia, adrenal insufficiency, or no true increased mortality above the baseline expected from the PWS diagnosis alone. However, other studies support an opposing view, that is, a beneficial role for GH therapy in improved ventilation responsiveness to carbon dioxide and improved sleep quality in children with PWS *(43,60,61)*. Until studies definitively address these issues, a pretreatment airway and sleep evaluation is recommended prior to, and possibly while receiving, GH therapy. Finally, GH treatment should be initiated by experienced centers and dosage of GH adjusted to maintain IGF-1 levels in the normal range. Children receiving GH therapy should be monitored for potential side-effects of GH, including glucose intolerance and worsening scoliosis.

Data in Childhood. In PWS children, GH treatment improves growth velocity and final height *(62)*. The use of GH in PWS is now approved by the U.S. Food and Drug Administration (FDA). Numerous studies have now shown that children with PWS respond to GH treatment with improvements in body composition (decreased fat mass and increased lean mass), improved bone mineral density, and increased resting energy expenditure (REE) associated with improved fatty acid oxidation (*39,43,61–66*). Improvements in physical strength, respiratory muscle hypotonia, and peripheral chemoreceptor sensitivity to carbon dioxide have also been reported with use of GH therapy *(43,44,61,62)*. One study has also reported a trend toward improvement in overall sleep quality, including reduction in the number of hypopnea and apnea events with administration of GH *(61)*. Finally, a few studies have found mild behavioral improvements, including reduction in depressive symptoms in those individuals older than 11 years of age; however, no significant change in intelligence quotient has been demonstrated with use of GH therapy *(61,67)*. Studies investigating the optimal dosage of growth hormone and use of growth hormone in adults with PWS are needed.

Sleep and Respiratory Abnormalities

PWS children commonly have excessive daytime sleepiness. The clinical and electrophysiologic patterns of their hypersomnolence include continuous hypersomnolence and/or periodic hypersomnolence (*68–72*). Interestingly, some PWS children without sleep-disordered breathing are hypersomnolent despite weight loss, and continuous positive airway pressure (CPAP) has not been able to fully correct this state of hypersomnolence. PWS children have a defective central respiratory drive, elevated hypercapnic arousal thresholds, abnormal ventilatory responses to both hypoxia and hypercapnia, absent peripheral chemoreceptor ventilatory responses, and abnormalities in rapid-eye-movement sleep (*73–78*). The etiology of the hypersomnolence and sleep-disordered breathing is not fully understood. One case of PWS associated with hypersomnolence has reported lower levels of orexin in the cerebrospinal fluid *(79)*. Orexin neurons in the lateral hypothalamus play a critical role in arousal and control of sleep. However, no detailed neuroanatomic mapping of the orexin neurons in PWS hypothalami has yet been done. All infants and children with PWS should undergo a sleep study before starting GH treatment; those with sleep-disordered breathing may benefit from additional weight reduction and CPAP. A few studies have shown that growth hormone treatment may improve respiratory muscle strength and the ventilatory response to carbon dioxide. These studies have also shown a trend toward improvement in number of hypopnea and apnea events *(43,60,61)*. Other larger, controlled studies are needed to address whether GH can improve these sleep abnormalities long-term.

Glucose Homeostasis in Prader-Willi Syndrome

Obesity is a strong risk factor for the development of type 2 diabetes. PWS individuals have an increased prevalence (7–20% compared with 5% in the general population) of early development of type 2 diabetes *(80, 81, 82)*. It is assumed that the etiology of type 2 diabetes in PWS is due to morbid obesity and concomitant hyperinsulinemia. However, the relationship between morbid obesity and development of type 2 diabetes appears to be different in PWS versus non-PWS individuals. In PWS children compared with body mass index (BMI)-matched controls, the insulin response to both a mixed meal and an oral glucose load is lower. Additionally, the first- and second-phase insulin secretions were significantly lower in PWS adults compared with obese controls during an intravenous glucose tolerance test (IVGTT). Finally, normal or increased sensitivity to exogenous insulin has been observed in PWS individuals (*83–85*). These findings suggest that the PWS group appears to be somewhat protected from obesity-associated insulin resistance *(86)*. Moreover, PWS patients were found to have higher hepatic insulin extraction and insulin clearance during basal and poststimulation conditions compared with obese controls. Finally, an absent pancreatic polypeptide response in PWS was noted, suggestive of vagal input abnormalities of the stomach and delayed gastric emptying *(87)*. The explanation for β-cell dysfunction in PWS is not fully understood at this time, but one hypothesis is that a decrease in vagal parasympathetic tone to the pancreas in PWS individuals leads to reduction in insulin secretion *(88)*. Another hypothesis includes the state of GH deficiency leading to a reduction in β-cell insulin secretion and increasing insulin sensitivity. In summary, glucose homeostasis in PWS individuals differs from that in non-PWS individuals. Exploration of the association among various genotypes in PWS and the presence or absence of glucose intolerance and diabetes has not been fully explored. Treatment of type 2 diabetes in PWS individuals requires weight reduction by dietary means and, sometimes, addition of an oral agent such as metformin, or insulin therapy.

Hypothalamic-Pituitary-Gonadal Axis in PWS

Simple obesity is commonly associated with early menarche, and it is postulated that a rise in leptin produced by the adipose tissue is a signal, which triggers the earlier onset of puberty. In contrast, PWS is most often associated with hypogonadism, which is prenatal in onset *(89)*. Males typically may have undescended testes, scrotal hypoplasia, and a small phallus, while females often have hypoplasia of the labia minora and clitoris *(90, 91)*. In both boys and girls with PWS, pubic and axillary hair development is normal or early as adrenal hormone function is unaffected *(84)*. True puberty, however, is delayed and usually incomplete *(90, 92)*. For example, adult males only sometimes have substantial facial and body hair, voice change, and male-type body habitus; females have amenorrhea and oligomenorrhea. Menarche in PWS females may occur as late as 30 to 40 years of age. In both males and females, sexual activity is rare, and infertility is common with few exceptions. Two case reports now exist of women with PWS giving birth to children: in one case, a mom with maternal disomy gave birth to an unaffected child, and in another case, a mom with deletion 15q11-q13 gave birth to a child with Angelman syndrome *(93, 94)*.

In addition to a hypothalamic defect in the regulation of gonadotropins manifesting as low levels of Luteinizing hormone (LH) and Follicle stimulating hormone (FSH), another etiology of hypogonadism in PWS is related to primary gonadal failure, which may be secondary to cryptorchidism (*84,92,95–97*). In one study, researchers examined the gonadal function of 38 PWS adults. The majority of PWS subjects demonstrated low LH and FSH levels, compatible with hypogonadotropic hypogonadism; 39.4% of subjects showed normal gonadotropins, and a small number of subjects demonstrated high gonadotropins, suggestive of gonadal failure *(98)*. Thus, factors regulating the hypothalamic-gonadal axis in PWS individuals are different from that of simple obesity, and the implications for other hormones such as leptin, insulin, and growth hormone in the modulation of reproduction in PWS is not yet fully understood.

Treatment for cryptorchidism in PWS males should occur before 2 years of age. Testosterone therapy at conservative doses is indicated to treat hypogonadism and prevent further reductions in bone mineral density that may lead to osteoporosis. Testosterone replacement should be started at age 13–14 years in males, with 50–75 mg depot-testosterone intramuscularly every 3–4 weeks or a testosterone patch daily; dosages are increased up to 150 mg every 3–4 weeks depending on blood testosterone levels. In females, estrogen treatment or birth control pills can increase breast size and result in menstrual cycles. The benefits of hormone replacement on cardiovascular outcomes and bone mineral density effects have not been well studied in the PWS population.

Neuroendocrine Control of Body Weight in Prader-Willi Syndrome

Ghrelin is an endogenous ligand of the growth hormone secretagogue receptor (GHSR), a hypothalamic G protein–coupled receptor *(99)*. Enteroendocrine cells (X/A-like cells) of the stomach are the major site of ghrelin synthesis, although a minor proportion of ghrelin synthesis occurs in other sites such as the hypothalamus, pituitary, duodenum, jejunum, and lung *(100)*. Circulating levels of ghrelin peak during fasting prior to a meal and fall after meals, suggesting a possible role in meal initiation *(101)*. Studies in rodents support the premise that ghrelin is involved in energy balance. In rats fed ad libitum, both intracerebroventricular and intraperitoneal administration of ghrelin potently stimulates food intake *(102)*. An effect of more physiologic levels of ghrelin on appetite and food intake in humans was studied recently. A randomized, double-blind, crossover study in human adults showed that ghrelin increased caloric consumption by $28 \pm 3.9\%$, ($p < 0.001$) *(103)*. Ghrelin levels are inversely related to body weight in humans *(104, 105)*, and ghrelin concentrations are higher during starvation *(104, 105)* and increase with weight loss *(106)*. Therefore, ghrelin may signal conservation of energy to prevent further weight loss and restore usual body weight.

Markedly elevated concentrations of ghrelin in both children and adults with PWS have been reported in several studies, which compared these individuals with obese controls and individuals with monogenic obesity defects in melanocortin 4 receptor (MC4R) or leptin (*107–109*). Because the human ghrelin gene on chromosome 3p26-25 is not located within the known deleted gene sequence that causes PWS, the exact cause of this elevation in ghrelin concentrations in PWS is not yet fully understood. The increased concentrations of ghrelin found in children with PWS may lead to stimulation of appetite through the hypothalamic neuropeptide Y (NPY)/agouti-related protein (AgRP) signaling pathways. Because ghrelin is thought to regulate GH secretion, and the majority of PWS children are GH-deficient, one might speculate that the increase in ghrelin concentration found in PWS children reflects a lack of feedback inhibition from GH. However, this theory is unlikely, given the finding that ghrelin concentrations are not elevated in subjects with GH deficiency, and GH therapy in these same individuals does not alter their levels of ghrelin *(110)*. It would be important to know whether most of the increase in ghrelin concentration in PWS is derived from the stomach or from other sources, such as the hypothalamus. Furthermore, because the assay used to measure ghrelin in these studies captures all ghrelin-like immunoreactive proteins, it is possible that the increase in ghrelin concentration is attributable not only to active acylated ghrelin protein but also to an increase in circulating fragments of ghrelin (possibly derived from degradation or alternative splicing or mutations of the ghrelin gene product), which presumably would be inactive. For instance, it is possible that PWS children may have altered processing of preproghrelin by prohormone convertase 2 (PC2) into the mature active peptide as supported by previous work that postulates a processing defect of vasopressin in some PWS subjects *(111)*. Therefore, it is possible that the increased ghrelin concentrations demonstrated in PWS children reflect mostly inactive hormone, which may explain why higher levels of GH are not observed in PWS children. A second possibility is that the defect in GH secretion in PWS children is not affected by GH secretagogues such as ghrelin *(45, 112)*. Alternatively, the elevated ghrelin levels in PWS may lead to lower GH levels through a paradoxical override inhibition, similar to that described before with continuous GH-releasing hormone stimulation of GH *(107, 113)*. Finally, abnormal parasympathetic vagal innervation of the stomach by abnormalities in the hypothalamus and brain stem may lead to hyperghrelinemia *(114)*.

This profound elevation in ghrelin may contribute to the obesity phenotype of PWS. Several case reports exist of PWS individuals who have undergone gastric bypass with improvement in weight, suggesting that gut hormones such as ghrelin may play a role in the PWS obesity phenotype (*115–117*). Nevertheless, preliminary short-term studies of suppression of ghrelin with octreotide or somatostatin have thus far shown no effect on body weight, food intake, or satiety *(118, 119)*. It is possible that longer-term suppression of ghrelin may be required to reduce body weight. Specific ghrelin antagonists may help to elucidate the role of hyperghrelinemia in PWS.

Other gut hormones have been evaluated in PWS. Cholecystokinin (CCK) is a hormone that induces satiety; it is made in the duodenum and secreted in response to food entering the intestine. PWS individuals have normal basal levels of CCK *(120, 121)*. However, one study showed that the usual positive correlation between fasting plasma fatty acids and CCK levels was missing in PWS subjects and, therefore, may signify a decreased response of CCK release in response to rising plasma fatty acid levels during a high-fat meal *(121)*. One additional satiety peptide studied in PWS is pancreatic polypeptide, another satiety-inducing hormone secreted from the intestine during meals. PWS individuals have been reported to have lower basal and meal-stimulated pancreatic polypeptide secretion *(87, 120, 122)*. One study demonstrated that short-term normalization of blood pancreatic polypeptide levels did not change food intake in PWS individuals *(123)*. Further study of gut satiety factors in PWS is warranted.

Insulin levels cannot explain the obese phenotype of PWS. In PWS individuals, a state of relative hypoinsulinemia occurs. For example, fasting insulin concentrations are lower in PWS compared with BMI-matched children *(42, 86, 124)*, and insulin sensitivity is increased *(86)*. Leptin levels in PWS subjects have been found to be appropriate for their degree of obesity and the same as weight-matched controls; therefore, leptin is not thought to play a major role in the PWS obese phenotype (*125–129*). Limitations to the conclusion that leptin and insulin signaling do not account for the obese phenotype of PWS include a lack of assessment of the sensitivity of neurons of the arcuate nucleus of the hypothalamus to respond appropriately to these signals. In several postmortem studies, the central circuitry of energy balance in PWS has been evaluated. One postmortem study found decreased NPY mRNA but not AgRP mRNA in PWS adults. Another postmortem study showed reduction in the PVN volume, an area of the brain that tends to reduce food intake and body weight. Finally, elevated circulating levels of γ-aminobutyric acid (GABA) have been shown in PWS individuals compared with age- and weight-matched controls *(130)*. These central hypothalamic changes may contribute also to the complex weight dysregulation and lack of satiety observed in PWS individuals.

Finally, one study involved sampling of abdominal fat tissue of PWS individuals compared with normal weight subjects *(131)*. Total lipid was extracted and fatty acid composition was measured by gas-liquid chromatography. Analysis of triglycerides from the PWS children revealed significantly lower percentages of c12:0 and c18:0 saturated fatty acids but noticeable elevation in long-chain polyunsaturated fatty acids. These changes were not due to dietary modifications. These findings may suggest an altered fatty acid metabolism in PWS individuals that warrants further investigation *(132)*.

Nutritional Management of Prader-Willi Syndrome

Several studies looking at body composition in PWS children by various methods [skinfold measurements, total body water, bioelectrical impedance analysis (BIA), deuterium dilution method] have demonstrated higher amounts of adipose tissue in PWS children compared with obese, non-PWS children *(131, 133)*. However, other studies have suggested that fat-free body mass (FFM)/kg body weight is similar in obese individuals and individuals with PWS and that increased FFM occurs with increased body weight; thus, individuals with PWS were not fatter than non-PWS obese individuals in some studies.

Analysis of the various components of total energy expenditure [basal metabolic rate (BMR), diet-induced thermogenesis (DIT), and physical activity] in individuals with PWS has been studied. Total energy expenditure, measured by doubly-labeled water, has been found to be decreased in individuals with PWS; most, but not all, of the decrease has been attributed to their small fat-free mass and reduced physical activity *(133)*. The BMR in PWS individuals (amount of energy to maintain physiologic function while resting) is normal when expressed per unit of body surface area (function of weight and height) or per kilogram of lean body mass *(125, 131, 133, 134)*. Therefore, the lower BMR demonstrated in some earlier studies has been attributed to the PWS individuals' lower FFM. DIT (the energy expended with the digestion and absorption of food) has not been studied in individuals with PWS. However, diet-induced thermogenesis has been found to be lower in many but not all studies of obese humans (*135–141*). In addition, a diet high in polyunsaturated relative to saturated fatty acids and a diet composed of unfamiliar foods have both been shown to result in relatively higher rates of DIT in normal-weight humans *(142, 143)*. Finally, the maximum DIT response occurs when the meal precedes exercise for lean men, but when the meal follows exercise for obese men *(141)*. Therefore, obese individuals may exhibit subtle changes in DIT. Finally, the contribution of physical activity to total energy expenditure in PWS individuals has been examined. These studies suggest that PWS individuals are less active in general, but there is a wide range of activity levels, which is a function of individual characteristics. Also, physical activity is as energy burning in PWS individuals as in normal individuals (*144–146*). Therefore, raising physical activity levels in individuals with PWS will increase their total energy expenditure, increase their lean body mass, and help in maintenance of body weight in general *(147, 148)*. Some authors have reported that a small amount of high-preference food may be used as an effective inducement for increased activity and exercise *(149)*.

Various case studies or intervention dietary studies have been conducted in children with PWS in attempt to induce weight loss. These studies include energy restriction with behavior management (*150–152*), hypocaloric diets (*153–156*), hypocaloric-protein sparing diets *(157, 158)*, energy-restricted ketogenic diets *(144, 159)*, and balanced macronutrient diets devoid of simple sugar *(160)*. Each of these dietary interventions required long-term intervention and resulted in only limited success.

The effects of gastric bypass in children with PWS have been described in the literature. One study reports outcomes in 11 children (7 boys, 4 girls) of mean age 13 years after gastric bypass surgery (n = 10) or gastroplasty (n = 1). Weight loss after gastric bypass was variable in these children, and an approximately 1 kg/month weight loss was demonstrated initially. However, a plateau in weight loss eventually occurred, and no reliable predictors of amount of weight loss were identified in this study. In this study, males usually did better than females, and the heavier the preoperative weight, the more weight postoperatively was lost. Normal linear growth was observed in these individuals, and no severe metabolic derangements occurred. One child did develop a postoperative wound infection and another developed acute congestive heart failure. As well, five children required revision of their gastric bypass *(115, 161)*. Another 15 young adult PWS subjects (BMI >35 with metabolic complications) after biliopancreatic diversion (BPD) were studied for 8.5 years by Marinari et al. *(162)*. These authors reported no perioperative complications and percent excess weight loss of 59% at 2 years, 56% at 3 years, and then progressive weight regain occurred. Percent excess weight loss at 10 years was 40% on average. Three cases showed good results, one showed a fair result, and three were failures. A correlation between weight loss at 5 years and lifestyle score was demonstrated. Better weight loss was shown in males. Decreases in comorbid conditions such as type 2 diabetes, hypercholesterolemia, and hypertension were also demonstrated. One patient who was unsuccessful at weight loss died at 9 years postoperatively from respiratory failure. The authors conclude that BPD should be considered for its value in prolonging and improving the PWS patient's life. Other case reports and case series of gastric bypass surgery in PWS have also been described, resulting in variable success rates *(117, 163)*.

Data collected on preschool and school-age children with PWS indicate that individuals with PWS at any age can lose weight on an energy-restricted diet of 7 kcal/cm/day *(156, 164)*. In addition, diets providing 8–11 kcal/cm/day have been reported to achieve weight maintenance *(156, 164)*. These energy goals translate into daily intakes of 600–800 kcal for young children with PWS and 800–1,300 kcal for older children and adults with PWS *(164)*. These energy goals are considerably lower than the caloric intake of normal children. Of note is that many group homes for those with PWS provide a diet consisting of 1,000 kcal/day *(165)*. The optimal macronutrient composition of the diet for individuals with PWS has not been well studied. Some authors suggest a diet consisting of approximately 25% protein, 50% carbohydrate, and 25% fat *(164)*. Limited data on the use of a ketogenic diet or protein-sparing modified fast suggests that hunger may be reduced by these particular diets *(157, 159)*; further research is needed in this area. Due to potential for insufficient intake of essential vitamins and minerals during prolonged periods of caloric restriction, a daily multivitamin is essential.

Pipes and Holm reported that early intervention is effective in preventing excessive weight gain *(166)*. In order to control weight effectively in PWS children, control of both dietary intake and behavior needs to occur. Parental and other caregiver (including school personnel) motivation is essential for successful weight control. Food-related behaviors are problematic for PWS individuals. Sneaking and gorging food is a common and serious problem. When given unlimited access to food, PWS individuals can consume massive amounts of food. Bray et al. reported ad libitum energy intake of unsupervised PWS individuals as reaching 5,167 ± 503 kcal/day *(84)*. As well, pica (consumption of food considered unappealing such as dog and cat food, garbage, etc.) is an additional concern. Families of individuals with PWS report other behaviors such as obsession with refrigerators and freezers, worrying about food (if there is enough, where the next meal will come from), and generalized preoccupation with food and eating *(156)*.

In general, nutrition education is essential to help individuals with PWS maintain a healthy weight. Initial instruction and weight measurements should occur weekly. Once weight maintenance goals are met and care providers feel comfortable with independent meal planning, nutritional intervention may be required only every 6 months. Small energy increases (100–200 kcal) should be added at any one time to minimize overshooting weight goals. Consistency with meal patterns and times for eating is important. Care providers should be taught about portion sizes; these are best described using common measurements such as cups, teaspoons, and fluid ounces or grams. At first, care providers may find it useful to record measurements for all daily food intake. The exchange system used by patients with diabetes also may be used to plan meals. For example, foods are divided into six groups: milk, meat, fruit, vegetable, bread, and fat. The portion size assigned to a food in each group provides equal amounts of protein, carbohydrate, fat, and calories. Therefore, foods within a group can be substituted or exchanged freely. Individualized menus should take into account different family lifestyles and be planned with a nutritionist on an ongoing basis. Consideration of food preferences is important; PWS individuals do have definite food preferences and will consistently choose a smaller amount of preferred food over a greater amount of lesser preferred food *(167)*. Also, individuals with PWS should play an active role in meal planning when possible. Daily exercise should also be part of the regular routine in order to enhance aerobic fitness and energy expenditure and help in maintenance of weight loss *(168)*. A reward system of points, verbal praise, and physical touch may enhance motivation for weight loss. Additional nutritional education resources are available from the Prader-Willi Syndrome Association (USA).

Ancillary Care

Effective management of PWS requires resources of a multidisciplinary team, including medical providers, physical therapist, speech therapist, occupational therapist, and other ancillary care providers. During infancy, hypotonia and muscle weakness should be managed with physical therapy (passive range of motion and placement of infant on mat in prone position to promote head lifting and pushing torso upward). Due to hypotonia, breastfeeding is rarely possible, and special feeding techniques, including special nipples and gavage feeding, may be required for weeks or months. Delayed motor milestones are common; the average age of sitting is 12 months and of walking is 24 months. Scoliosis, presumed to be related to hypotonia, is also common in PWS individuals. Clinical screening for scoliosis should occur at all routine visits and if present should prompt further evaluation by a scoliosis x-ray series and referral to an orthopedist. Also, speech therapy is frequently indicated for speech and language delay. PWS individuals commonly have poor articulation and can demonstrate slurred and/or nasal-sounding speech. Teeth may erupt late *(169)*, and enamel hypoplasia *(160)* may predispose PWS individuals to early caries. Therefore, routine preventative dental care is important in this population. Finally, strabismus caused by muscle weakness frequently occurs, and all children with PWS should have a formal ophthalmologic examination between ages 1 and 3 years.

During childhood, dietary guidance should be provided by a nutritionist experienced with PWS. Efforts to restrict caloric intake and limit food access requires constant supervision and consistency in setting limits. The dietary changes necessitated by caring for a child with PWS impacts on the household functioning; for example, limitation of second helpings, eating low-energy, low-fat foods, a lack of snack food at home, eating at a consistent time, and locking of food occurs. Some parents avoid parties, family gatherings, and restaurants due to the stress of monitoring their child's intake.

Most PWS individuals exhibit cognitive delays with the majority being mildly retarded (mean IQ 60–70) *(170, 171)*. The vast majority of PWS individuals require placement in a special educational classroom or special assistance in a regular classroom. As adults, most PWS individuals can read, write, and do simple arithmetic. Particular relative strengths have been noted in reading and vocabulary, visual-spatial skills (especially skills with jigsaw puzzles), and long-term memory, while weaknesses are typically seen in arithmetic, sequential processing, and short-term memory.

Worsening behavioral difficulties including temper tantrums, oppositional behavior, stubbornness, and compulsive behaviors like skin and/or rectal picking may emerge during childhood *(172, 173)*. A true psychosis also may occur in 5–10% of individuals with PWS and typically begins in young adulthood *(174, 175)*. Additionally, some of the repetitive behaviors in PWS such as insisting on sameness and "just-right" behaviors overlap with those seen in autism *(176)*. Behavioral management, including a strict routine, structure, limits, "time-outs," and positive rewards are useful techniques for these families to implement *(177)*. Additionally, psychotherapy with use of fluoxetine, antipsychotics, and topiramate may improve compulsive eating and help with other obsessive-compulsive type behaviors. Finally, parents of children with PWS have increased marital and family discord and stress levels, and it is important to offer families professional counseling if indicated *(178)*

LONG-TERM PROGNOSIS

Life expectancy is decreased in individuals with PWS (20–30 years), and few individuals live past 50 years of age. An annual mortality rate of about 3% per year is seen in this population *(179)*. A few individuals in the National PWS Association (USA) database are reported to be in their sixties currently. The major causes of death are secondary to obesity and include respiratory failure with cor pulmonale, type 2 diabetes mellitus, and arteriosclerosis. Because of autonomic dysfunction manifesting as a high pain threshold and abnormal temperature regulation, warning signs of illness may be absent, such as pain and fever and stomach pain. Other health issues seen in adults with PWS include scoliosis, hypoventilation, recurrent respiratory infections/aspiration, choking, sleep apnea, hypertension, osteoporosis, and leg ulceration *(72)*. Often, adults have behavior abnormalities (tantrums and stubbornness) that prevent them from living in the community at large and retaining a job. Group homes that operate with resources of a multidisciplinary team and emphasize control of diet and behavior management tend to be successful *(33)*. Additionally, most PWS adults who are successfully employed are in sheltered workshops that provide a structured environment that is free from all sources of potentially edible food items. Many PWS individuals have good fine-motor skills, and thus assembly work, office work, and laboratory work are potentially well-suited career choices for them. Finally, it is often beneficial for families to work with an attorney specializing in working with families of the disabled to develop a will ensuring that continuation of funds will be available to their disabled survivors. Further community resources for these families are available through the Prader-Willi Syndrome Association in the United States.

FUTURE STUDIES AND THERAPIES

A lack of detailed understanding of the neuroendocrine control of appetite and obesity in PWS currently hampers progress into design of antiobesity drugs. However, some strides have been made. It is possible that specific ghrelin antagonists may have an effect in PWS-related obesity. In addition, recent evidence points to central melanocortin agonists being able to block ghrelin-mediated feeding. Therefore, potential combinatorial therapy with a ghrelin antagonist and melanocortin agonist may ameliorate hyperghrelinemia effects in PWS. These studies provide some hope, but many questions still remain unanswered. For example, what may be the contribution of central versus peripheral ghrelin receptor effects on body weight regulation in PWS? At what age does the hyperghrelinemia in PWS begin? What may be the potential side-effects (suppression of GH axis or cardiovascular implications) of using a ghrelin antagonist? Finally, how might central pathways regulate body weight in PWS? One study revealed a significant reduction in total number of cells and of oxytocin-containing cells of the paraventricular nucleus (PVN), an important hypothalamic area contributing to the control of body weight and appetite *(3)*. These central abnormalities may contribute to the peripheral abnormalities of hyperghrelinemia by the fact that projections from the PVN to the brain stem and vagus nerve are involved in energy homeostasis circuitry. Additionally, because the arcuate nucleus sends projections to the PVN in the control of feeding, it is possible that the target CNS pathways in PWS will not respond normally to pharmacologic interventions *(180)*.

CONCLUSION

The study of PWS is likely to elucidate further understanding of the control of weight regulation in humans in general:

1. PWS individuals demonstrate abnormal partitioning of body fat and lean mass, which may be due partially to hypothalamic abnormalities in growth hormone and insulin secretion. Study of PWS may lead to further understanding of partitioning of body fat and lean mass.
2. Evidence points to abnormalities in the autonomic system (lower vagal parasympathetic tone) in PWS and, therefore, studies of PWS will likely lead to further understanding of the autonomic nervous system's contribution to the control of energy homeostasis.
3. The genetics of PWS is very complex; there is loss of a gene in this disorder that plays a vital role in the defense of body fat. Further investigation of the genetics of PWS may lead to understanding of new genetic pathways in the regulation of body weight.
4. Some evidence points to alterations in fatty acid metabolism in individuals with PWS. Further research is needed to understand these metabolic changes and how these alterations may play a role in other forms of obesity.

ACKNOWLEDGMENTS

This work was supported by NIH grant 1K23-RR-021979 to A.M.H. We thank Dr. Robert Nicholls for generously providing a figure illustrating human chromosome 15q11-q13.

REFERENCES

1. Prader A, Labhart A, Willi H. Ein Syndrom von Adipositas, Kleinwuchs, Kryptorchismus und Oligophrenie nach myotoniertigem Zustand im Neugeborenalter. Schweiz Med Wochenschr 1956;86:1260–1261.
2. Cassidy SB, Dykens E, Williams CA. Prader-Willi and Angelman syndromes: sister imprinted disorders. Am J Med Genet 2000;97:136–146.
3. Swaab DF. Prader-Willi syndrome and the hypothalamus. Acta Paediatr 1997;423(Suppl):50–54.
4. DiMario FJ Jr, Dunham B, Burleson JA, Moskovitz J, Cassidy SB. An evaluation of autonomic nervous system function in patients with Prader-Willi syndrome. Pediatrics 1994;93:76–81.
5. Hudgins L, Cassidy SB. Hand and foot length in Prader-Willi syndrome. Am J Med Genet 1991;41:5–9.
6. Nicholls RD, Knepper JL. Genome organization, function, and imprinting in Prader-Willi and Angelman syndromes. Annu Rev Genomics Hum Genet 2001;2:153–175.
7. Nicholls RD, Saitoh S, Horsthemke B. Imprinting in Prader-Willi and Angelman syndromes. Trends Genet 1998;14:194–200.
8. Ohta T, Gray TA, Rogan PK, et al. Imprinting-mutation mechanisms in Prader-Willi syndrome. Am J Hum Genet 1999;64:397–413.

9. Schulze A, Hansen C, Baekgaard P, Blichfeldt S, Petersen MB, Tommerup N, Brondum-Nielsen K. Clinical features and molecular genetic analysis of a boy with Prader-Willi syndrome caused by an imprinting defect. Acta Paediatr 1997;86:906–910.
10. Runte M, Huttenhofer A, Gross S, Kiefmann M, Horsthemke B, Buiting K. The IC-SNURF-SNRPN transcript serves as a host for multiple small nucleolar RNA species and as an antisense RNA for UBE3A. Hum Mol Genet 2001;10:2687–2700.
11. Niinobe M, Koyama K, Yoshikawa K. Cellular and subcellular localization of necdin in fetal and adult mouse brain. Dev Neurosci 2000;22:310–319.
12. Muscatelli F, Abrous DN, Massacrier A, Boccaccio I, Le Moal M, Cau P, Cremer H. Disruption of the mouse Necdin gene results in hypothalamic and behavioral alterations reminiscent of the human Prader-Willi syndrome. Hum Mol Genet 2000;9:3101–3110.
13. Lee S, Kozlov S, Hernandez L, Chamberlain SJ, Brannan CI, Stewart CL, Wevrick R. Expression and imprinting of MAGEL2 suggest a role in Prader-willi syndrome and the homologous murine imprinting phenotype. Hum Mol Genet 2000;9:1813–1819.
14. Yoshikawa K. Cell cycle regulators in neural stem cells and postmitotic neurons. Neurosci Res 2000;37:1–14.
15. Schule B, Albalwi M, Northrop E, et al. Molecular breakpoint cloning and gene expression studies of a novel translocation t(4;15)(q27;q11.2) associated with Prader-Willi syndrome. BMC Med Genet 2005;6:18.
16. Gallagher RC, Pils B, Albalwi M, Francke U. Evidence for the role of PWCR1/HBII-85 C/D box small nucleolar RNAs in Prader-Willi syndrome. Am J Hum Genet 2002;71:669–678.
17. Yang T, Adamson TE, Resnick JL, et al. A mouse model for Prader-Willi syndrome imprinting-centre mutations. Nat Genet 1998;19:25–31.
18. Gabriel JM, Merchant M, Ohta T, Jet al. A transgene insertion creating a heritable chromosome deletion mouse model of Prader-Willi and angelman syndromes. Proc Natl Acad Sci USA 1999;96:9258–9263.
19. Tsai TF, Jiang YH, Bressler J, Armstrong D, Beaudet AL. Paternal deletion from Snrpn to Ube3a in the mouse causes hypotonia, growth retardation and partial lethality and provides evidence for a gene contributing to Prader-Willi syndrome. Hum Mol Genet 1999;8:1357–1364.
20. Goldstone AP. Prader-Willi syndrome: advances in genetics, pathophysiology and treatment. Trends Endocrinol Metab 2004;15:12–20.
21. Gerard M, Hernandez L, Wevrick R, Stewart CL. Disruption of the mouse necdin gene results in early post-natal lethality. Nat Genet 1999;23:199–202.
22. Ren J, Lee S, Pagliardini S, Gerard M, Stewart CL, Greer JJ, Wevrick R. Absence of Ndn, encoding the Prader-Willi syndrome-deleted gene necdin, results in congenital deficiency of central respiratory drive in neonatal mice. J Neurosci 2003;23:1569–1573.
23. Holm VA, Cassidy SB, Butler MG, Hanchett JM, Greenswag LR, Whitman BY, Greenberg F. Prader-Willi syndrome: consensus diagnostic criteria. Pediatrics 1993;91:398–340.
24. Gunay-Aygun M, Schwartz S, Heeger S, O'Riordan MA, Cassidy SB. The changing purpose of Prader-Willi syndrome clinical diagnostic criteria and proposed revised criteria. Pediatrics 2001;108:E92.
25. Ledbetter DH, Mascarello JT, Riccardi VM, Harper VD, Airhart SD, Strobel RJ. Chromosome 15 abnormalities and the Prader-Willi syndrome: a follow-up report of 40 cases. Am J Hum Genet 1982;34:278–285.
26. Nicholls RD, Knoll JH, Butler MG, Karam S, Lalande M. Genetic imprinting suggested by maternal heterodisomy in nondeletion Prader-Willi syndrome. Nature 1989;342:281–285.
27. Robinson WP, Bottani A, Xie YG, Balakrishman J, Binkert F, Machler M, Prader A, Schinzel A. Molecular, cytogenetic, and clinical investigations of Prader-Willi syndrome patients. Am J Hum Genet 1991;49:1219–1234.

28. Mascari MJ, Gottlieb W, Rogan PK, et al. The frequency of uniparental disomy in Prader-Willi syndrome. Implications for molecular diagnosis. N Engl J Med 1992;326:1599–607.
29. Reis A, Dittrich B, Greger V, Buiting K, et al. Imprinting mutations suggested by abnormal DNA methylation patterns in familial Angelman and Prader-Willi syndromes. Am J Hum Genet 1994;54:741–747.
30. Buiting K, Saitoh S, Gross S, Dittrich B, Schwartz S, Nicholls RD, Horsthemke B. Inherited microdeletions in the Angelman and Prader-Willi syndromes define an imprinting centre on human chromosome 15. Nat Genet 1995;9:395–400.
31. Butler MG, Meaney FJ Standards for selected anthropometric measurements in Prader-Willi syndrome. Pediatrics 1991;88:853–860.
32. Wollmann HA, Schultz U, Grauer ML, Ranke MB. Reference values for height and weight in Prader-Willi syndrome based on 315 patients. Eur J Pediatr 1998;157:634–642.
33. Greenswag LR. Adults with Prader-Willi syndrome: a survey of 232 cases. Dev Med Child Neurol 1987;29:145–152.
34. Costeff H, Holm VA, Ruvalcaba R, Shaver J. Growth hormone secretion in Prader-Willi syndrome. Acta Paediatr Scand 1990;79:1059–1062.
35. Cappa M, Grossi A, Borrelli P, Ghigo E, Bellone J, Benedetti S, Carta D, Loche S. Growth hormone (GH) response to combined pyridostigmine and GH-releasing hormone administration in patients with Prader-Labhard-Willi syndrome. Horm Res 1993;39:51–55.
36. Angulo M, Castro-Magana M, Mazur B, Canas JA, Vitollo PM, Sarrantonio M. Growth hormone secretion and effects of growth hormone therapy on growth velocity and weight gain in children with Prader-Willi syndrome. J Pediatr Endocrinol Metab 1996;9:393–400.
37. Grosso S, Cioni M, Buoni S, Peruzzi L, Pucci L, Berardi R. Growth hormone secretion in Prader-Willi syndrome. J Endocrinol Invest 1998;21:418–422.
38. Grugni G, Guzzaloni G Moro D, Bettio D, De Medici C, Morabito F. Reduced growth hormone (GH) responsiveness to combined GH-releasing hormone and pyridostigmine administration in the Prader-Willi syndrome. Clin Endocrinol (Oxf) 1998;48:769–775.
39. Lindgren AC, Hagenas L, Muller J, Blichfeldt S, Rosenborg M, Brismar T, Ritzen EM. Growth hormone treatment of children with Prader-Willi syndrome affects linear growth and body composition favourably. Acta Paediatr 1998;87:28–31.
40. Thacker MJ, Hainline B, St Dennis-Feezle L, Johnson NB, Pescovitz OH. Growth failure in Prader-Willi syndrome is secondary to growth hormone deficiency. Horm Res 1998;49:216–220.
41. Corrias A, Bellone J, Beccaria L, et al. GH/IGF-I axis in Prader-Willi syndrome: evaluation of IGF-I levels and of the somatotroph responsiveness to various provocative stimuli. Genetic Obesity Study Group of Italian Society of Pediatric Endocrinology and Diabetology. J Endocrinol Invest 2000;23:84–89.
42. Eiholzer U, Stutz K, Weinmann C, Torresani T, Molinari L, Prader A. Low insulin, IGF-I and IGFBP-3 levels in children with Prader-Labhart-Willi syndrome. Eur J Pediatr 1998;157:890–893.
43. Carrel AL, Myers SE, Whitman BY, Allen DB. Growth hormone improves body composition, fat utilization, physical strength and agility, and growth in Prader-Willi syndrome: A controlled study. J Pediatr 1999;134:215–221.
44. Burman P, Ritzen EM, Lindgren AC. Endocrine dysfunction in Prader-Willi syndrome: a review with special reference to GH. Endocr Rev 2001;22:787–799.
45. Grugni G, Guzzaloni G, Morabito F. Impairment of GH responsiveness to GH-releasing hexapeptide (GHRP-6) in Prader-Willi syndrome. J Endocrinol Invest 2001;24:340–348.
46. Brambilla P, Bosio L, Manzoni P, Pietrobelli A, Beccaria L, Chiumello G. Peculiar body composition in patients with Prader-Labhart-Willi syndrome. Am J Clin Nutr 1997;65:1369–1374.
47. Eiholzer U, Blum WF, Molinari L. Body fat determined by skinfold measurements is elevated despite underweight in infants with Prader-Labhart-Willi syndrome. J Pediatr 1999;134:222–225.

48. Bekx MT, Carrel AL, Shriver TC, Li Z, Allen DB. Decreased energy expenditure is caused by abnormal body composition in infants with Prader-Willi Syndrome. J Pediatr 2003;143:372–376.
49. Carrel AL, Moerchen V, Myers SE, Bekx MT, Whitman BY, Allen DB. Growth hormone improves mobility and body composition in infants and toddlers with Prader-Willi syndrome. J Pediatr 2004;145:744–749.
50. Eiholzer U, L'Allemand D, Schlumpf M, Rousson V, Gasser T, Fusch C. Growth hormone and body composition in children younger than 2 years with Prader-Willi syndrome. J Pediatr 2004;144:753–758.
51. Nagai T, Obata K, Tonoki H, et al. Cause of sudden, unexpected death of Prader-Willi syndrome patients with or without growth hormone treatment. Am J Med Genet 2005;136:45–48.
52. Sacco M, Di Giorgio G. Sudden death in Prader-Willi syndrome during growth hormone therapy. Horm Res 2005;63:29–32.
53. Schrander-Stumpel CT, Curfs LM, Sastrowijoto P, Cassidy SB, Schrander JJ, Fryns JP. Prader-Willi syndrome: causes of death in an international series of 27 cases. Am J Med Genet 2004;124:333–338.
54. Vogels A, Van Den Ende J, Keymolen K, Mortier G, Devriendt K, Legius E, Fryns JP. Minimum prevalence, birth incidence and cause of death for Prader-Willi syndrome in Flanders. Eur J Hum Genet 2004;12:238–240.
55. Van Vliet G, Deal CL, Crock PA, Robitaille Y, Oligny LL. Sudden death in growth hormone-treated children with Prader-Willi syndrome. J Pediatr 2004;44:129–131.
56. Oiglane E, Ounap K, Bartsch O, Rein R, Talvik T. Sudden death of a girl with Prader-Willi syndrome. Genet Couns 2002;3:459–464.
57. Eiholzer U, Nordmann Y, L'Allemand D. Fatal outcome of sleep apnoea in PWS during the initial phase of growth hormone treatment. A case report. Horm Res 2002;58(Suppl 3):24–26.
58. Nordmann Y, Eiholzer U, l'Allemand D, Mirjanic S, Markwalder C. Sudden death of an infant with Prader-Willi syndrome–not a unique case? Biol Neonate 2002;82:139–141.
59. Schrander-Stumpel C, Sijstermans H, Curfs L, Fryns JP. Sudden death in children with Prader-Willy syndrome: a call for collaboration. Genet Couns 1998;9:231–232.
60. Lindgren AC, Hellstrom LG, Ritzen EM, Milerad J. Growth hormone treatment increases CO(2) response, ventilation and central inspiratory drive in children with Prader-Willi syndrome. Eur J Pediatr 1999;158:936–940.
61. Haqq AM, Stadler DD, Jackson RH, Rosenfeld RG, Purnell JQ, LaFranchi SH. Effects of growth hormone on pulmonary function, sleep quality, behavior, cognition, growth velocity, body composition, and resting energy expenditure in Prader-Willi syndrome. J Clin Endocrinol Metab 2003;88:2206–2212.
62. Carrel AL, Myers SE, Whitman BY, Allen DB. Benefits of long-term GH therapy in Prader-Willi syndrome: a 4-year study. J Clin Endocrinol Metab 2002;87:1581–1585.
63. Lindgren AC, Ritzen EM. Five years of growth hormone treatment in children with Prader-Willi syndrome. Swedish National Growth Hormone Advisory Group. Acta Paediatr Suppl 1999;88: 109–111.
64. Eiholzer U, l'Allemand D. Growth hormone normalises height, prediction of final height and hand length in children with Prader-Willi syndrome after 4 years of therapy. Horm Res 2000 ;53:185–192.
65. Myers SE, Carrel AL, Whitman BY, Allen DB; Sustained benefit after 2 years of growth hormone on body composition, fat utilization, physical strength and agility, and growth in Prader-Willi syndrome. J Pediatr 2000;137:42–49.
66. Carrel AL, Myers SE, Whitman BY, Allen DB. Sustained benefits of growth hormone on body composition, fat utilization, physical strength and agility, and growth in Prader-Willi syndrome are dose-dependent. J Pediatr Endocrinol Metab 2001;14:1097–1105.

67. Whitman BY, Myers S, Carrel A, Allen D. The behavioral impact of growth hormone treatment for children and adolescents with Prader-Willi syndrome: a 2-year, controlled study. Pediatrics 2002;109:E35.
68. Clarke DJ, Waters J, Corbett JA. Adults with Prader-Willi syndrome: abnormalities of sleep and behaviour. J R Soc Med 1989; 82:21–24.
69. Vela-Bueno A, Kales A, Soldatos CR, Dobladez-Blanco B, Campos-Castello J, Espino-Hurtado P, Olivan-Palacios J. Sleep in the Prader-Willi syndrome. Clinical and polygraphic findings. Arch Neurol 1984;41:294–296.
70. Gau SF, Soong WT, Liu HM, et al. Kleine-Levin syndrome in a boy with Prader-Willi syndrome. Sleep 1996;19:13–17.
71. Vgontzas AN, Bixler EO, Kales A, Centurione A, Rogan PK, Mascari M, Vela-Bueno A. Daytime sleepiness and REM abnormalities in Prader-Willi syndrome: evidence of generalized hypoarousal. Int J Neurosci 1996;87:127–139.
72. Butler JV, Whittington JE, Holland AJ, Boer H, Clarke D, Webb T. Prevalence of, and risk factors for, physical ill-health in people with Prader-Willi syndrome: a population-based study. Dev Med Child Neurol 2002;44:248–255.
73. Schluter B, Buschatz D, Trowitzsch E, Aksu F, Andler W. Respiratory control in children with Prader-Willi syndrome. Eur J Pediatr 1997;156:65–68.
74. Livingston FR, Arens R, Bailey SL, Keens TG, Ward SL. Hypercapnic arousal responses in Prader-Willi syndrome. Chest 1995;108:1627–1631.
75. Nixon GM, Brouillette RT. Sleep and breathing in Prader-Willi syndrome. Pediatr Pulmonol 2002;34:209–217.
76. Arens R, Gozal D, Omlin KJ, Livingston FR, Liu J, Keens TG, Ward SL. Hypoxic and hypercapnic ventilatory responses in Prader-Willi syndrome. J Appl Physiol 1994;77:2224–2230.
77. Gozal D, Arens R, Omlin KJ, Ward SL, Keens TG. Absent peripheral chemosensitivity in Prader-Willi syndrome. J Appl Physiol 1994;77:2231–2236.
78. Manni R, Politini L, Nobili L, et al. Hypersomnia in the Prader Willi syndrome: clinical-electrophysiological features and underlying factors. Clin Neurophysiol 2001;112:800–805.
79. Mignot E, Lammers GJ, Ripley B, Oet al. The role of cerebrospinal fluid hypocretin measurement in the diagnosis of narcolepsy and other hypersomnias. Arch Neurol 2002;59:1553–1562.
80. Martin BC, Warram JH, Krolewski AS, Bergman RN, Soeldner JS, Kahn CR. Role of glucose and insulin resistance in development of type 2 diabetes mellitus: results of a 25-year follow-up study. Lancet 1992;340:925–929.
81. Donaldson MD, Chu CE, Cooke A, Wilson A, Greene SA, Stephenson JB. The Prader-Willi syndrome. Arch Dis Child 1994;70:58–63.
82. Cassidy SB. Prader-Willi syndrome. Curr Probl Pediatr 1984;14:1–55.
83. Landwirth J, Schwartz AH, Grunt JA. Prader-Willi syndrome. Am J Dis Child 1968;116:211–217.
84. Bray GA, Dahms WT, Swerdloff RS, Fiser RH, Atkinson RL, Carrel RE. The Prader-Willi syndrome: a study of 40 patients and a review of the literature. Medicine (Baltimore) 1983;62:59–80.
85. Sareen C, Ruvalcaba RH, Kelley VC. Some aspects of carbohydrate metabolism in Prader-Willi syndrome. J Ment Defic Res 1975;19:113–119.
86. Schuster DP, Osei K, Zipf WB. Characterization of alterations in glucose and insulin metabolism in Prader-Willi subjects. Metabolism 1996;45:1514–1520.
87. Zipf WB, O'Dorisio TM, Cataland S, Dixon K. Pancreatic polypeptide responses to protein meal challenges in obese but otherwise normal children and obese children with Prader-Willi syndrome. J Clin Endocrinol Metab 1983;57:1074–1080.
88. Berthoud HR, Powley TL. Morphology and distribution of efferent vagal innervation of rat pancreas as revealed with anterograde transport of Dil. Brain Res 1991;553:336-341.

89. Lee PD. Disease management of Prader-Willi syndrome. Expert Opin Pharmacother 2002;3: 1451–1459.
90. Cassidy SB, Ledbetter DH. Prader-Willi syndrome. Neurol Clin 1989;7:37–54.
91. Cassidy SB. Prader-Willi syndrome. J Med Genet 1997;34:917–923.
92. Jeffcoate WJ, Laurance BM, Edwards CR, Besser GM. Endocrine function in the Prader-Willi syndrome. Clin Endocrinol (Oxf) 1980;12:81–89.
93. Akefeldt A, Tornhage CJ, Gillberg C. A woman with Prader-Willi syndrome gives birth to a healthy baby girl. Dev Med Child Neurol 1999;41:789–790.
94. Schulze A, Mogensen H, Hamborg-Petersen B, Graem N, Ostergaard JR, Brondum-Nielsen K. Fertility in Prader-Willi syndrome: a case report with Angelman syndrome in the offspring. Acta Paediatr 2001;90:455–459.
95. Hamilton CR Jr, Scully RE, Kliman B. Hypogonadotropinism in Prader-Willi syndrome. Induction of puberty and sperm altogenesis by clomiphene citrate. Am J Med 1972;52:322–329.
96. Wannarachue N, Ruvalcaba RH. Hypogonadism in Prader-Willi syndrome. Am J Ment Defic 1975;79:592–603.
97. Garty B, Shuper A, Mimouni M, Varsano I, Kauli R. Primary gonadal failure and precocious adrenarche in a boy with Prader-Labhart-Willi syndrome. Eur J Pediatr 1982;139:201–203.
98. Grugni G, Marabito F, Crino A. Gonadal function and its disorders in simple obesity and in Prader-Willi Syndrome. In: Eiholzer U, ed. Prader-Willi syndrome as a model for obesity. Zurich: Karger; 2003:140–155.
99. Kojima M, Hosoda H, Date Y, Nakazato M, Matsuo H, Kangawa K. Ghrelin is a growth-hormone-releasing acylated peptide from stomach. Nature 1999;402:656–660.
100. Ariyasu H, Takaya K, Tagami T, et al. Stomach is a major source of circulating ghrelin, and feeding state determines plasma ghrelin-like immunoreactivity levels in humans. J Clin Endocrinol Metab 2001;86:4753–4758.
101. Cummings DE, Purnell JQ, Frayo RS, Schmidova K, Wisse BE, Weigle DS. A preprandial rise in plasma ghrelin levels suggests a role in meal initiation in humans. Diabetes 2001;50:1714–1749.
102. Wren AM, Small CJ, Ward HL, et al. The novel hypothalamic peptide ghrelin stimulates food intake and growth hormone secretion. Endocrinology 2000;141:4325–4328.
103. Wren AM, Seal LJ, Cohen MA, et al. Ghrelin enhances appetite and increases food intake in humans. J Clin Endocrinol Metab 2001;86:5992.
104. Shiiya T, Nakazato M, Mizuta M, et al. Plasma ghrelin levels in lean and obese humans and the effect of glucose on ghrelin secretion. J Clin Endocrinol Metab 2002;87:240–244.
105. Tschop M, Weyer C, Tataranni PA, Devanarayan V, Ravussin E, Heiman ML. Circulating ghrelin levels are decreased in human obesity. Diabetes 2001;50:707–709.
106. Cummings DE, Weigle DS, Frayo RS, Breen PA, Ma MK, Dellinger EP, Purnell JQ. Plasma ghrelin levels after diet-induced weight loss or gastric bypass surgery. N Engl J Med 2002;346:1623–1630.
107. Cummings DE, Clement K, Purnell JQ, et al. Elevated plasma ghrelin levels in Prader Willi syndrome. Nat Med 2002;8:643–644.
108. DelParigi A, Tschöp M, Heiman ML, et al. High circulating ghrelin: a potential cause for hyperphagia and obesity in prader-willi syndrome. J Clin Endocrinol Metab 2002;87:5461–5464.
109. Haqq AM, Farooqi IS, O'Rahilly S, et al. Serum ghrelin levels are inversely correlated with body mass index, age, and insulin concentrations in normal children and are markedly increased in Prader-Willi syndrome. J Clin Endocrinol Metab 2003;88:174–178.
110. Janssen JA, van der Toorn FM, Hofland LJ, et al. Systemic ghrelin levels in subjects with growth hormone deficiency are not modified by one year of growth hormone replacement therapy. Eur J Endocrinol 2001;145:711–716.

111. Gabreels BA, Swaab DF, de Kleijn DP, et al. Attenuation of the polypeptide 7B2, prohormone convertase PC2, and vasopressin in the hypothalamus of some Prader-Willi patients: indications for a processing defect. J Clin Endocrinol Metab 1998;83:591–599.
112. Cappa M, Raguso G, Palmiotto T, et al. The growth hormone response to hexarelin in patients with Prader-Willi syndrome. J Endocrinol Invest 1998;21:501–505.
113. Rittmaster RS, Loriaux DL, Merriam GR. Effect of continuous somatostatin and growth hormone-releasing hormone (GHRH) infusions on the subsequent growth hormone (GH) response to GHRH. Evidence for somatotroph desensitization independent of GH pool depletion. Neuroendocrinology 1987;45:118–122.
114. Date Y, Murakami N, Toshinai K, Matsukura S, Niijima A, Matsuo H, Kangawa K, Nakazato M. The role of the gastric afferent vagal nerve in ghrelin-induced feeding and growth hormone secretion in rats. Gastroenterology 2002;23:1120–1128.
115. Soper RT, Mason EE, Printen KJ, Zellweger H. Gastric bypass for morbid obesity in children and adolescents. J Pediatr Surg 1975;10:51–58.
116. Counts D. An adult with Prader-Willi syndrome and anorexia nervosa: a case report. Int J Eat Disord 2001;30:231–233.
117. Kobayashi J, Kodama M, Yamazaki K, Morikawa O, Murano S, Kawamata N, Kawamura I. Gastric bypass in a Japanese man with Prader-Willi syndrome and morbid obesity. Obes Surg 2003;13:803–805.
118. Haqq AM, Stadler DD, Rosenfeld RG, et al. Circulating ghrelin levels are suppressed by meals and octreotide therapy in children with Prader-Willi syndrome. J Clin Endocrinol Metab 2003;88: 3573–3576.
119. Tan TM, Vanderpump M, Khoo B, Patterson M, Ghatei MA, Goldstone AP. Somatostatin infusion lowers plasma ghrelin without reducing appetite in adults with Prader-Willi syndrome. J Clin Endocrinol Metab 2004;89:4162–4165.
120. Tomita T, Greeley G Jr, Watt L, Doull V, Chance R. Protein meal-stimulated pancreatic polypeptide secretion in Prader-Willi syndrome of adults. Pancreas 1989;4:395–400.
121. Butler MG, Carlson MG, Schmidt DE, Feurer ID, Thompson T. Plasma cholecystokinin levels in Prader-Willi syndrome and obese subjects. Am J Med Genet 2000;95:67–70.
122. Zipf WB, O'Dorisio TM, Cataland S, Sotos J. Blunted pancreatic polypeptide responses in children with obesity of Prader-Willi syndrome. J Clin Endocrinol Metab 1981;52:1264–1266.
123. Zipf WB, O'Dorisio TM, Berntson GG. Short-term infusion of pancreatic polypeptide: effect on children with Prader-Willi syndrome. Am J Clin Nutr 1990;51:162–166.
124. Lindgren AC, Hagenas L, Ritzen EM. Growth hormone treatment of children with Prader-Willi syndrome: effects on glucose and insulin homeostasis. Swedish National Growth Hormone Advisory Group. Horm Res 1999;51:157–161.
125. Goldstone AP, Brynes AE, Thomas EL, et al. Resting metabolic rate, plasma leptin concentrations, leptin receptor expression, and adipose tissue measured by whole-body magnetic resonance imaging in women with Prader-Willi syndrome. Am J Clin Nutr 2002;75:468–475.
126. Bueno G, Moreno LA, Pineda I, et al. Serum leptin concentrations in children with Prader-Willi syndrome and non-syndromal obesity. J Pediatr Endocrinol Metab 2000;13:425–4230.
127. Butler MG, Moore J, Morawiecki A, Nicolson M. Comparison of leptin protein levels in Prader-Willi syndrome and control individuals. Am J Med Genet 1998;75:7–12.
128. Lindgren AC, Marcus C, Skwirut C, Elimam A, Hagenas L, Schalling M, Anvret M, Lonnqvist F. Increased leptin messenger RNA and serum leptin levels in children with Prader-Willi syndrome and nonsyndromal obesity. Pediatr Res 1997;42:593–596.
129. Weigle DS, Ganter SL, Kuijper JL, Leonetti DL, Boyko EJ, Fujimoto WY. Effect of regional fat distribution and Prader-Willi syndrome on plasma leptin levels. J Clin Endocrinol Metab 1997;82:566–570.

130. Ebert MH, Schmidt DE, Thompson T, Butler MG. Elevated plasma gamma-aminobutyric acid (GABA) levels in individuals with either Prader-Willi syndrome or Angelman syndrome. J Neuropsychiatry Clin Neurosci 1997;9:75–80.
131. Nelson R, Huse D, Holman R, Kimbrough B, Wahner H, Callaway C, Hayles A. Nutrition, metabolism, body composition and response to the ketogenic diet in Prader-Willi Syndrome. In: Holm VA, ed. Prader-Willi syndrome. Baltimore: University Park Press; 1981:105–120.
132. Johnsen S, Crawford JD, Haessler HA. Fasting hyperlipogenesis: an inborn error of energy metabolism in Prader-Willi syndrome. Pediatr Res 1967;1:291.
133. Schoeller DA, Levitsky LL, Bandini LG, Dietz WW, Walczak A. Energy expenditure and body composition in Prader-Willi syndrome. Metabolism 1988;37:115–120.
134. van Mil EA, Westerterp KR, Gerver WJ, Curfs LM, Schrander-Stumpel CT, Kester AD, Saris WH. Energy expenditure at rest and during sleep in children with Prader-Willi syndrome is explained by body composition. Am J Clin Nutr 2000;71:752–756.
135. Steiniger J, Karst H, Noack R, Steglich HD. Diet-induced thermogenesis in man: thermic effects of single protein and carbohydrate test meals in lean and obese subjects. Ann Nutr Metab 1987;31:117–125.
136. Schutz Y, Bessard T, Jequier E. Diet-induced thermogenesis measured over a whole day in obese and nonobese women. Am J Clin Nutr 1984;40:542–552.
137. Jequier E, Schutz Y. New evidence for a thermogenic defect in human obesity. Int J Obes 1985 (Suppl 2):1–7.
138. Jequier E. Energy metabolism in human obesity. Soz Praventivmed 1989;34:58–62.
139. Thorne A. Diet-induced thermogenesis. An experimental study in healthy and obese individuals. Acta Chir Scand Suppl 1990;558:6–59.
140. Matsumoto T, Miyawaki C, Ue H, Kanda T, Yoshitake Y, Moritani T. Comparison of thermogenic sympathetic response to food intake between obese and non-obese young women. Obes Res 2001;9:78–85.
141. Segal KR, Gutin B. Thermic effects of food and exercise in lean and obese women. Metabolism 1983;32:581–589.
142. van Marken Lichtenbelt WD, Mensink RP, Westerterp KR. The effect of fat composition of the diet on energy metabolism. Z Ernahrungswiss 1997;36:303–305.
143. Westerterp-Plantenga MS, Van den Heuvel E, Wouters L, Ten Hoor F. Diet-induced thermogenesis and cumulative food intake curves as a function of familiarity with food and dietary restraint in humans. Physiol Behav 1992;51:457–465.
144. Nardella MT, Sulzbacher SI, Worthington-Roberts BS. Activity levels of persons with Prader-Willi syndrome. Am J Ment Defic 1983;87:498–505.
145. Davies PS, Joughin C. Using stable isotopes to assess reduced physical activity of individuals with Prader-Willi syndrome. Am J Ment Retard 1993;98:349–353.
146. Curfs LM, Hoondert V, van Lieshout CF, Fryns JP. Personality profiles of youngsters with Prader-Willi syndrome and youngsters attending regular schools. J Intellect Disabil Res 1995;39(Pt 3):241–248.
147. Eiholzer U, Nordmann Y, l'Allemand D, Schlumpf M, Schmid S, Kromeyer-Hauschild K. Improving body composition and physical activity in Prader-Willi Syndrome. J Pediatr 2003;142:73–78.
148. Schlumpf M, Eiholzer U, Gygax M, Schmid S, van der Sluis I, l'Allemand D. A daily comprehensive muscle training programme increases lean mass and spontaneous activity in children with Prader-Willi syndrome after 6 months. J Pediatr Endocrinol Metab 2006;19:65–74.
149. Caldwell ML, Taylor RL, Bloom SR. An investigation of the use of high- and low-preference food as a reinforcer for increased activity of individuals with Prader-Willi syndrome. J Ment Defic Res 1986;30:347–354.
150. Heiman MF. The management of obesity in the post-adolescent developmentally disabled client with Prader-Willi syndrome. Adolescence 1978;13:291–296.

151. Altman K, Bondy A, Hirsch G. Behavioral treatment of obesity in patients with Prader-Willi syndrome. J Behav Med 1978;1:403–412.
152. Kriz JS, Cloninger BJ. Management of a patient with Prader-Willi syndrome by a dental-dietary team. Spec Care Dentist 1981;1:179–182.
153. Evans PR. Hypogenital dystrophy with diabetic tendency. Guy's Hospital Reports 1964;113:207–222.
154. Jancar J. Prader-Willi syndrome. (Hypotonia, obesity, hypogonadism, growth and mental retardation). J Ment Defic Res 1971;15:20–29.
155. Juul J, Dupont A. Prader-Willi syndrome. J Ment Defic Res 1967;11:12–22.
156. Holm VA, Pipes PL. Food and children with Prader-Willi syndrome. Am J Dis Child 1976;130:1063–1067.
157. Bistrian BR, Blackburn GL, Stanbury JB. Metabolic aspects of a protein-sparing modified fast in the dietary management of Prader-Willi obesity. N Engl J Med 1977;296:774–779.
158. Collier SB, Walker WA Parenteral protein-sparing modified fast in an obese adolescent with Prader-Willi syndrome. Nutr Rev 1991;49:235–238.
159. Nelson R, Hayles A, Novak L, Margie J, Vernet J. Ketogenic diet and Prader-Willi syndrome. Am J Clin Nutr 1970;23:667.
160. Coplin SS, Hine J, Gormican A. Out-patient dietary management in the Prader-Willi syndrome. J Am Diet Assoc 1976;68:330–334.
161. Anderson AE, Soper RT, Scott DH. Gastric bypass for morbid obesity in children and adolescents. J Pediatr Surg 1980;15:876–881.
162. Marinari GM, Camerini G, Novelli GB, et al. Outcome of biliopancreatic diversion in subjects with Prader-Willi Syndrome. Obes Surg 2001;11:491–495.
163. Dietz WH. Genetic syndromes. In: Bjorntorp P, Brodoff BN, eds. Obesity. Philadelphia: Lippincott; 1992:589–593.
164. Stadler DD. Nutritional Management. In: Greenswag LR, ed. Management of Prader-Willi syndrome. Second ed. New York: Springer-Verlag, 1995:88–114.
165. Hoffman CJ, Aultman D, Pipes P. A nutrition survey of and recommendations for individuals with Prader-Willi syndrome who live in group homes. J Am Diet Assoc 1992;92:823–830, 833.
166. Pipes PL, Holm VA. Weight control of children with Prader-Willi syndrome. J Am Diet Assoc 1973;62:520–524.
167. Caldwell ML, Taylor RL. A clinical note on food preference of individuals with Prader-Willi syndrome: the need for empirical research. J Ment Defic Res 1983;27:45–49.
168. Silverthorn KH, Hornak JE. Beneficial effects of exercise on aerobic capacity and body composition in adults with Prader-Willi syndrome. Am J Ment Retard 1993;97:654–658.
169. Foster SC. Prader-Willi syndrome: report of cases. J Am Dent Assoc 1971;83:634–638.
170. Curfs LM, Fryns JP. Prader-Willi syndrome: a review with special attention to the cognitive and behavioral profile. Birth Defects Orig Artic Ser 1992;28:99–104.
171. Dykens EM, Hodapp RM, Walsh K, Nash LJ. Profiles, correlates, and trajectories of intelligence in Prader-Willi syndrome. J Am Acad Child Adolesc Psychiatry 1992;31:1125–1130.
172. Dykens EM, Hodapp RM, Walsh K, Nash LJ. Adaptive and maladaptive behavior in Prader-Willi syndrome. J Am Acad Child Adolesc Psychiatry 1992;31:1131–1136.
173. Dykens EM, Leckman JF, Cassidy SB. Obsessions and compulsions in Prader-Willi syndrome. J Child Psychol Psychiatry 1996;37:995–1002.
174. Clarke DJ. Prader-Willi syndrome and psychoses. Br J Psychiatry 1993;163:680–684.
175. Clarke D. Prader-Willi syndrome and psychotic symptoms: 2. A preliminary study of prevalence using the Psychopathology Assessment Schedule for Adults with Developmental Disability checklist. J Intellect Disabil Res 1998;42:451–454.
176. Greaves N, Prince E, Evans DW, Charman T. Repetitive and ritualistic behaviour in children with Prader-Willi syndrome and children with autism. J Intellect Disabil Res 2006;50:92–100.

177. Goldberg DL, Garrett CL, Van Riper C, Warzak WJ. Coping with Prader-Willi syndrome. J Am Diet Assoc 2002;102:537–542.
178. Couper RT, Couper JJ. Prader-Willi syndrome. Lancet 2000;356:673–675.
179. Whittington JE, Holland AJ, Webb T, Butler J, Clarke D, Boer H. Population prevalence and estimated birth incidence and mortality rate for people with Prader-Willi syndrome in one UK Health Region. J Med Genet 2001;38:792–798.
180. Cone RD, Cowley MA, Butler AA, Fan W, Marks DL, Low MJ. The arcuate nucleus as a conduit for diverse signals relevant to energy homeostasis. Int J Obes Relat Metab Disord 2001;25(Suppl 5):S63–67.
181. Cavaille J, Buiting K, Kiefmann M, et al. Identification of brain-specific and imprinted small nucleolar RNA genes exhibiting an unusual genomic organization. Proc Natl Acad Sci USA 2000;97:14311–14316.

12 Antipsychotic Medication–Induced Weight Gain and Risk for Diabetes and Cardiovascular Disease

John W. Newcomer

CONTENTS

Abstract

Compared with the general population, individuals with schizophrenia demonstrate an increased prevalence of obesity, type 2 diabetes mellitus (T2DM), and cardiovascular disease (CVD), with related increases in mortality. Increased adiposity is associated with decreases in insulin sensitivity, leading to increased risk of hyperglycemia and hyperlipidemia. Current evidence supports the hypothesis that treatment with antipsychotic medications is associated with increased risk for weight gain, insulin resistance, hyperglycemia, dyslipidemia, and T2DM. Key studies in this emerging literature are summarized, including case reports, observational studies, retrospective database analyses, and controlled experimental studies. Treatment with different antipsychotic medications is associated with variable effects on body weight, ranging from modest increases (e.g., ≤1 kg) with ziprasidone and with aripiprazole, to larger

From: *Contemporary Endocrinology: Energy Metabolism and Obesity: Research and Clinical Applications*
Edited by: P. A. Donohoue © Humana Press Inc., Totowa, NJ

increases during treatment with agents such as olanzapine and clozapine (e.g., 4–10 kg). Substantial evidence indicates that increases in adiposity are associated with decreases in insulin sensitivity in persons with and without psychiatric disease. The effects of increasing adiposity, as well as other effects, may contribute to increases in plasma glucose and lipids observed during treatment with certain antipsychotics. Treatment with certain antipsychotic medications is associated with metabolic adverse events that can increase risk for metabolic syndrome and related conditions such as prediabetes, T2DM, and CVD.

Key Words: adverse effects, antipsychotic medications, cardiovascular disease, dyslipidemia, hyperglycemia, metabolic syndrome, type 2 diabetes mellitus.

INTRODUCTION

There is substantial concern about the medical risk faced by patients with major mental disorders such as schizophrenia. A recent study compared the mortality of public mental health patients in multiple U.S. states with the mortality of their state general populations for 1997 through 2000. In all states, mental health clients had a higher relative risk of death compared with the general populations of their states, died at younger ages, and lost decades of potential life when compared with the corresponding general populations, with the largest risks attributed to patients with major mental illnesses like schizophrenia and bipolar disorder. In all states, cardiovascular disease (CVD) was found to be the leading cause of death in mentally ill patients. In states with data for both outpatient and inpatient populations where total mortality could be calculated, persons with major mental illness were observed to lose an average of more than 25 years of potential life, primarily due to early coronary heart disease mortality *(1)*. Persons with schizophrenia have previously been reported to have standardized mortality ratios for various natural causes of death that range from 1.8 to 4.4 *(2)*, with lower-end estimates of at least a 50% increased risk of death from medical causes *(3)*, and with a 20% shorter life span compared with the general population *(4)*. An earlier meta-analysis of 18 studies looking at causes of death in patients with major mental illness indicated that CVD (including cerebrovascular events, coronary artery disease, and peripheral vascular disease) is the leading cause of death in patients with schizophrenia *(5)*. CVD continues to be the leading contributor to mortality in persons with major mental illnesses like schizophrenia, with some evidence that standardized mortality rates have increased over the past decade *(1, 6)*.

The Framingham Heart Study *(7)* and other large, population-based studies have identified key modifiable risk factors for developing CVD. These key risk factors include obesity, smoking, hyperglycemia, hypertension, and dyslipidemia. These risk factors may be more than additive, so that having more than one of these risks can multiply the odds of developing CVD *(7)*. The thesis underlying a growing body of research in this area is that patients with major mental disorders suffer an increase in the prevalence of CVD due to an increased prevalence of these key modifiable risk factors.

METABOLIC CONTRIBUTIONS TO MEDICAL RISK

Obesity is a predictor of CVD risk as well as an important contributor to risk for the development of several of the other modifiable risk factors mentioned above. For example, as body mass index (BMI) increases, there is an increase in the relative risk for a number of medical conditions, including especially type 2 diabetes mellitus (T2DM) *(8)*. The relationship between increasing adiposity, particularly central adiposity, and increased risk for CVD and T2DM can be explained in part by the relationship between adiposity and insulin resistance.

Increases in adiposity are associated with decreases in insulin sensitivity *(9)*, initially resulting in a compensatory increase in insulin secretion by pancreatic β-cells. Insulin resistance and associated hyperinsulinemia are associated with a number of disturbances in physiology that are commonly referred to as the *insulin resistance syndrome (10)*. The insulin resistance syndrome includes key pathophysiologic changes that contribute to CVD risk: disturbances in glucose metabolism, disturbances in uric acid metabolism, disturbances in lipid metabolism, with a characteristic dyslipidemia including increases in fasting plasma triglyceride, hypertension, increases in inflammatory markers, and increased risk of clotting (*10–13*). Increases in insulin resistance and related increases in free fatty acid levels may be detected clinically as an increase in fasting plasma triglyceride levels, with recent interest in the use of plasma triglyceride as an indicator of clinically significant insulin resistance. While overweight or obese individuals (BMI ≥25) are reported to have an approximately 50% probability of clinically significant insulin resistance, those who additionally have fasting plasma triglyceride levels >130 mg/dl have a 70% probability of clinically significant insulin resistance *(14)*.

The insulin resistance syndrome is associated with risk for illnesses such as hypertension, sleep breathing disorder, nonalcoholic fatty liver disease, certain types of cancers, and polycystic ovarian syndrome *(15)*. Patients with the insulin resistance syndrome are at particular risk for the development of T2DM (*11–13*), which in turn is associated with increased risk for macrovascular disease, as well as microvascular diseases such as retinopathy, nephropathy, or neuropathy *(16)*. The effect of diabetes on CVD risk is substantial; approximately 20% of individuals with diabetes mellitus will develop coronary heart disease (CHD) or have a recurrent CHD event within 10 years, equivalent to the risk of recurrent CHD events in persons with a prior myocardial infarction *(17)*.

The combined disturbance in glucose and lipid metabolism and other changes that characterize the insulin resistance syndrome have become an important target of public health efforts. With the public health goal of targeting risk reduction in particularly vulnerable persons, specific threshold levels of abdominal adiposity (measured as waist circumference), fasting plasma triglyceride, high-density lipoprotein (HDL) cholesterol, glucose, and blood pressure have been used to define the metabolic syndrome *(18, 19)* (Table 12.1). Although there is debate about the added value of the metabolic syndrome construct over and above the predictive validity of individual insulin resistance markers, there is established interest in the value of individual metabolic syndrome elements as indicators of risk for CVD and T2DM *(20, 21)*. In men, metabolic syndrome is associated with a 25–50% increased risk of CVD disease and mortality *(22)*. Metabolic syndrome increases CVD risk more in men than in women, but it is highly predictive of T2DM in both genders *(19)*. Consistent with recent interest in focusing on individual metabolic syndrome criteria rather than only on the overall syndrome, the presence of even one metabolic syndrome criterion is associated with an increase in CVD risk, with risk increasing progressively with increasing numbers of additional metabolic syndrome risk factors *(23, 24)*.

Table 12.1
Modified National Cholesterol Education Program criteria for metabolic syndrome

Presence of three or more criteria:	
1. Abdominal obesity (waist circumference)	
Men	>40 inches
Women	>35 inches
2. Fasting triglycerides	≥150 mg/dl
3. High-density lipoprotein	
Men	<40 mg/dl
Women	<50 mg/dl
4. Blood pressure	≥130/85 mm Hg or on antihypertensives
5. Fasting glucose	110 mg/dl* or on insulin or hypoglycemic medication

Source: Information in the table was derived from multiple sources *(72–75,125–130)*.
Note: To increase awareness of insulin resistance–related CVD risk factors, the U.S. National Cholesterol Education Program Adult Treatment Panel III (ATP III) *(18)* created criteria for the *metabolic syndrome* (MS). MS is two to three times more common among antipsychotic-treated patients with schizophrenia than in the general population. Because MS components are not equally associated with CHD (e.g., waist circumference may add little risk beyond low HDL) and important CHD risk factors (e.g., LDL, smoking, age, family history) are not included in the MS definition, some have argued that the MS "diagnosis" may be less informative than the sum of its parts *(12)*. Nonetheless, in psychiatry and other specialties, the concept has usefully driven cross-discipline collaboration.
*The 2004 NHLBI/AHA modified definition uses a fasting glucose cutoff of ≥100 mg/dl.

METABOLIC RISK IN A MAJOR MENTAL DISORDER

Metabolic risk factors like obesity and T2DM are 1.5 to 2.0 times more common in schizophrenia than in the general population *(25)*. In the largest sample to date, funded by the National Institute of Mental Health and encompassing more than 50 diverse sites across the United States, investigators compared baseline metabolic characteristics of fasting subjects with schizophrenia entering the Clinical Antipsychotic Trials of Intervention Effectiveness (CATIE) study to characteristics of age-matched persons in the general population based on data from the National Health and Nutrition Examination Survey (NHANES) III *(26)*. Metabolic syndrome was found to be present in 41% of schizophrenia patients overall, including 51.6% of women and 36.0% of men with schizophrenia, while healthy women and men had rates of 25.1% and 19.7%, respectively. Men and women with schizophrenia had a higher prevalence of almost all criteria for metabolic syndrome, including increased prevalence of the waist circumference, triglyceride, high-density lipoprotein, and blood pressure criteria, as well as more impaired fasting blood glucose in women with schizophrenia compared with the aged-matched general population NHANES controls. The only exception to the rule that CATIE schizophrenia subjects generally had a higher prevalence of all metabolic syndrome criteria was that men with schizophrenia entering the CATIE study had a similar prevalence of abnormal fasting blood glucose (measured here with the more recent American Diabetes Association cutoff of ≥100 mg/dl). This may be related to the compensatory hyperinsulinemia that can buffer changes in plasma glucose.

Despite the increased prevalence of metabolic syndrome criteria in the baseline CATIE sample, this large study also revealed a low prevalence of appropriate treatment for these conditions, for example, with 88% of patients with dyslipidemia receiving no lipid-lowering medications *(27)*. Reduced access to medical treatment along with challenges associated with the treatment of chronic medical conditions in schizophrenia have increased interest in the prevention of cardiometabolic risk in this population. The well-established impact of psychotropic agents on body weight and the growing evidence of antipsychotic treatment effects on other metabolic risk factors has contributed to increased interest in the potential adverse effects of antipsychotic medication.

ANTIPSYCHOTIC MEDICATION OVERVIEW

Second-generation antipsychotic (SGA) medications accounted for approximately 90% of more than 40 million prescriptions for antipsychotics written in the United States in 2005, more than twice the number of antipsychotic prescriptions written prior to the introduction of the five first-line U.S.-marketed SGAs (risperidone, olanzapine, quetiapine, ziprasidone. and aripiprazole) *(28)*. SGAs are currently U.S. Food and Drug Administration (FDA)-approved for treatment of schizophrenia and bipolar disorder in adults but are prescribed in increasing numbers for behavioral disturbances in children *(29)*, to nursing home residents *(30)*, and by nonpsychiatric physicians *(31)*. Nearly half of prescriptions are for off-label indications *(32)*. A reduced propensity to cause neurologic adverse events, broadly termed *extrapyramidal side effects* (EPS) that include reversible drug-induced parkinsonism and the sometimes-irreversible movement disorder tardive dyskinesia, has supported the perception of increased safety for SGAs in comparison to first-generation antipsychotic (FGA) agents. However, growing evidence of the effect of certain SGAs to induce clinically significant weight gain and dyslipidemia and the association of these SGAs with risk for T2DM and CVD has emerged as an important safety concern.

Chlorpromazine was introduced in 1954 and followed by the approval of other FGA medications. These agents improved symptoms of psychosis sufficiently to allow many psychiatric patients to live outside of custodial institutions. However, these drugs offered limited efficacy for many patients, and their aggressive blockade of D_2 dopamine receptors is associated with parkinsonism and other motor side effects. Often termed *atypical* or *second generation* because of evidence of greater efficacy and reduced EPS, clozapine was approved in 1990 for treatment-resistant schizophrenia. Broader use was limited by the perception of risk of agranulocytosis and the need for frequent white blood cell monitoring. Over the next decade, five new SGAs were introduced in the United States with anticipation that each might possess clozapine-like efficacy without the risks associated with clozapine itself. These SGA agents all share the property of D_2 receptor antagonism that is common to FGAs, but SGAs bind with different affinity or intrinsic activity to the D_2 receptor and/or interact with specific $5HT_2$ serotonin receptors, and they are associated with a reduced risk of EPS at clinically relevant doses. Clozapine remains the only agent with well-established effectiveness for treatment-resistant schizophrenia, but utilization continues to be relatively low based on factors that include tolerability concerns. Meanwhile, the differential efficacy of other SGAs relative to each other and FGAs continues to be debated. Available trials, most sponsored by industry, indicate that some SGAs may be modestly more efficacious than FGAs, with modest efficacy differences among SGAs in some but not all studies *(33)*.

EVIDENCE OF ANTIPSYCHOTIC EFFECTS ON METABOLIC RISK

The general preference for SGAs over FGAs has been driven to a large extent by the neurologic safety advantages offered by SGAs. However, evidence of adverse metabolic disturbances associated with specific SGAs, including weight gain, dyslipidemia, and the risk of T2DM *(34)*, has tempered this generalized enthusiasm and led to a more detailed evaluation of risks associated with individual SGA agents. Most data on the association between SGAs and metabolic risk comes from studies of schizophrenia. Growing concerns about the impact of antipsychotics on metabolic risk prompted the American Diabetes Association, along with the American Psychiatric Association, the American Association of Clinical Endocrinologists, and the North American Association for the Study of Obesity, to review all available evidence and issue a consensus statement *(35)* that noted the relationship between certain SGAs and the development of weight gain and risk for diabetes and dyslipidemia. The report concluded that clozapine and olanzapine treatment were associated with the greatest weight gain potential among SGAs, with consistent evidence for increased risk of T2DM and dyslipidemia. The report concluded that there was intermediate weight gain potential with risperidone and quetiapine, with discrepant results concerning the risk of diabetes and dyslipidemia with these agents. The report indicated that available evidence suggested minimal risk of weight gain with aripiprazole and ziprasidone, with no evidence of risk for diabetes or dyslipidemia. It is worth noting that statements about the risk associated with specific medications are largely based on analyses of mean data, leading to the caveat that individual response to medications may vary, and that metabolic risk can be associated with any condition in which substantial weight gain occurs *(34)*.

EVIDENCE OF ANTIPSYCHOTIC EFFECTS ON WEIGHT AND ADIPOSITY

Clinical trials consistently indicate that mean weight gain and incidence of clinically significant weight gain varies across available SGA agents, with greater than placebo-level effects on weight observed for all currently available agents in the United States (Fig. 12.1). However, a review of weight gain in various placebo-controlled trials and head-to-head comparisons indicates that the relative incidence and magnitude of weight gain is not equal among antipsychotic medications *(34)*. Clozapine, olanzapine, and low-potency FGAs are associated with the greatest mean weight increases, risperidone and quetiapine with intermediate mean weight gain, and ziprasidone and aripiprazole with smaller weight increases. The risks of weight gain with antipsychotic therapy have been evaluated in short-term and long-term trials. In short-term trials, treatment with various antipsychotics has been shown to produce a wide range of changes in mean body weight, from <1 kg to >4 kg. For example, estimated mean weight gain for a patient treated with clozapine, olanzapine, risperidone, or ziprasidone ranges from 4.45, 4.15, 2.10, to 0.4 kg respectively over 10 weeks of treatment *(36)*. Reported means

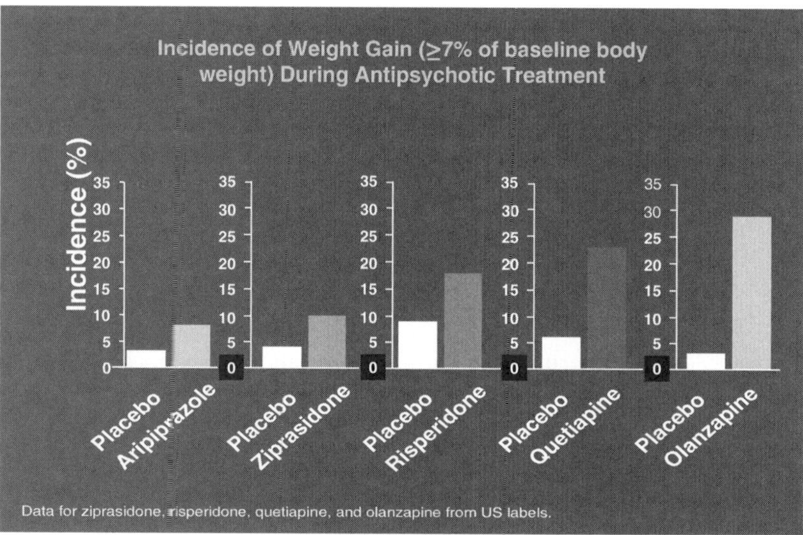

Fig. 12.1 Weight gain liability of antipsychotic drugs. Clinical trials consistently indicate weight gain variability across available antipsychotics. Shown is the percentage of patients gaining ≥7% of pretreatment body weight reported on labels for U.S. marketed SGAs. Clozapine (not shown) and olanzapine are associated with the greatest weight gain, risperidone and quetiapine with intermediate weight gain, and ziprasidone and aripiprazole with limited or no weight gain. Low-potency first-generation antipsychotics are also associated with intermediate weight gain. A 5-kg gain in weight after age 18 years doubles the risk of T2DM *(125)*, suggesting that the weight gain associated with some antipsychotic medications is a clinically significant risk factor for T2DM.

have most commonly been based on last-observation-carried-forward (LOCF) analyses that underestimate observed case (OC) effects. Over long-term trials of 52 weeks or greater, using data pooled from multiple clinical trials *(37)*, aripiprazole (*38–42*) and ziprasidone (*36,43–45*) were associated with a mean weight gain of approximately 1 kg over 1 year (LOCF); amisulpride with a gain of ~1.5 kg over 1 year *(46)*; quetiapine and risperidone (*47–50*) with approximately 2–3.5 kg over 1 year (LOCF and OC, respectively); and olanzapine with a gain of >6 kg over 1 year (using pooled doses from 2.5–17.5 mg/day, LOCF), with a mean gain of approximately 12 kg in patients who received olanzapine at doses between 12.5 and 17.5 mg/day (LOCF) *(51, 52)*. In clinical practice, it is not uncommon to see patients who have gained 50–100 lb during the first year of treatment, particularly during their first exposure to antipsychotic medication. Weight gain may slow and stabilize after the first year, although longer-term increases have also been reported *(53, 54)* and near linear weight increases over 5 years of treatment have been reported in some cohorts *(55)*.

The results of prospective randomized comparisons of individual agents have been consistent with the results of these estimates for individual agents from the pivotal trials. For example, after 6 months of treatment with amisulpride (n = 189) and olanzapine (n = 188), olanzapine was associated with a significantly greater mean increase in body weight (3.9 kg vs. 1.6 kg, $p < 0.01$) *(56)*. In a recent OC analysis of long-term weight gain on olanzapine in first-episode patients with schizophrenia, mean weight increases of more than 15 kg over 1 year of treatment were observed in the olanzapine treatment condition (in contrast with 10 kg, LOCF) *(53)*. The Clinical Antipsychotic Trials of Intervention Effectiveness (CATIE) study is a major prospective trial sponsored by the U.S. National Institute of Mental Health that was designed to assess the efficacy of the second-generation antipsychotic agents olanzapine, quetiapine, risperidone, and ziprasidone, with perphenazine included as a first-generation agent. The trial included 1,493 patients with schizophrenia at 57 sites in the United States. The primary outcome measure was time to all-cause discontinuation. This measure aimed to integrate patients' and clinicians' judgments of efficacy, safety, and tolerability into a global measure of effectiveness *(57)*. Secondary outcome measures include assessment of the reasons for discontinuation (e.g., lack of efficacy vs. intolerability due to side effects, the latter including weight gain and metabolic disturbances). Consistent with the ADA Consensus Statement and multiple industry-funded trials to date, the CATIE phase I study indicated that patients in the olanzapine group experienced more weight gain than patients in other treatment groups, with an average increase of 2 lb (0.9 kg) per month of treatment *(57)*. Additionally, a higher percentage of patients in the olanzapine group (30%) gained more than 7% of their baseline weight compared with the other medications in the study (on which between 7% and 16% of patients gained >7% of their baseline weight).

Importantly, recent studies suggest that switching from a medication with higher weight gain liability to a lower weight gain liability may produce significant reductions in body weight and BMI. Although none of the available SGAs can be considered weight-loss drugs, ziprasidone and perphenazine treatment in the CATIE I trial were associated with weight loss, most likely related to a removal of a previous antipsychotic treatment prior to being started on ziprasidone or perphenazine that had been contributing to weight gain or weight maintenance. Patients randomized to ziprasidone experienced significant weight loss (0.73 kg). Similar effects (1.37 kg loss after 26 weeks of treatment) have been reported in post hoc analyses conducted in a trial where patients switched from previous medications to aripiprazole *(58)*. In CATIE phase 2T (tolerability arm), in which patients who had discontinued their antipsychotic in phase I due to efficacy or tolerability concerns were randomly assigned to double-blind treatment with a different antipsychotic, weight differences between the antipsychotics were also pronounced *(59)*. Patients randomized to olanzapine gained a mean of 1.3 lb per month, whereas patients receiving ziprasidone had a mean loss of 1.7 lb per month. Risperidone and quetiapine treated subjects both experienced no mean weight change during phase 2T. Also consistent with previous studies, in CATIE 2T more patients receiving olanzapine gained >7% of their baseline weight (27%) than patients on other study medications (13% for risperidone and quetiapine; 6% for ziprasidone). Discontinuations during CATIE 2T due to weight gain or metabolic side effects varied across the assigned medications, with 0% discontinuing ziprasidone versus 5% with risperidone, 8% with olanzapine, and 10% with quetiapine. Of those patients who had gained >7% of their body weight in CATIE phase 1 who were randomized to ziprasidone in phase 2T, 42% lost more than 7% of their body weight; 20% of those randomized to risperidone lost more than 7% of their body weight; and 7% of patients randomized to quetiapine lost 7% of their body weight. None of the patients who gained >7% of their body weight in phase 1 who were randomized to olanzapine in phase 2T lost more than 7%. In terms of mean changes, among the group who had gained significant weight (>7%) in phase 1 who were then randomized in phase 2T, patients assigned to ziprasidone lost a mean of 11.3 lb, those on risperidone lost a mean of 1.4 lb, and patients on quetiapine experienced no significant weight change, while those patients randomized to olanzapine gained a mean of 2.1 lb.

EVIDENCE OF ANTIPSYCHOTIC EFFECTS ON METABOLIC RISK

A range of evidence suggests that treatment with certain antipsychotic medications is associated with an increased risk for insulin resistance, hyperglycemia, and T2DM compared with no treatment or treatment with alternative antipsychotics *(60)*. However, interpretation of the literature has been complicated by reports that patients with major mental disorders like schizophrenia have an increased prevalence of abnormalities in glucose regulation (e.g., insulin resistance) before the initiation of antipsychotic therapy *(61)*. However, these early studies did not control for age, body weight, adiposity, ethnicity, or diet, and one can readily hypothesize that differences in key factors such as diet and activity level between psychotic patients and control subjects contribute to at least some of the observed abnormalities. A recent study in 26 hospitalized first-episode antipsychotic-naive patients with schizophrenia found that 15% of these patients had impaired fasting glucose *(62)*. The schizophrenia patients (vs. controls) had significantly higher fasting plasma glucose (95.8 vs. 88.2 mg/dl), insulin (9.8 vs. 7.7 U/ml) and cortisol (499.4 vs. 303.2 nmol/L) values compared with control subjects matched for lifestyle and anthropometric measures. The elevated plasma cortisol levels observed in this sample probably contributed to some of the increase in insulin resistance and plasma glucose concentrations. However, hypercortisolemia is not typically observed in patients with schizophrenia during chronically antipsychotic treatment *(63)*, so this study may have overestimated the degree of insulin resistance and hyperglycemia that can be expected to persist past the acute psychotic episode and/or agitated condition that led to hospitalization. This group also reported increases in intraabdominal fat in drug-naive patients, in contrast with other larger samples showing no differences in drug-naive patients (*64–66*). However, this patient sample had an uncharacteristically long period of untreated illness and a higher mean age than most reported samples of first-episode patients *(67)*. It remains unclear whether this is a generalized finding in drug-naive samples. In any case, these studies complement earlier reports (see Refs. 68 and 69 for review) that patients with schizophrenia and other major mental disorders may have an increased risk for insulin resistance and T2DM independent of their exposure to antipsychotic medications.

There are now approximately 1,000 reports in the published literature concerning antipsychotic medications and metabolic risk. This literature has previously been reviewed in detail elsewhere *(34)* and will be briefly reviewed below. Concern about SGA-associated hyperglycemia began with case reports of new-onset T2DM, exacerbation of existing diabetes, diabetic ketoacidosis (DKA), and death in relatively young patients treated with clozapine and olanzapine *(70, 71)*. Most cases were detected within several months of initiating drug treatment, and hyperglycemia often improved rapidly after drug discontinuation. Less often, new-onset T2DM has been reported with other SGAs (*72–75*). Currently, only one case report of DKA associated with aripiprazole has been published, and no reports have associated amisulpride or ziprasidone with DKA *(76)*. Of note, the case involving aripiprazole occurred in a 34-year-old African-American woman with a 10-year history of T2DM without previously reported episodes of DKA. Four days prior to admission, aripiprazole 30 mg/day was added to her ongoing regimen of olanzapine 20 mg/day. One case of rhabdomyolysis, hyperglycemia, and pancreatitis has been associated with ziprasidone treatment *(77)*.

Pharmacoepidemiology studies in health care databases overall suggest increased risk for incident diabetes and dyslipidemia in treated patients compared with nonpatient groups, with a variable pattern of differential risk across agents but relatively consistent evidence of increased risk with clozapine and olanzapine *(34)*. A number of these reported observational analyses have used large administrative or health plan databases to test the strength of the association between treatment with specific antipsychotic medications and the presence of T2DM (*78–94*). Their common approach has been to identify the association within a database between the use of specific antipsychotic medications and the presence of ≥ 1 surrogate indicator of T2DM [e.g., prescription of an oral hypoglycemic medication, relevant International Classification of Diseases, Ninth Revision (ICD-9) codes]. A recent case-control study in a large claims database reported an association between incident hyperlipidemia and treatment with FGAs and all tested SGAs except aripiprazole *(95)*. Approximately two-thirds of these studies report findings suggesting that drugs associated with greater weight gain were also associated with an increased risk for T2DM compared with either no treatment, conventional treatment, or a drug associated with less weight gain. The other one-third of studies reported to date have generally detected no difference between groups or a nonspecific increase in the association for all treated groups compared with untreated controls. However, these studies have a number or methodological limitations, including relying on surrogate markers for the presence of diabetes, without direct measures of metabolism.

To clarify these findings, a recent meta-analyses *(96)* of 14 studies (11 retrospective, 5 case-control) (*79–83,85,87–93,94*) examined the association of diabetes incidence among patients treated with atypical antipsychotics compared with conventional or no antipsychotic treatment. All of the included studies were retrospective analyses of existing databases, with 11 retrospective cohort studies representing the vast majority of patients (n = 232,871) and 5 case-control studies (n = 40,084) of large health care plans (Medicaid, Blue Cross/Blue Shield, Veterans Affairs, etc.). Six studies (n = 122,270) included only schizophrenia diagnoses, while 10 studies included patients with various psychotic illnesses (n = 150,685). Data were available for clozapine, olanzapine, quetiapine, and risperidone. Meta-analyses on the association of diabetes incidence among patients treated with atypical antipsychotics were performed using conventional antipsychotics or no antipsychotic treatment as the comparator groups. All odds ratios (ORs), relative risks (RRs), and hazard ratios (HRs), included in the meta-analyses were adjusted for a variety of covariates, most commonly treatment duration, age, and gender. This analysis indicated that clozapine was consistently associated with increased risk for diabetes [vs. conventionals: OR, 1.37; 95% confidence interval (CI), 1.25–1.52; vs. no antipsychotics: OR, 7.44; 95% CI, 1.59–34.75]. Olanzapine was also associated with increased risk for diabetes (vs. conventionals: OR, 1.26; 95% CI, 1.10–1.46; vs. no antipsychotic: OR, 2.31; 95% CI, 0.98–5.46).

Neither risperidone (vs. conventional: OR, 1.07; 95% CI, 1.00–1.13; vs. no antipsychotic: OR, 1.20; 95% CI, 0.51–2.85), nor quetiapine (vs. conventional: OR, 1.22; 95% CI, 0.92–1.61; vs. no antipsychotic: OR, 1.00; 95% CI, 0.83–1.20) was associated with an increased diabetes risk. The results of this quantitative analysis of the association between atypical antipsychotic use and incident diabetes in large real-world databases suggests that the risk of diabetes varies among atypical antipsychotics, ranging from increases in risk relative to multiple comparators to no increase in risk for diabetes relative to any tested comparator.

More scientifically rigorous confirmation of the link between antipsychotic medications and metabolic abnormalities comes from a growing number of short- and long-term randomized controlled trials. However, clinical trials are often too short to capture most incident T2DM. Notably, one 14-week trial reported incident hyperglycemia (fasting blood sugar (FBS) >125) in 6 of 28 clozapine, 4 of 26 olanzapine, 3 of 22 risperidone, and 1 of 25 haloperidol-treated patients *(97)*. A naturalistic study reported that 36.6% of clozapine-treated patients developed T2DM over a 5-year period *(55)*. More commonly, clinical trials can be used to detect clinically significant changes in indicators of insulin resistance, rather than frank diabetes.

At least five studies have reported statistically significant increases in plasma insulin levels during olanzapine treatment (*98–102*), suggesting increased insulin resistance, and two of these studies reported a significant increase in calculated insulin resistance from baseline during olanzapine therapy ($p < 0.05$) *(100, 101)*. Two studies reported elevated insulin levels in 31% to 71% of patients receiving olanzapine treatment ($p < 0.05$) *(102, 103)*. Howes and colleagues reported a prospective assessment of clozapine's effects on insulin resistance, measured by oral glucose tolerance test, in 20 schizophrenia patients switched to clozapine from a variety of other medications *(104)*. There was no control group. After a mean 2.5 ± 0.95 months of treatment, mean fasting glucose level increased by 0.55 mmol/L ($t = -2.9, df = 19, p = 0.01$), and mean 2-h glucose level increased by 1.4 mmol/L ($t = -3.5, df = 19, p = 0.002$). There was no significant change in insulin level ($t = 0.128, df = 14, p = 0.9$) or insulin resistance level measured by the homeostasis model assessment ($t = -0.9, df = 14, p = 0.37$). Mean body mass index increased by 0.82 kg/m^2, although this was not statistically significant ($t = -1.325, df = 17, p = 0.2$).

A nonblinded crossover study of 15 schizophrenia patients examined the effects of olanzapine or risperidone on weight and fasting lipid profile after 3 months of treatment *(105)*. BMI decreased from 25.7 ± 3.1 kg/m^2 to 24.2 ± 3.1 kg/m^2 in the group switched to risperidone and increased from 24.8 ± 4.0 kg/m^2 to 25.9 ± 4.3 kg/m^2 in the group switched to olanzapine ($p = 0.015$). Plasma triglycerides decreased from 211.8 ± 134.9 to 125.8 ± 90.8 mg/dl in patients switched to risperidone and increased from 112.4 ± 76.3 to 196.7 ± 154.8 mg/dl in patients switched to olanzapine ($p = 0.001$).

A randomized, double-blind trial in 157 schizophrenia patients consisted of an 8-week fixed-dose period and a 6-week variable-dose period of treatment with clozapine, olanzapine, risperidone, or haloperidol *(97)*. There were significant increases from baseline in mean glucose levels at the end of the 6-week variable-dose period in patients who received olanzapine ($n = 22$; $p < 0.02$) and at the end of the 8-week fixed-dose period in patients who received clozapine ($n = 27$; $p < 0.01$) or haloperidol ($n = 25$; $p < 0.03$). The authors indicated that a trend-level difference was seen between treatments at the end of the 8-week fixed-dose period ($p = 0.06$) but not at the end of the 6-week variable-dose phase. Mean cholesterol levels were increased at the end of the 6-week variable-dose period in patients who received olanzapine ($p < 0.01$) and at the end of the 8-week fixed-dose period in patients who received clozapine or olanzapine ($p < 0.02$ and $p < 0.04$, respectively). However, interpretation was complicated by baseline and end-point body weights in some groups that are not consistent with those seen in clinical practice or clinical trials.

A randomized, double-blind, 6-week study comparing olanzapine and ziprasidone therapy in 269 inpatients with acute exacerbation of schizophrenia or schizoaffective disorder assessed glucose, insulin, and lipid parameters *(106)*. Significant increases from baseline in median fasting plasma insulin levels ($p < 0.0001$) and homeostasis model assessment insulin resistance ($p < 0.0001$) were observed with olanzapine therapy. Median body weight increased by 7.2 lb (3.3 kg) from baseline with olanzapine treatment compared with 1.2 lb (0.5 kg) with ziprasidone, and median body weight was significantly higher in the olanzapine group at end point ($p < 0.0001$). In this relatively young sample that demonstrated significant compensatory hyperinsulinemia, plasma glucose in the olanzapine-treated subjects did not increase significantly despite increased insulin resistance. In a 6-month, blinded follow-up study comparing olanzapine ($n = 71$) and ziprasidone ($n = 62$) therapy in patients with schizophrenia or schizoaffective disorder *(107)*, statistically significant increases from baseline in median fasting glucose and insulin levels were seen with olanzapine therapy. No statistically significant changes were observed with ziprasidone after 6 months of treatment.

The comparative effects of olanzapine and ziprasidone were again assessed in a 28-week prospective, randomized, double-blind study *(108, 109)*; 277 schizophrenia patients were randomized to olanzapine 10–20 mg/day (mean 15.27 ± 4.52 mg/day), and 271 to ziprasidone 80–160 mg/day (mean 115.96 ± 39.91 mg/day) at a standardized initial dose of each, with any further clinically determined dose changes performed using standardized increments. The proportion of patients with treatment-emergent hyperglycemia (≥ 126 mg/dl during treatment) did not differ significantly between the two groups (olanzapine, 11.5%; ziprasidone, 7.4%; $p = 0.159$). However, 35% of olanzapine-treated patients versus 5% of ziprasidone-treated patients experienced weight gain, defined in this report as a $\geq 7\%$ increase over baseline weight ($p < 0.001$), with mean weight gain of 3.06 ± 6.87 kg in the olanzapine group and -1.12 ± 4.70 kg in the ziprasidone group. The olanzapine group versus the ziprasidone group showed, respectively, a $+5.04 \pm 30.24$ versus -0.18 ± 21.42 mg/dl change in fasting glucose ($p = 0.38$), a $+3.1 \pm 36.74$ versus -12.76 ± 31.32 mg/dl change in total cholesterol ($p = 0.002$), a $+34.54 \pm 105.4$ versus -21.26 ± 96.54 mg/dl change in triglyceride level ($p < 0.001$), a $+0.77 \pm 29.8$ versus -10.44 ± 25.91 mg/dl change in low-density lipoprotein (LDL; $p = 0.02$), and a -2.32 ± 10.05 versus 0.77 ± 9.67 mg/dl change in HDL.

A 6-week, placebo-controlled study of aripiprazole treatment in schizophrenia patients examined changes in fasting blood glucose *(38)*. Pooling data from three aripiprazole groups (10 mg/day, 15 mg/day, or 20 mg/day) showed minimal mean changes in blood glucose from baseline (-0.37 mg/dl; $n = 120$), similar to those observed with placebo (-5.03 mg/dl; $n = 34$). Comparable effects on fasting serum glucose with aripiprazole and placebo have also been seen in patients with bipolar I disorder *(110)*. Long-term schizophrenia trials have demonstrated similar effects. In a 26-week relapse prevention study involving patients with chronic stable schizophrenia *(40)*, no clinically significant change from baseline was observed in fasting glucose levels of aripiprazole-treated patients or placebo-treated patients (aripiprazole: +0.13 mg/dl change; placebo: +2.1 mg/dl). In a 26-week randomized study of patients with schizophrenia comparing weight change and metabolic indices during treatment with olanzapine versus aripiprazole *(58)*, the olanzapine-treated group experienced statistically significant differences in mean changes in triglycerides (+79.4 mg/dl vs. −6.5 mg/dl, respectively), HDL (−3.39 mg/dl vs. +3.61 mg/dl, respectively), and more patients on olanzapine raised their total cholesterol to >200 at end point (38% vs. 19% on aripiprazole).

A 6-week randomized study of atypical antipsychotics in 56 schizophrenia patients (clozapine, olanzapine, quetiapine, and risperidone; each $n = 14$) found significant changes from baseline in triglyceride levels with quetiapine therapy (11.64 mg/dl; $p < 0.05$) *(111)*. However, this mean increase was approximately 3 times less than that observed in clozapine recipients (36.28 mg/dl; $p < 0.01$) or olanzapine recipients (31.23 mg/dl; $p < 0.01$) *(111)*. No significant increase from baseline in triglyceride levels was observed in risperidone-treated patients ($p = 0.76$).

Consistent with this literature, the CATIE phase 1 study indicated differences in the metabolic effects associated with different antipsychotic medications (Table 12.2) *(57)*. In this study, olanzapine-treated patients experienced the greatest increase in total cholesterol (exposure adjusted mean increase 9.4 mg/dl), triglycerides (exposure adjusted mean increase 40.5 mg/dl), and glycosylated hemoglobin (exposure adjusted mean increase 0.4 mg/dl), with statistically significant differences between treatment groups in each of these indices. Ziprasidone treatment, in contrast, was associated with a decrease in total cholesterol (exposure adjusted mean decrease 8.2), triglycerides (exposure adjusted mean decrease 16.5), and glycosylated hemoglobin (exposure adjusted mean decrease 0.11). Notably, no significant between-group effects were observed on plasma glucose.

CATIE phase 2T results further illustrated the metabolic effects of the various antipsychotics (Table 12.3) *(59)*. In phase 2T, olanzapine was associated with increases in total cholesterol (exposure adjusted mean increase of 17.5) and triglyceride (exposure adjusted mean increase of 94.1) whereas risperidone and ziprasidone treatment were associated with decreases in these parameters. Comparison of the CATIE phase 1 and 2T data illustrate an interesting pattern, relevant to the interpretation of other clinical trial data. In CATIE phase 1, where patients could be randomized to agents that they were previously treated with in the immediate past, those randomized to olanzapine experienced an approximately 40 mg/dl exposure adjusted mean increase in plasma triglyceride. In CATIE phase 2T, where patients previously on a specific antipsychotic could not be randomized to the same agent, those randomized to olanzapine experienced a 94 mg/dl exposure adjusted mean increase in plasma triglyceride. The results of metabolic results of CATIE reported to date are consistent with the growing literature of randomized clinical trials in this area and shed useful light on the interpretation of metabolic risk during antipsychotic treatment.

Table 12.2
Changes in weight, lipids, and glucose measures in phase I of the CATIE study

Assessment, Change	*Olanzapine (N = 336)*	*Perphenazine (N = 261)*	*Quetiapine (N = 337)*	*Risperidone (N = 341)*	*Ziprasidone (N = 185)*
Weight (lb/month)					
Mean (SE)	2.0 (0.3)	−0.2 (0.2)	0.5 (0.2)	0.4 (0.3)	−0.3 (0.3)
Triglycerides (mg/dL)					
Mean (SE)	42.9 (8.4)	8.3 (11.5)	19.2 (10.6)	−2.6 (6.3)	−18.1 (9.4)
Exp-Adj Mean (SE)	40.5 (8.9)	9.2 (10.1)	21.2 (9.2)	−2.4 (9.1)	−16.5 (12.2)
Cholesterol (mg/dL)					
Mean (SE)	9.7 (2.1)	0.5 (2.3)	5.3 (2.1)	−2.1 (1.9)	−9.2 (5.2)
Exp-Adj Mean (SE)	9.4 (2.4)	1.5 (2.7)	6.6 (2.4)	−1.3 (2.4)	−8.2 (3.2)
HbA1c (%)					
Mean (SE)	0.41 (0.09)	0.10 (0.06)	0.05 (0.05)	0.08 (0.04)	−0.10 (0.14)
Exp-Adj Mean (SE)	0.4 (0.07)	0.09 (0.09)	0.04 (0.08)	0.07 (0.08)	0.11 (0.09)
Blood Glucose (mg/dL)					
Mean (SE)	15.0 (2.8)	5.2 (2.0)	6.8 (2.5)	6.7 (2.0)	2.3 (3.9)
Exp-Adj Mean (SE)	13.7 (2.5)	5.4 (2.8)	7.5 (2.5)	6.6 (2.5)	2.9 (3.4)

Exp-Adj Mean = Exposure-adjusted mean (least-squares mean from an ANCOVA adjusting for whether the patient had an exacerbation in the preceding 3 months and for duration of exposure to the study drug in phase 1)

Source: Lieberman JA, Stroup TS, McEvoy JP, et al. Effectiveness of antipsychotic drugs in patients with chronic schizophrenia. N Engl J Med 2005;353:1209–1223.

CLINICAL SIGNIFICANCE OF MEDICATION-RELATED METABOLIC EFFECTS

Reports of excess diabetes and CVD risk in schizophrenia predate the introduction of antipsychotic drugs *(68)*, and schizophrenia patients experience lifestyle changes (smoking, poor diet, low physical activity) that may contribute to weight gain, T2DM, and CVD. With limited studies of drug-naive patients and/or nonpsychiatric controls, it has been difficult to precisely quantify the relative contributions of medication, illness, and lifestyle on SGA-associated metabolic risk. Despite these uncertainties, the weight gain and other metabolic effects associated with antipsychotic treatment can be predicted to have a major clinical significance.

Using clinical trial data that established the efficacy of clozapine for the prevention of suicide, Fontaine and colleagues *(59)* estimated that approximately 492 suicide deaths per 100,000 patients with schizophrenia could be prevented over 10 years with the use of clozapine; however, based on projections from the Framingham Heart Study data, a 10-kg weight gain due to antipsychotic treatment could potentially result in an additional 416 deaths per 100,000 over 10 years for those with baseline BMIs of 27. This result highlights the significant contribution of weight gain to potential mortality in patients with schizophrenia and provocatively suggests that lives saved via antipsychotic treatment may be offset by deaths due to treatment-induced weight gain. A recent analysis of baseline CATIE data can similarly be used to estimate the

Table 12.3
Changes in weight, lipids, and glucose in the CATIE tolerability pathway (phase 2T)

Assessment, Change	*Olanzapine (N = 108)*	*Risperidone (N = 104)*	*Quetiapine (N = 95)*	*Ziprasidone (N = 137)*
Weight (lb/month)				
Mean (SE)	1.3 (0.6)	−0.2 (0.4)	0.1 (0.6)	−1.7 (0.5)
Triglycerides (mg/dL)				
Mean (SE)	69.6 (19.7)	−27.7 (13.8)	15.5 (16.8)	−29.1 (10.3)
Exp-Adj Mean (SE)	94.1 (21.8)	−5.2 (21.6)	39.3 (22.1)	−3.5 (20.9)
Cholesterol (mg/dL)				
Mean (SE)	17.9 (3.3)	−2.6 (3.9)	4.8 (3.8)	−12.5 (3.5)
Exp-Adj Mean (SE)	17.5 (5.2)	−3.1 (5.2)	6.5 (5.3)	−10.7 (5.1)
HbA1c (%)				
Mean (SE)	0.52 (0.30)	0.10 (0.16)	0.23 (0.28)	0.09 (0.06)
Exp-Adj Mean (SE)	0.97 (0.3)	0.49 (0.3)	0.61 (0.3)	0.46 (0.3)
Blood Glucose (mg/dL)				
Mean (SE)	14.8 (4.0)	8.4 (4.3)	−0.2 (4.3)	−1.1 (3.9)
Exp-Adj Mean (SE)	13.8 (5.9)	6.9 (5.8)	1.2 (6.0)	0.8 (5.6)

Exp-Adj Mean = Exposure-adjusted mean (ANCOVA least squares mean adjusting for whether the patient had an exacerbation in the preceding 3 months and duration of exposure to phase 1 study drug [olanzapine: N = 89; quetiapine: N = 81; risperidone: N = 85; ziprasidone: N = 106])

clinical significance of metabolic conditions that are often induced by antipsychotic treatment conditions *(112)*. Goff and colleagues calculated the 10-year risk for coronary heart disease in treated patients compared with age-matched controls from the general population, noting increased prevalence of cigarette smoking (68% vs. 35%), diabetes (13% vs. 3%), hypertension (27% vs. 17%), and dyslipidemia, supporting the result that cardiac risk was significantly elevated in treated patients. Metabolic risk associated with certain SGAs may be of particular significance. In a recent 10-year naturalistic study of patients treated with clozapine, the 10-year mortality rate from coronary heart disease was 9% and the rate of new-onset T2DM was 43% *(113)*, significantly higher than that reported in general population samples.

PATHOPHYSIOLOGY

In brief, the pathophysiology of antipsychotic-induced or exacerbated metabolic disturbance appears to be complex and may include both adiposity-related and adiposity-independent pathways *(114)*. Increasing adiposity is directly associated with insulin resistance, dyslipidemia, and increased risk for T2DM and CVD, so that any treatment that causes significant weight gain could potentially increase these outcomes. Differences in weight gain associated with antipsychotic agents likely reflects their order of risk for insulin resistance and dyslipidemia *(25, 63, 68, 115)*. However, about one-quarter of reported antipsychotic-associated T2DM cases occurred without substantial weight gain, DKA has sometimes observed during SGA treatment, and a relatively rapid onset and offset of hyperglycemia and dyslipidemia can occur during challenge and dechallenge with some SGAs. These observations suggest the possibility of direct, adiposity-independent drug effects on β-cell functioning and/or alteration of insulin receptor function or insulin signaling that could supplement drug effects on adiposity. Consistent with these hypotheses, investigators have reported defects in β-cell response to insulin resistance in dogs treated with olanzapine and not risperidone *(116)*, as well as acute (within 2 h) onset of dose-dependent insulin resistance in rats treated with olanzapine and clozapine but not ziprasidone, risperidone, or quetiapine *(117)*.

PREVENTION AND MANAGEMENT OF ANTIPSYCHOTIC-INDUCED CVD RISK

The problem of antipsychotic-induced weight gain, dyslipidemia, and risk for hyperglycemia and CVD argues for the use of lower-risk medications whenever possible and also underscores the need for additional antipsychotic medication options with low risk for metabolic adverse events. In addition, there is a need for increased attention to patient education, informed consent, and risk/benefit analysis in selection of pharmacotherapy. Metabolic risks associated with treatment also reinforce the need to ensure appropriate medical care for psychiatric patients, particularly the use of existing public health guidelines (*18,118–120*) concerning the prevention and treatment of T2DM, hypertension, and CVD. Much progress remains to be accomplished in this area. A recent study of nearly 1,500 patients with schizophrenia from 52 diverse U.S. sites reported nontreatment rates of 30.2% for T2DM, 62.4% for hypertension, and 88% for dyslipidemia *(27)*.

Monitoring guidelines for SGA-treated patients recommend assessment of personal and family medical history (e.g., obesity, diabetes, hypertension, CVD) at or near baseline when starting antipsychotic therapy and serial assessment of weight (BMI), waist circumference, blood pressure, fasting plasma glucose, and fasting lipid profile *(26)*. Other recommendations include considering switching at-risk patients who gain 5% or more of their baseline body weight to an antipsychotic with less weight liability and referral to a primary care provider (PCP) or appropriate specialist for patients who develop T2DM, hypertension, or dyslipidemia. Patients and caregivers should be educated regarding the signs and symptoms of diabetes, including the symptoms of DKA. The cognitive and motivational impairments associated with serious mental illness may create the need for engagement of families and/or case-workers to assist with recommended follow-up, referrals, and monitoring. Management of patients taking SGAs often requires collaboration between a psychiatrist and PCP or specialist, but because of inadequate service integration, patients with serious mental illness may not receive general medical care or may receive inadequate care *(121)*.

Adherence to therapeutic lifestyle changes recommended for CVD risk management is a major challenge for patients with or without psychiatric disorders. Pharmacologic approaches to reversing SGA-induced weight gain including amantadine, nizatidine (histamine-2 receptor antagonist), naltrexone, topiramate, fluvoxamine, fluoxetine, reboxetine, metformin, and sibutramine have been studied in small trials, with modest and variable weight reductions reported; there is currently inadequate evidence to support any particular pharmacologic approach (*122–124*).

CONCLUSION

Substantial evidence indicates that certain SGAs can contribute to weight gain, dyslipidemia, and the risk of T2DM and CVD. There is an unmet need for additional metabolically safe and effective antipsychotics. Weight-sparing antipsychotic agents should be first-line treatment choices for new patients whenever available. In addition, weight-sparing agents should be preferred switch options for patients with emergent or long-standing adverse metabolic risk profiles. Psychiatrists should be encouraged to monitor for metabolic side effects of antipsychotic agents and the knowledge about when to refer, and PCPs and relevant specialists should be encouraged to aggressively treat metabolic risk factors in this at-risk population. Given the challenges in managing metabolic complications in patients with severe illnesses like schizophrenia, the increased availability of metabolically favorable medications remains an important public health priority.

ACKNOWLEDGMENTS

John W. Newcomer, M.D., has no significant financial conflict of interest in compliance with the Washington University School of Medicine Conflict of Interest Policy. Dr. Newcomer receives grant support from The National Institute of Mental Health (NIMH), The National Alliance for Research on Schizophrenia and Depression (NARSAD), Sidney R. Baer Jr. Foundation, Janssen Pharmaceutica, Pfizer, Inc., Wyeth, and Bristol-Myers Squibb. Dr. Newcomer is a consultant for Janssen Pharmaceutica, Pfizer, Inc., Bristol-Myers Squibb, AstraZeneca Pharmaceuticals, GlaxoSmithKline, Organon, Solvay, and Wyeth. Dr. Newcomer serves on the Data Safety Monitoring Committee for Organon, and Dr. Newcomer has received royalties for a Metabolic Screening Form from Compact Clinicals. Dr. Newcomer is supported in part by NIMH R01 MH072912 and R01 MH63985. I thank Glenn Floyd for his editorial assistance on this chapter.

REFERENCES

1. Colton CW, Manderscheid RW. Congruencies in increased mortality rates, years of potential life lost, and causes of death among public mental health clients in eight states. Prev Chronic Dis 2006;3:A42.
2. Allebeck P, Schizophrenia: a life-shortening disease. Schizophr Bull 1989;15:81–89.
3. Harris EC, Barraclough B. Excess mortality of mental disorder. Br J Psychiatry 1998;173:11–53.
4. Newman SC, Bland RC. Mortality in a cohort of patients with schizophrenia: a record linkage study. Can J Psychiatry 1991;36:239–245.
5. Brown S. Excess mortality of schizophrenia. A meta-analysis. Br J Psychiatry 1997;171: 502–508.
6. Osby U, Correia N, Brandt L, et al. Time trends in schizophrenia mortality in Stockholm county, Sweden: cohort study. BMJ 2000; 321:483–484.
7. Wilson PW, D'Agostino RB; Levy D, et al. Prediction of coronary heart disease using risk factor categories. Circulation 1998;97:1837–1847.
8. Willett WC, Dietz WH, Colditz GA. Guidelines for healthy weight. N Engl J Med 1999;341:427–434.
9. Banerji MA, Lebowitz J, Chaiken RL, et al. Relationship of visceral adipose tissue and glucose disposal is independent of sex in black NIDDM subjects. Am J Physiol 1997;273:E425–432.
10. Reaven G. Syndrome X: 10 years after. Drugs 1999;58(Suppl 1):19–20; discussion 75–82.
11. Steinberg HO, Baron AD. Vascular function, insulin resistance and fatty acids. Diabetologia 2002;45:623–634.

12. Caballero AE. Endothelial dysfunction in obesity and insulin resistance: a road to diabetes and heart disease. Obes Res 2003;11:1278–1289.
13. Reaven GM. Banting lecture 1988. Role of insulin resistance in human disease. Diabetes 1988;37:1595–1607.
14. McLaughlin T, Abbasi F, Cheal K, et al. Use of metabolic markers to identify overweight individuals who are insulin resistant. Ann Intern Med 2003;139:802–809.
15. Reaven GM. Why Syndrome X? From Harold Himsworth to the insulin resistance syndrome. Cell Metab 2005;1:9–14.
16. American Diabetes Association, Diagnosis and classification of diabetes mellitus. Diabetes Care 2006;29(Suppl 1):S43–48.
17. Haffner SM, Lehto S, Ronnemaa T, et al. Mortality from coronary heart disease in subjects with type 2 diabetes and in nondiabetic subjects with and without prior myocardial infarction. N Engl J Med 1998;339:229–234.
18. National Cholesterol Education Program, Executive Summary of The Third Report of The National Cholesterol Education Program (NCEP) Expert Panel on Detection, Evaluation, and Treatment of High Blood Cholesterol in Adults (Adult Treatment Panel III). JAMA 2001;285:2486–2497.
19. Grundy SM, Brewer Jr HB, Cleeman JI, et al. Definition of metabolic syndrome: Report of the National Heart, Lung, and Blood Institute/American Heart Association conference on scientific issues related to definition. Circulation 2004;109:433–438.
20. Reaven GM. The metabolic syndrome: is this diagnosis necessary? Am J Clin Nutr 2006;83: 1237–1247.
21. American Diabetes Association. The Cardiometabolic Risk Initiative. Available at: http://www.diabetes.org/for-health-professionals-and-scientists/cardiometabolic-risk.jsp.
22. Eberly LE, Prineas R, Cohen JD, et al. Metabolic syndrome: risk factor distribution and 18-year mortality in the multiple risk factor intervention trial. Diabetes Care 2006;29:123–130.
23. Sattar N, Gaw A, Scherbakova O, et al. Metabolic syndrome with and without C-reactive protein as a predictor of coronary heart disease and diabetes in the West of Scotland Coronary Prevention Study. Circulation 2003;108:414–419.
24. Ridker PM, Buring JE, Cook NR, et al. C-reactive protein, the metabolic syndrome, and risk of incident cardiovascular events: an 8-year follow-up of 14 719 initially healthy American women. Circulation 2003;107:391–397.
25. American Diabetes Association, Consensus development conference on antipsychotic drugs and obesity and diabetes. J Clin Psychiatry 2004;65:267–272.
26. McEvoy JP, Meyer JM, Goff DC, et al. Prevalence of the metabolic syndrome in patients with schizophrenia: Baseline results from the Clinical Antipsychotic Trials of Intervention Effectiveness (CATIE) schizophrenia trial and comparison with national estimates from NHANES III. Schizophr Res 2005;80:19–32.
27. Nasrallah HA, Meyer JM, Goff DC, et al. Low rates of treatment for hypertension, dyslipidemia and diabetes in schizophrenia: data from the CATIE schizophrenia trial sample at baseline. Schizophr Res 2006;86:15–22.
28. IMS Health. Perspectives NS. 2006. Available at http://www.imshealth.com.
29. Olfson M, Blanco C, Liu L, et al. National trends in the outpatient treatment of children and adolescents with antipsychotic drugs. Arch Gen Psychiatry 2006;63:679–685.
30. Briesacher BA, Limcangco MR, Simoni-Wastila L, et al. The quality of antipsychotic drug prescribing in nursing homes. Arch Intern Med 2005;165:1280–1285.
31. Van Brunt DL, Gibson PJ, Ramsey JL, et al. Outpatient use of major antipsychotic drugs in ambulatory care settings in the United States, 1997-2000. MedGenMed 2003;5:16.
32. Verispan. Physician drug & diagnosis audit (PDDA). 2006. Available at http://www.verispan.com/products/product details.php?id=38j2rzrc6s.

33. Davis JM, Chen N, Glick ID. A meta-analysis of the efficacy of second-generation antipsychotics. Arch Gen Psychiatry 2003;60:553–564.
34. Newcomer JW. Second-generation (atypical) antipsychotics and metabolic effects: a comprehensive literature review. CNS Drugs 2005;19(Suppl 1):1–93.
35. American Diabetes Association. Consensus development conference on antipsychotic drugs and obesity and diabetes. Diabetes Care 2004;27:596–601.
36. Allison DB, Mentore JL, Heo M, et al. Antipsychotic-induced weight gain: a comprehensive research synthesis. Am J Psychiatry 1999;156:1686–1696.
37. Newcomer JW, Haupt DW. The metabolic effects of antipsychotic medications. Can J Psychiatry 2006;51:480–491.
38. Marder SR, McQuade RD, Stock E, et al. Aripiprazole in the treatment of schizophrenia: safety and tolerability in short-term, placebo-controlled trials. Schizophr Res 2003;61:123–136.
39. Kasper S, Lerman MN, McQuade RD, et al. Efficacy and safety of aripiprazole vs. haloperidol for long-term maintenance treatment following acute relapse of schizophrenia. Int J Neuropsychopharmacol 2003;6:325–337.
40. Pigott TA, Carson WH, Saha AR, et al. Aripiprazole for the prevention of relapse in stabilized patients with chronic schizophrenia: a placebo-controlled 26-week study. J Clin Psychiatry 2003;64: 1048–1056.
41. McQuade RD, Jody D, Kujawa M, et al. Long-term weight effects of aripiprazole versus olanzapine. Poster presented at the American Psychiatric Association (APA) Annual Meeting, San Francisco, 2003.
42. Bristol-Myers Squibb. Abilify. Package insert. 2004. Bristol-Myers Squibb. New York, NY.
43. Daniel DG, Zimbroff DL, Potkin SG, et al. Ziprasidone 80 mg/day and 160 mg/day in the acute exacerbation of schizophrenia and schizoaffective disorder: a 6-week placebo-controlled trial. Ziprasidone Study Group. Neuropsychopharmacology 1999;20:491–505.
44. Hirsch SR, Kissling W, Baumi J, et al. A 28-week comparison of ziprasidone and haloperidol in outpatients with stable schizophrenia. J Clin Psychiatry 2002;63:516–523.
45. Pfizer. Geodon (ziprasidone HCl). Package insert. 2004. Available at http://www.pfizer.com/download/uspi_geodon.pdf.
46. Leucht S, Wagenpfeil S, Hamann J, et al. Amisulpride is an "atypical" antipsychotic associated with low weight gain. Psychopharmacology (Berl) 2004;173 112–115.
47. Jones AM, Rak IW, Raniwalla J. Weight changes in patients treated with quetiapine. Poster presented at the 153rd Annual Meeting of the American Psychiatric Association Chicago, IL, May 13–18, 2000.
48. AstraZeneca. Seroquel (quetiapine). Package insert. 2004. Available at http:/www.fda.gov/medwatch/SAFETY/2004/Seroquel-lbl.pdf.
49. Janssen Pharmaceutica Products, L.P. Risperdal (risperidone). Package insert. 2003. Available at http://www.risperdal.com/files/risperdal.pdf.
50. Csernansky JG, Mahmoud R, Brenner R. A comparison of risperidone and haloperidol for the prevention of relapse in patients with schizophrenia. N Engl J Med 2002;346:16–22.
51. Nemeroff CB. Dosing the antipsychotic medication olanzapine. J Clin Psychiatry 1997;58(Suppl 10):45–49.
52. Kinon B.J. The routine use of atypical antipsychotic agents: maintenance treatment. J Clin Psychiatry 1998;59(Suppl 19):18–22.
53. Zipursky RB, Gu H, Green AI, et al. Course and predictors of weight gain in people with first-episode psychosis treated with olanzapine or haloperidol. Br J Psychiatry 2005;187:537–543.
54. Gentile S. Long-term treatment with atypical antipsychotics and the risk of weight gain: a literature analysis. Drug Saf 2006;29:303–319.
55. Henderson DC, Cagliero E, Gray C, et al. Clozapine, diabetes mellitus, weight gain, and lipid abnormalities: A five-year naturalistic study. Am J Psychiatry 2000;157:975–981.

56. Mortimer A, Martin S, Loo H, et al. A double-blind, randomized comparative trial of amisulpride versus olanzapine for 6 months in the treatment of schizophrenia. Int Clin Psychopharmacol 2004;19:63–69.
57. Lieberman JA, Stroup TS, McEvoy JP, et al. Effectiveness of antipsychotic drugs in patients with chronic schizophrenia. N Engl J Med 2005;353:1209–1223.
58. McQuade RD, Stock E, Marcus R, et al. A comparison of weight change during treatment with olanzapine or aripiprazole: results from a randomized, double-blind study. J Clin Psychiatry 2004;65(Suppl 18):47–56.
59. Stroup TS, Lieberman JA, McEvoy JP, et al. Effectiveness of olanzapine, quetiapine, risperidone, and ziprasidone in patients with chronic schizophrenia following discontinuation of a previous atypical antipsychotic. Am J Psychiatry 2006;163:611–622.
60. Casey DE, Haupt DW, Newcomer JW, et al. Antipsychotic-induced weight gain and metabolic abnormalities: implications for increased mortality in patients with schizophrenia. J Clin Psychiatry 2004;65(Supp 7):4–18.
61. Kasanin J. The blood sugar curve in mental disease. Arch Neuro Psychiatry 1926;16:414–419.
62. Ryan MC, Collins P, Thakore JH. Impaired fasting glucose tolerance in first-episode, drug-naive patients with schizophrenia. Am J Psychiatry 2003;160:284–289.
63. Newcomer JW, Haupt DW, Fucetola R, et al. Abnormalities in glucose regulation during antipsychotic treatment of schizophrenia. Arch Gen Psychiatry 2002;59:337–345.
64. Ryan MC, Flanagan S, Kinsella U, et al. The effects of atypical antipsychotics on visceral fat distribution in first episode, drug-naive patients with schizophrenia. Life Sci 2004;74:1999–2008.
65. Arranz B, Rosel P, Ramirez N, et al. Insulin resistance and increased leptin concentrations in noncompliant schizophrenia patients but not in antipsychotic-naive first-episode schizophrenia patients. J Clin Psychiatry 2004;65:1335–1342.
66. Zhang ZJ, Yao ZJ, Liu W, et al. Effects of antipsychotics on fat deposition and changes in leptin and insulin levels. Magnetic resonance imaging study of previously untreated people with schizophrenia. Br J Psychiatry 2004;184:58–62.
67. Reynolds GP. Metabolic syndrome and schizophrenia. Br J Psychiatry 2006;188:86; author reply 86–87.
68. Haupt DW, Newcomer JW. Abnormalities in glucose regulation associated with mental illness and treatment. J Psychosom Res 2002;53:925–933.
69. Haupt DW, Newcomer JW. Hyperglycemia and antipsychotic medications. J Clin Psychiatry 2001;62(Suppl 27):15–26.
70. Koller E, Schneider B, Bennett K, et al. Clozapine-associated diabetes. Am J Med 2001;111:716–723.
71. Koller EA, Doraiswamy PM. Olanzapine-associated diabetes mellitus. Pharmacotherapy 2002;22:841–852.
72. Herran A, de Santiago A, Sandoya M, et al. Determinants of smoking behaviour in outpatients with schizophrenia. Schizophr Res 2000;41:373–381.
73. Ucok A, Polat A, Bozkurt O, et al. Cigarette smoking among patients with schizophrenia and bipolar disorders. Psychiatry Clin Neurosci 2004;58:434–437.
74. Dixon L, Postrado L, Delahanty J, et al. The association of medical comorbidity in schizophrenia with poor physical and mental health. J Nerv Ment Dis 1999;187:496–502.
75. Cassidy F, Ahearn E, Carroll BJ. Elevated frequency of diabetes mellitus in hospitalized manic-depressive patients. Am J Psychiatry 1999;156:1417–1420.
76. Church CO, Stevens DL, Fugate SE. Diabetic ketoacidosis associated with aripiprazole. Diabet Med 2005;22:1440–1443.
77. Yang SH, McNeely MJ. Rhabdomyolysis, pancreatitis, and hyperglycemia with ziprasidone. Am J Psychiatry 2002;159:1435.

78. Lund BC, Perry PJ, Brooks JM, et al. Clozapine use in patients with schizophrenia and the risk of diabetes, hyperlipidemia, and hypertension: a claims-based approach. Arch Gen Psychiatry 2001;58:1172–1176.
79. Caro JJ, Ward A, Levinton C, et al. The risk of diabetes during olanzapine use compared with risperidone use: a retrospective database analysis. J Clin Psychiatry 2002;63:1135–1139.
80. Farwell W, Stump T, Wang J, et al. Do olanzapine and risperidone cause weight gain and diabetes? The International Journal of Neuropsychopharmacology 2002;5:049.
81. Gianfrancesco FD, Grogg AL, Mahmoud RA, et al. Differential effects of risperidone, olanzapine, clozapine, and conventional antipsychotics on type 2 diabetes: findings from a large health plan database. J Clin Psychiatry 2002;63:920–930.
82. Koro CE, Fedder DO, L'Italien GJ, et al. Assessment of independent effect of olanzapine and risperidone on risk of diabetes among patients with schizophrenia: population based nested case-control study. BMJ 2002;325:243.
83. Sernyak MJ, Leslie DL, Alarcon RD, et al. Association of diabetes mellitus with use of atypical neuroleptics in the treatment of schizophrenia. Am J Psychiatry 2002;159:561–566.
84. Wang PS, Glynn RJ, Ganj DA, et al. Clozapine use and risk of diabetes mellitus. J Clin Psychopharmacol 2002;22: 236–243.
85. Buse JB, Cavazzoni P, Hornbuckle K, et al. A retrospective cohort study of diabetes mellitus and antipsychotic treatment in the United States. J Clin Epidemiol 2003;56:164–170.
86. Citrome L, Jaffe A, Levine J, et al. Antipsychotic medication treatment and new prescriptions for insulin and oral hypoglycemics. Eur Neuropsychopharmacol 2003;13(suppl 4):S306.
87. Fuller MA, Shermock KM, Secic M, et al. Comparative study of the development of diabetes mellitus in patients taking risperidone and olanzapine. Pharmacotherapy 2003;23:1037–1043.
88. Gianfrancesco F, White R, Wang RH, et al. Antipsychotic-induced type 2 diabetes: evidence from a large health plan database. J Clin Psychopharmacol 2003;23:328–335.
89. Grogg A, Markowitz J, Mahmoud RA. Risk of diabetes in medical patients prescribed atypical antipsychotics. Abstract presented at the 156th Annual Meeting of the American Psychiatric Association, San Francisco, CA, May 17–22, 2003.
90. Citrome L, Jaffe A, Levine J, et al. Relationship between antipsychotic medication treatment and new cases of diabetes among psychiatric inpatients. Psychiatr Serv 2004;55:1006–1013.
91. Lambert BL, Chou CH, Chang KY, et al. Antipsychotic exposure and type 2 diabetes among patients with schizophrenia: a matched case-control study of California Medicaid claims. Pharmacoepidemiol Drug Saf 2005;14:417–425.
92. Leslie DL, Rosenheck RA. Incidence of newly diagnosed diabetes attributable to atypical antipsychotic medications. Am J Psychiatry 2004;161:1709–1711.
93. Ollendorf DA, Joyce AT, Rucker M. Rate of new-onset diabetes among patients treated with atypical or conventional antipsychotic medications for schizophrenia. MedGenMed 2004;6:5.
94. Sumiyoshi T, Roy A, Anil AE, et al. A comparison of incidence of diabetes mellitus between atypical antipsychotic drugs: a survey for clozapine, risperidone, olanzapine, and quetiapine. J Clin Psychopharmacol 2004;24:345–348.
95. Olfson M, Marcus SC, Corey-Lisle P, et al. Hyperlipidemia following treatment with antipsychotic medications. Am J Psychiatry 2006;163:1821–1825.
96. Newcomer JW, Rasgon N, Craft S, et al. Insulin resistance and metabolic risk during antipsychotic treatment. Presented at the annual American Psychiatric Association symposium Insulin Resistance and Metabolic Syndrome in Neuropsychiatry, Atlanta, GA, 2005.
97. Lindenmayer JP, Czobor P, Volovka J, et al. Changes in glucose and cholesterol levels in patients with schizophrenia treated with typical or atypical antipsychotics. Am J Psychiatry 2003;160: 290–296.
98. Cuijpers P, Smit F. Excess mortality in depression: a meta-analysis of community studies. J Affect Disord 2002;72:227–236.

99. Sikich L, Hamer RM, Bashford RA, et al. A pilot study of risperidone, olanzapine, and haloperidol in psychotic youth: a double-blind, randomized, 8-week trial. Neuropsychopharmacology 2004;29: 133–145.
100. Visser M, Pahor M, Tylavsky F, et al. One- and two-year change in body composition as measured by DXA in a population-based cohort of older men and women. J Appl Physiol 2003;94:2368–2374.
101. Gallagher D, Ruts E, Visser M, et al. Weight stability masks sarcopenia in elderly men and women. Am J Physiol Endocrinol Metab 2000;279:E366–375.
102. Barak Y, Shamir E, Weizman R. Would a switch from typical antipsychotics to risperidone be beneficial for elderly schizophrenic patients? A naturalistic, long-term, retrospective, comparative study. J Clin Psychopharmacol 2002;22:115–120.
103. Goldberg RJ. Weight variance associated with atypical neuroleptics in nursing home dementia patients. J Am Med Dir Assoc 2001;2:26–28.
104. Howes OD, Bhatnagar A, Gaughran FP, et al. A prospective study of impairment in glucose control caused by clozapine without changes in insulin resistance. Am J Psychiatry 2004;161:361–363.
105. Su KP, Wu PL, Pariante CM. A crossover study on lipid and weight changes associated with olanzapine and risperidone. Psychopharmacology (Berl) 2005;183:383–386.
106. Glick ID, Romano SJ, Simpson G, et al. Insulin resistance in olanzapine- and ziprasidone-treated patients: results of a double-blind, controlled 6-week trial. Presented at the Annual Meeting of the American Psychiatric Association, New Orleans, LA, 2001.
107. Simpson G, Weiden P, Pigott TA, et al. Ziprasidone vs olanzapine in schizophrenia: 6-month continuation study. Eur Neuropsychopharmacol 2002;2(Suppl 3):S310.
108. Breier A, Berg PH, Thakore JH, et al. Olanzapine versus ziprasidone: results of a 28-week double-blind study in patients with schizophrenia. Am J Psychiatry 2005;162:1879–1887.
109. Hardy TA, Poole-Hoffmann V, Lu Y, et al. Fasting glucose and lipid changes in patients with schizophrenia treated with olanzapine or ziprasidone. Poster presented at the 42nd Annual Meeting of the American College of Neuropsychopharmacology, San Juan, Puerto Rico, 2003.
110. Keck PE Jr, Marcus R, Tourkodimitris S, et al. A placebo-controlled, double-blind study of the efficacy and safety of aripiprazole in patients with acute bipolar mania. Am J Psychiatry 2003;160:1651–1658.
111. Atmaca M, Kuloglu M, Tezcan E, et al. Serum leptin and triglyceride levels in patients on treatment with atypical antipsychotics. J Clin Psychiatry 2003;64:598–604.
112. Goff DC, Sullivan LM, McEvoy JP, et al. A comparison of ten-year cardiac risk estimates in schizophrenia patients from the CATIE study and matched controls. Schizophr Res 2005;80: 45–53.
113. Henderson DC, Nguyen DD, Copeland PM, et al. Clozapine, diabetes mellitus, hyperlipidemia, and cardiovascular risks and mortality: results of a 10-year naturalistic study. J Clin Psychiatry 2005;66:1116–1121.
114. Bergman RN, Ader M. Atypical antipsychotics and glucose homeostasis. J Clin Psychiatry 2005;66:504–514.
115. Henderson DC, Cagliero E, Copeland PM, et al. Glucose metabolism in patients with schizophrenia treated with atypical antipsychotic agents: a frequently sampled intravenous glucose tolerance test and minimal model analysis. Arch Gen Psychiatry 2005;62:19–28.
116. Ader M, Kim SP, Catalono KJ, et al. Metabolic dysregulation with atypical antipsychotics occurs in the absence of underlying disease: a placebo-controlled study of olanzapine and risperidone in dogs. Diabetes 2005;54:862–871.
117. Houseknecht KL, Robertson AS, Zavadowski W, et al. Acute effects of atypical antipsychotics on whole-body insulin resistance in rats: implications for adverse metabolic effects. Neuropsychopharmacology 2007;32:289–297.

118. Grundy SM, Hansen B, Smith Jr SC et al. Clinical management of metabolic syndrome: report of the American Heart Association/National Heart, Lung, and Blood Institute/American Diabetes Association conference on scientific issues related to management. Circulation 2004;109(4):551–556.
119. National Diabetes Association and National Institute of Diabetes Digestive and Kidney Disease. The prevention or delay of type 2 diabetes. Diabetes Care 2002;25:742–749.
120. U.S. Department of Health and Human Services. The seventh report of the joint national committee of prevention, detection, evaluation and treatment of high blood pressure. NIH publication 04-5230. Washington, DC: U.S. Department of Health and Human Services; 2004.
121. Horvitz-Lennon M, Kilbourne AM, Pincus HA. From silos to bridges: meeting the general health care needs of adults with severe mental illnesses. Health Aff (Millwood) 2006;25:659–669.
122. Hester EK, Thrower MR. Current options in the management of olanzapine-associated weight gain. Ann Pharmacother 2005,39:302–310.
123. Schwartz TL, Nihalani N, Virk S, et al. Psychiatric medication-induced obesity: treatment options. Obes Rev 2004;5:233–238.
124. Henderson DC, Copeland PM, Daley TB, et al. A double-blind, placebo-controlled trial of sibutramine for olanzapine-associated weight gain. Am J Psychiatry 2005;162:954–962.
125. Fagiolini A, Frank A, Scott JA, et al. Metabolic syndrome in bipolar disorder: findings from the Bipolar Disorder Center for Pennsylvanians. Bipolar Disord 2005;7:424–430.
126. Hennekens CH, Hennekens AR, Hollar D, et al. Schizophrenia and increased risks of cardiovascular disease. Am Heart J 2005;150:1115–1121.
127. McElroy SL, Frye MA, Suppes T, et al. Correlates of overweight and obesity in 644 patients with bipolar disorder. J Clin Psychiatry 2002;63:207–213.
128. Davidson S, Judd F, Jolley D, et al. Cardiovascular risk factors for people with mental illness. Aust N Z J Psychiatry 2001;35:196–202.
129. Kilbourne AM, Cornelius JR, Han X, et al. Burden of general medical conditions among individuals with bipolar disorder. Bipolar Disord 2004;6:368–373.
130. Koro CE, Fedder DO, L'Italien GJ, et al. An assessment of the independent effects of olanzapine and risperidone exposure on the risk of hyperlipidemia in schizophrenic patients. Arch Gen Psychiatry 2002;59:1021–1026.

13 Treatment of Insulin Resistance in Youth: The Role of Metformin

Molly Emott and Michael Freemark

CONTENTS

Abstract

The authors review the pathogenesis and diagnostic evaluation of insulin resistance in obesity and the polycystic ovary syndrome. They discuss the benefits and risks of lifestyle intervention and pharmacotherapy and present a tailored approach to pharmacotherapy in high risk adolescents.

Key Words: obesity, polycystic ovary syndrome, metformin, antipsychotics, fatty liver disease, thiazolidinedione, orlistat

From: *Contemporary Endocrinology: Energy Metabolism and Obesity: Research and Clinical Applications*
Edited by: P. A. Donohoue © Humana Press Inc., Totowa, NJ

INTRODUCTION

The significance of insulin resistance continues to evolve and broaden as our generation bears witness to an increased prevalence of both type 2 diabetes mellitus (T2DM) and the polycystic ovarian syndrome (PCOS) and their metabolic and cardiovascular comorbidities. Insulin resistance is the cornerstone of disease progression in both conditions and is a well-established independent risk factor for cardiovascular disease. Much attention is now focused on identifying subjects with insulin resistance so as to study possible therapeutic interventions. Metformin has been shown to delay the onset of diabetes, blunt weight gain, improve cardiovascular risk profiles, and promote ovulation in patients with obesity, impaired glucose tolerance, and PCOS. Our goals in this chapter are to review our current understanding of insulin resistance in obesity and PCOS, to discuss the mechanism of action and safety profile of metformin, and to explore its use as a means of treating insulin resistance and preventing future morbidity and mortality.

INSULIN RESISTANCE AND METABOLIC COMPLICATIONS

In simple terms, insulin resistance is a state of altered glucose homeostasis: target tissues (adipocytes, skeletal muscle, and hepatocytes) are less responsive to insulin, and the pancreas must secrete increasing amounts in order to exert hypoglycemic and antilipolytic effects. Insulin resistance is not necessarily uniform throughout the body, however, and various tissues can maintain hormone sensitivity. In obesity and PCOS, insulin resistance may be a primary pathophysiologic state; alternatively, hyperinsulinism may in some cases precede obesity and insulin resistance, the latter serving as an adaptive, protective response to prevent ongoing weight gain *(1)*.

Regardless, the state of insulin resistance does not exist in isolation or without consequence (Fig. 13.1). Metabolic complications of insulin resistance include dyslipidemia, hepatic dysfunction, reproductive and menstrual disorders, type 2 diabetes, hypertension, and atherosclerotic cardiovascular disease. Pancreatic dysfunction begins with islet cell hypertrophy and increased β-cell mass. Subsequently, there may be altered first-phase insulin secretion and processing, a decline in insulin production, and, ultimately, deposition of amyloid in islet cells, rendering them dysfunctional.

In children, obesity and insulin resistance (IR) may cause important changes in linear growth and pubertal development *(2,3)*. Increased rates of linear growth and bone maturation may reflect increased sensitivity of target tissues to growth hormone, resulting from insulin-induced increases in growth hormone receptors, and increased levels of free insulin-like growth factor 1 (IGF-1), resulting from decreased levels of IGF binding proteins 1 and 2. Androgen excess may exacerbate this process: excess insulin and IGF-1 act in concert with adrenocorticotropin hormone and luteinizing hormone (LH) to stimulate p450 17-hydroxylase activity and production of androgens from the adrenal gland and ovary, respectively. Free androgen levels are also higher due to insulin suppression of sex hormone binding globulin. The increased androgens feed back on the pituitary axis to increase the frequency of gonadotropin-releasing hormone (GnRH) pulses and the ratio of LH to follicle-stimulating hormone (FSH), which in turn increases ovarian thecal androgen production. In prepubertal children, this hormonal milieu manifests as premature adrenarche; in pubertal children, it manifests as anovulation and hirsutism in girls and gynecomastia in boys as androstenedione is aromatized to estrone in adipose tissue.

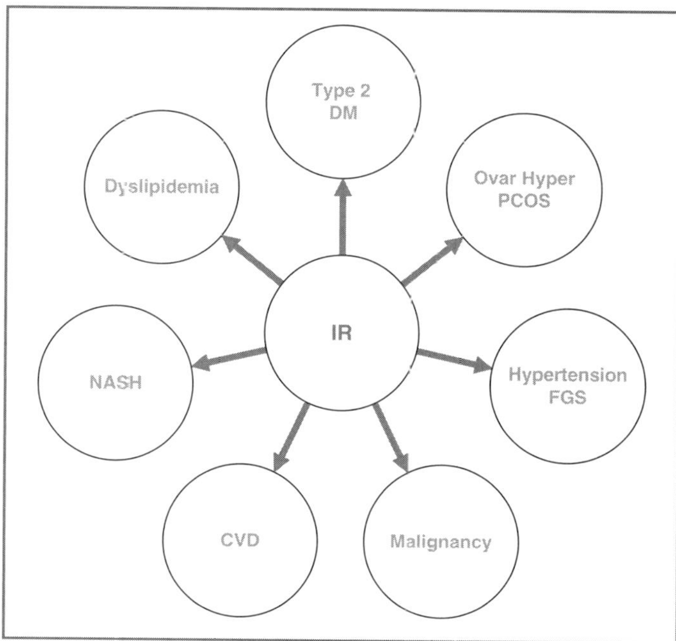

Fig. 13.1 Metabolic complications of insulin resistance (IR). Type 2 DM, type 2 diabetes mellitus; ovar hyper, ovarian hyperandrogenism; PCOS, polycystic ovary syndrome; NASH, nonalcoholic steatohepatitis; FGS, focal glomerulosclerosis; CVD, cardiovascular disease.

Many of the other consequences of hyperinsulinemia and insulin resistance can be grouped together under the rubric of the metabolic syndrome, the incidence of which correlates with the severity of insulin resistance and the presence of which conveys an increased risk of cardiovascular disease (*3–6*). The pathogenic mechanism of atherogenesis is complex and involves direct and indirect effects of insulin resistance and hyperglycemia on endothelial tissues, mediated by hormones, growth factors, vasoactive agents, cytokines, oxygen radicals, and cellular adhesion molecules *(7)*. Dyslipidemia in the form of hypertriglyceridemia and low plasma high-density lipoprotein (HDL) levels is due to decreased lipoprotein lipase activity, increased release of free fatty acids, decreased suppression of very-low-density lipoprotein (VLDL) release from the liver, and increased metabolic clearance of HDL *(8)*. Systolic hypertension is frequently seen in patients with obesity and insulin resistance; proposed mechanisms including resistance to insulin's vasodilatory induction of nitric oxide synthase and generation of nitric oxide *(9, 10)*.

Nonalcoholic fatty liver disease, steatohepatitis, and gallstones may develop as a consequence of dyslipidemia. Renal dysfunction in the form of glomerulomegaly and focal segmental glomerulosclerosis has also been linked with obesity and hyperinsulinemia, facilitated by concurrent hypertension *(11)*. Certain malignancies occur at higher frequencies in obese adults, possibly a consequence of hyperinsulinemia and increases in circulating free IGF-1 and sex steroids *(12)*. Given the enormity of the complications associated with decreased insulin sensitivity, it is clear that early identification and intervention are necessary to prevent what is already being seen as a health care crisis.

RISK FACTORS FOR INSULIN RESISTANCE

A definitive biochemical pathway of insulin resistance has yet to be fully elucidated. Theories as to its pathogenesis, discussed below, are more easily conceptualized against a background of known risk factors for insulin resistance that may begin in utero (Fig. 13.2) (reviewed in Ref. *3*). Infants of diabetic mothers and infants born small for gestational age are prime examples *(13)*. The prevalence of diabetes in Pima Indian children is most strongly predicted by exposure to maternal diabetes in utero. Paradoxically, children who are born thin but gain weight rapidly during childhood are also at increased risk for insulin resistance and for adult-onset cardiovascular disease *(14)*. Pubertal status is itself a risk factor as surges in growth hormone oppose the actions of insulin and may unmask disease in those with other predispositions. In Caucasians and African Americans, Tanner stage III marks the peak in insulin resistance, with return to prepubertal levels by Tanner V; in Hispanic children, however, this pubertal influence may not be as strong, or may be overshadowed by high levels of body fat and positive family histories of T2DM *(15)*. Family history, and similarly, ethnic background are clearly crucial. In a population of Mexican children and adolescents, among the best predictors of insulin sensitivity was family history. Hispanic, Native American, and Pacific Island background seem to pose the greatest risk, followed by African American descent and Caucasian heritage (*3,15–17*). Part of this disparity is likely due to the higher prevalence of obesity among the former ethnicities *(17, 18)*. Ethnic differences in the adaptive response of β-cells likely play an important role as well *(18)*.

Other risk factors for insulin resistance include genetic syndromes (Prader-Willi, Bardet-Biedl, leprechaunism, etc.), drugs (especially glucocorticoids and some of the newer atypical antipsychotics), and hormonal disorders resulting in hyperandrogenism, of which PCOS is the most common example and is discussed in detail below. Obesity, however, is by far the most prevalent and, importantly, most modifiable risk factor. Indeed, the majority of pediatric and adult patients with T2DM are obese or overweight,

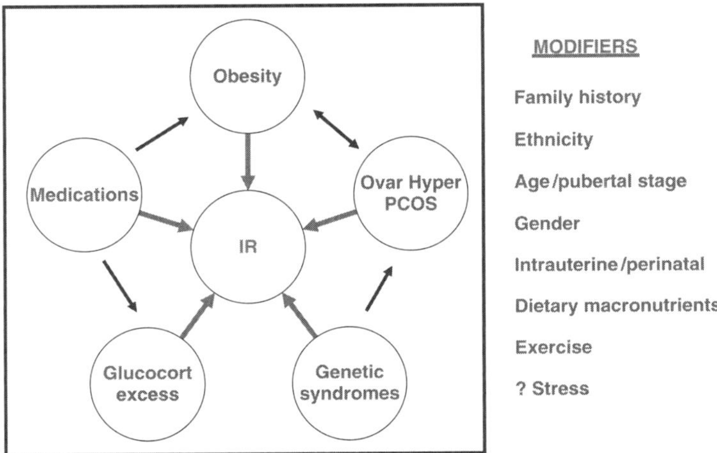

Fig. 13.2 Risk factors for the development of insulin resistance (IR). Ovar hyper, ovarian hyperandrogenism; Glucocort, glucocorticoid.

and insulin sensitivity correlates inversely with body mass index (BMI) and percentage body fat *(3, 4, 19, 20)*. In a study of 167 severely obese (defined as BMI higher than the 95% for age and sex) children and adolescents, 21–25% had impaired glucose tolerance, and 4% had "silent" T2DM *(19)*. Adolescents with BMI >95th percentile for age and gender have increased prevalence of fasting hyperglycemia, hyperinsulinemia, impaired glucose tolerance, hypertriglyceridemia, increased C-reactive protein, and systolic hypertension, while those with BMI between 85th and 95th percentile are at higher risk for insulin resistance and dyslipidemia *(19)*.The risk of progressing to T2DM has been estimated to be 40-fold higher for adult women with the highest population BMIs than for those with the lowest (reviewed in Refs. 3 and 20) Clearly, as America's youth have gotten fatter—approximately one-seventh of 15 year olds in the United States are considered obese according to recent NHANES data—the incidence and prevalence of T2DM in children and adolescents has increased, and it now accounts for up to 30% of diabetes diagnoses in 11–18 year olds. Although the notion of the all-encompassing "obesity gene" remains popular, in fact only 5% of obese individuals can be diagnosed with a specific syndromal or genetic abnormality. However, despite the rarity of these syndromes, genetic predisposition—in the form of polygenic polymorphisms—is still thought to account for almost half of a child's tendency toward overweight. Overlaying such predisposition is a growing understanding of the effect of the American fast-food diet—which now accounts for 10% of energy intake in children—on nutritional status, weight, and risk for insulin resistance and diabetes (*21–23*). The energy-dense, highly palatable fast-food meals have high glycemic indices and high saturated fat to carbohydrate ratios, factors that both exaggerate insulin response to food and prolong postprandial hyperinsulinemia, resulting in rebound hypoglycemia and increased energy intake at later meals *(21)*. A prolonged diet of palatable food has also been shown in experimental animals to be associated with increases in hunger signals (neuropeptide Y and orexins) and a resistance to increased satiety signals (leptin, insulin, cholecystokinin), perhaps through a direct effect of high-fat diets on intracellular pathways and on passage of insulin across the blood-brain barrier. In addition, the rewarding effect of foods high in sugar and fat via activation of the opioid system likely plays a role in superseding the satiety signals: a drive for pleasure overrides the body's sense of energy homeostasis.

DIAGNOSING INSULIN RESISTANCE

Many children and adolescents with insulin resistance are asymptomatic, and the majority have normal fasting glucose levels *(19)*. These findings, combined with growing evidence that pancreatic β-cell dysfunction occurs early in the process of hyperinsulinemia and insulin resistance, warrants the use of proactive, clinic-friendly primary screening tools for insulin resistance so as to prevent unfavorable sequelae and enable ongoing epidemiologic research. The gold standard for diagnosis has been the euglycemic insulin clamp, where insulin is infused at a constant rate and glucose requirements needed to maintain euglycemia correspond with insulin sensitivity. For obvious reasons this method and the intravenous glucose tolerance test are cumbersome for use outside the academic setting. Although measurement of individual variables known to correlate with insulin resistance, such as blood pressure, lipid levels (importantly fasting triglyceride and HDL), glucose, insulin, and hepatic enzymes, are helpful, it is fasting insulin and glucose levels that correlate best with insulin resistance in multiple models. An oral glucose tolerance test with serial glucose and insulin levels can provide useful information regarding insulin secretion as well as sensitivity and glucose tolerance. Alternatively, glucose tolerance can be assessed imperfectly with fasting glucose and insulin levels and a fingerstick blood glucose 2 h after a 75-g carbohydrate load *(3)*. Insulin sensitivity can be estimated (imperfectly) using the homeostasis model assessment (HOMA), which employs basal glucose and insulin or c-peptide concentrations to estimate β-cell function and insulin resistance. The original model (HOMA1) is a simple equation {HOMA = [fasting plasma insulin (uU/ml) × fasting plasma glucose (mmol)]/22.5}, whereas the HOMA2 is a computer model. The Quantitative Insulin Sensitivity Check Index {QUICKI = 1/[log fasting insulin (uU/ml) + log fasting glucose (mmol)]}, is identical to the simple form of the HOMA except that it uses a log transformation of the insulin glucose product *(24)*. Some investigators argue that QUICKI is better able than HOMA to discriminate insulin resistance in various groups of patients and that its correlation with the insulin clamp is superior *(25)*. The Composite Insulin Sensitivity Index (CISI) takes into account whole-body insulin sensitivity in the both basal and glucose-stimulated state *(26)*. Each of these measures has been validated as a useful tool.

PATHOGENESIS OF INSULIN RESISTANCE IN OBESITY

The pathogenesis of insulin resistance in children and adolescents with obesity but without underlying genetic or hypothalamic abnormalities is under active research (Fig. 13.3). We know that insulin binding to its receptor and postreceptor phosphorylation steps are reduced in target tissues in insulin-resistant states but do not exactly know why. Visceral adipose deposition—as opposed to gluteal or subcutaneous—contributes to insulin resistance in obese patients, at least in Caucasian populations. However, the severity of insulin resistance and rates of type 2 diabetes are higher in African American children and adults than in Caucasians for a given level of visceral fat. Adipocyte cytokines such as tumor necrosis factor α (TNF-α) and interleukin-6 (IL-6) are known to be overexpressed in obese states *(27)* and are thought to mediate resistance in adipocyte cells, in part by interfering with glucose and free fatty acid uptake via paracrine downregulation of GLUT4 gene expression, the major insulin-responsive glucose transporter. The cytokines may cause downregulation of lipoprotein lipase and increase lipolysis and thereby increase the circulating concentrations and delivery of free fatty acids to the portal circulation. This is thought to be particularly important in abdominal adipocytes that are more lipolytically active at baseline *(27)*. Concomitantly, there is reduced expression of adiponectin, which increases insulin sensitivity in skeletal muscle and liver cells. Elevated free fatty acids facilitate hepatic triglyceride deposition, resulting in fatty liver and possible steatohepatitis; triglyceride accumulation may impede insulin uptake, action, and clearance, a state of "lipotoxicity" that is exacerbated by direct effects of the aforementioned cytokines and by hyperinsulinemia itself, which is known to downregulate insulin receptors and desensitize postreceptor pathways. The end result is an increase in hepatic glucose and triglyceride output, the former most likely due to increased gluconeogenesis although

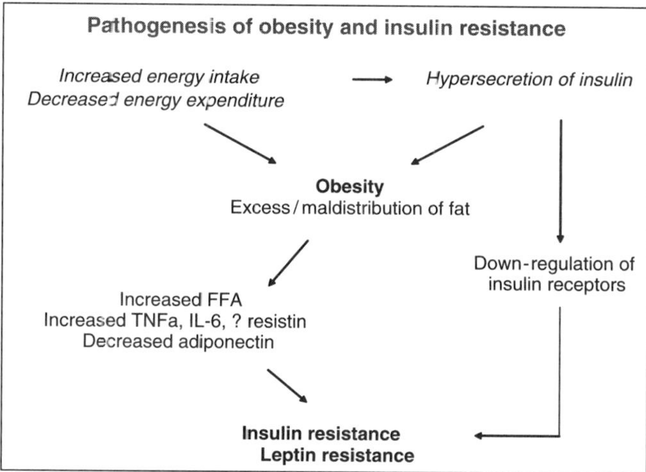

Fig. 13.3 Pathogenesis of obesity and insulin resistance. FFA, free fatty acids; TNFα, tumor necrosis factor α; IL-6, interleukin-6.

possibly related to glycogenolysis as well. Myocytes also demonstrate fatty accumulation, the by-products of which impair glucose uptake through inhibition of insulin signaling, glucose transporter 4 expression, translocation, and activity. The reduction in glucose transport and increases in hepatic glucose production trigger a rise in glucose concentrations, which signals the pancreas to secrete increasing amounts of insulin.

Certain races and ethnic groups with normal insulin sensitivity hypersecrete insulin in response to an oral glucose challenge *(1, 17)*. Elevated insulin levels predispose to fat storage and weight gain and reduce the expression of insulin receptors, thus facilitating or sustaining the development of obesity and insulin resistance. Leptin levels rise in response to the accumulation of white adipose tissue. However, peripheral and central resistance to leptin may exacerbate the resistance to insulin in peripheral tissues and blunt the effect of leptin on food intake and weight gain. In healthy, nonobese adults, cerebrospinal fluid (CSF) levels of insulin and leptin correspond closely with those in the plasma. Insulin binds to its receptors, densely populated in the arcuate and ventromedial hypothalamic nuclei, and acts to curb appetite and decrease energy intake, as demonstrated by the hyperphagia and obesity seen in studies of central nervous system (CNS)-specific insulin receptor knockout mice; parallel effects are seen with leptin *(21)*. In obese states, there is evidence of decreased CNS transport of insulin and leptin and possibly decreased postreceptor signaling; thus, CNS resistance to insulin and leptin exacerbates the hyperphagic state, the obese phenotype, and peripheral metabolic dysfunction.

INSULIN RESISTANCE AND PCOS

Functional adrenal and ovarian hyperandrogenism due to abnormal regulation/hyperresponsiveness of cytochrome P450c17 (possibly related to abnormal serine phosphorylation) has been postulated to be an underlying abnormality of the hormonal dysregulation seen in PCOS. Ibanez et al. *(28)* studied pubertal girls with a history of premature adrenarche and found exaggerated production of ovarian and adrenal androgen synthesis compared with Tanner stage and bone-age matched controls. They also found significant elevations in insulin levels before and during pubertal development in lean girls with premature adrenarche. Subsequent investigations have found both an intrinsic defect in insulin action independent of obesity and hyperandrogenism (possibly related to abnormal serine phosphorylation of the receptor) as well as primary β-cell dysfunction in PCOS. As many as 40% of adults and adolescents with PCOS have impaired glucose tolerance, and at least 7.5% meet criteria for the diagnosis of T2DM. Multiple studies have confirmed the relationship between PCOS and hyperinsulinemia, a finding that marks the disease as a metabolic as well as a reproductive risk *(29)*. In 1997, Dunaif et al. *(29)* found that both obese and lean women with PCOS had significantly increased insulin responses to an oral glucose tolerance test (OGTT) compared with age- and weight-matched ovulatory hyperandrogenic controls. Glucose responses, however, were significantly increased only in obese women with PCOS, with 20% of their cohort meeting criteria for T2DM. This finding supports the previous discussion of the effect of obesity on glucose tolerance and demonstrates a synergistic negative effect of both obesity and PCOS on insulin sensitivity. It is estimated that 10% of cases of impaired glucose tolerance in premenopausal women can be attributed to PCOS-related insulin resistance and hyperinsulinemia.

PHARMACOLOGIC APPROACHES TO THE TREATMENT OF INSULIN RESISTANCE AND PREVENTION OF TYPE 2 DIABETES

The American Diabetes Association and National Institute of Diabetes, Digestive and Kidney Diseases presented a position statement in January 2003 entitled "The Prevention or Delay of Type 2 Diabetes" *(30)*. The ADA identified five conditions pertaining to a disease that would warrant attempting its prevention: 1) significant public health implications; 2) good understanding of early warning signs and natural history; 3) a safe test that predicts progression/development of predisease state; 4) safe, effective methods of prevention; 5) economical implications of identifying and implementing preventive measures. The first three conditions are easily satisfied by T2DM and its onset in adolescence. We have already addressed the validity of various diagnostic tests. The fourth and fifth conditions have been studied in adults and to a lesser degree in children, though critical questions remain unanswered.

Lifestyle intervention can delay or prevent the development of T2DM in adults. For example, the Finnish Diabetes Prevention Study randomly assigned 522 at-risk adults (middle-aged, overweight, with impaired glucose tolerance (IGT)) to individualized intensive lifestyle counseling with the goals of dietary modification and weight loss or standard care *(31)*. Based on annual OGTTs conducted over a period of 4 years, 11% of patients in the intervention group versus 23% in the control group developed diabetes; this translates into a 58% relative risk reduction (based on cumulative incidence) and a number needed to treat of 8 to prevent one case in 4 years. Similar findings (reviewed in Ref. 20) were reported in the Malmo study (63% reduction in type 2 diabetes/5 years), the DaQing study (36% reduction in 6 years), and the Diabetes Prevention Program (described below).

However, effective lifestyle intervention typically has required intensive counseling, individualized programming, and frequent meetings with study staff, making it expensive and very time consuming. For example, in the Finnish study, dietary advice was tailored to each subject on the basis of 3-day food records completed 4 times per year. Each subject in the intervention group had seven sessions with a nutritionist during the first year of the study and one session every 3 months thereafter. The subjects also received individual guidance on increasing their level of physical activity.

Standard, population-based lifestyle counseling has not been nearly as effective as intensive lifestyle intervention, and there is very limited information about the long-term success of lifestyle intervention in children. Small studies demonstrate that dietary/exercise/counseling regimens can be quite successful in reducing weight in highly motivated children *(32, 32a)*; their efficacy in reducing risks for type 2 diabetes and other complications is unclear. Moreover, other studies and extensive clinical experience indicates that standard or intensive lifestyle intervention is not universally successful. This has prompted clinicians to seek therapeutic approaches that could complement the effect of lifestyle intervention and reduce the risks of type 2 diabetes and other long-term complications.

In theory, a number of criteria should be met before recommending the use of a pharmacologic agent for the treatment of insulin resistance: a) the severity of insulin resistance should place the subject at high risk for glucose intolerance, hepatic or renal dysfunction, and/or cardiovascular disease; b) the response to lifestyle intervention should be inadequate or incomplete; c) the drug selected for therapy should exert biological actions that counteract insulin resistance and/or prevent or reverse its complications; d) experimental animal data should show beneficial effects of the drug on insulin action and/or glucose tolerance; e) human clinical studies in the target population should show both short- and long-term benefits that reduce the severity or risks of complications; f) the drug's benefits should outweigh its short- and long-term risks; and g) the economic costs of the drug for individuals and for society at large should be acceptable. Pharmacologic interventions would be particularly important if delaying therapy might worsen long-term outcome. As described below, the drug metformin meets the minimal criteria for short- and long-term use in adolescents and adults and can therefore be recommended as an adjunct to lifestyle intervention for selected individuals.

METFORMIN: MECHANISMS OF ACTION

Most studies show that metformin (Fig. 13.4), a biguanide in use for almost 50 years, inhibits hepatic gluconeogenesis and that it is primarily this effect that accounts for its ability to reduce plasma glucose concentrations *(10, 33, 34)*. The mechanisms accounting for the decreased conversion of pyruvate, lactate, glycerol, and amino acids to glucose are under active investigation; they include: a) a direct effect of metformin on the insulin receptor, resulting in increased insulin receptor kinase activity and subsequent activation of insulin-receptor substrate-2, a key mediator of glucose handling in the liver *(34)*; b) an indirect effect upon the insulin receptor via inhibition of tyrosine phosphatases that inhibit the insulin receptor kinase *(35)*; c) increased phosphorylation and activation of AMP-induced protein kinase (AMPK), mediated by mitochondria-derived reactive nitrogen species, which appears to be required for inhibition of hepatocyte glucose production *(36, 37)*; d) inhibition of mitochondrial respiratory chain oxidation; e) decreased mRNA expression of genes coding peptides involved in gluconeogenesis *(36)*; f) suppression of dipeptidyl peptidase IV activity,

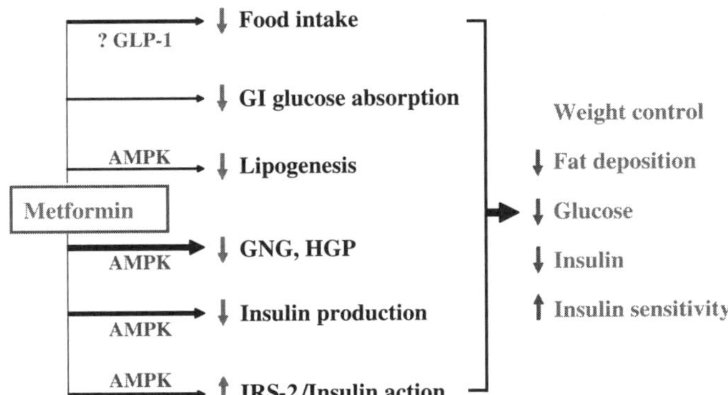

Fig. 13.4 Mechanisms of action and functional benefits of metformin. GLP-1, glucagon-like peptide 1; AMPK, AMP-activated protein kinase; GI, gastrointestinal; GNG, gluconeogenesis; HGP, hepatic glucose production; IRS, insulin receptor substrate.

possibly allowing for more potent insulinotropic effects of gut-derived hormones *(38)*; and g) possible decreased intestinal absorption of glucose related to metformin concentrations in the small intestine *(10)*.

Metformin effects on glycogenolysis are less clear but may also play a role in lowering systemic glucose levels, as does increased peripheral glucose uptake by skeletal muscle. The latter effect can be attributed to direct insulin receptor and AMPK activation, as well as to increased numbers of glucose transporters 1 and 4 in the plasma membrane and increased efficiency with which they transport glucose *(10)*.

Metformin also has favorable effects on lipids, thus reducing lipotoxicity as well as glucotoxicity; the drug reduces LDL concentrations in PCOS and increased HDL levels in the Diabetes Prevention Program. The dyslipidemia seen with insulin resistance includes hypertriglyceridemia, increased low-density lipoprotein, and decreased high-density lipoprotein. As discussed previously, the elevated free fatty acids seen with obesity likely contribute to insulin resistance and exacerbate increased hepatic glucose production. Although most studies support the finding that metformin decreases plasma levels of free fatty acid, there is debate as to its effect on free fatty acid oxidation. Stimulation of AMPK inactivates acetyl-CoA carboxylase, resulting in decreased levels of malonyl-CoA and decreased de novo fatty acid biosynthesis with increased flow through the oxidative pathway *(36)*. AMPK also suppresses a lipogenic transcription factor, SREBP-1, and thus production of target genes that mediate lipid synthesis. However, increased free fatty oxidation is known to inhibit glycolytic enzymes and ultimately reduces glucose uptake and oxidation. Nonetheless, the beneficial effects of metformin on lipid metabolism, may account for its observed cardiovascular protective effects *(39)*. Other cardioprotective mechanisms include increased fibrinolysis and reduced thrombogenic tendencies with decreased platelet aggregation, possible improvement in diabetic cardiomyopathy related to enhanced intracellular calcium handling, and potential antihypertensive action via increased artery relaxation *(10)*.

Weight stabilization or mild weight loss is commonly seen with metformin; as much as 80–90% of the weight loss may reflect a reduction in adipose tissue *(33)*. Reductions in lipogenesis and increased rates of fatty acid oxidation may play roles. There is no observed change in resting energy expenditure or physical activity, but appetite and caloric intake are decreased. A possible mechanism is an increase in the half-life of GLP-1, an appetite suppressant *(38, 40)*. A recent study suggests that metformin may reduce hypothalamic expression of neuropeptide Y *(40a)*.

METFORMIN USE IN OBESITY-RELATED INSULIN RESISTANCE

The Diabetes Prevention Program, published in 2002, was the first study to conduct a head-to-head comparison of lifestyle intervention with pharmacologic therapy, namely metformin *(41)*. In this landmark trial, 3,234 nondiabetic adults (≥25 years of age) with impaired fasting glucose (IFG) or impaired glucose tolerance (IGT) were randomized to placebo, metformin, or an intensive lifestyle modification program. The former two arms were given "routine" lifestyle modification information, which included annual oral and written instructions on healthy eating and exercise habits. Those in the intensive arm received specialized counseling and training; patients had meetings with a case manager 16 times over the first 6 months and then monthly thereafter, with additional group meetings and supervised exercise sessions twice weekly. In both routine and intensive groups, free use of exercise facilities was offered. Development of diabetes was based on ADA criteria on two separate occasions, and data was analyzed by intention to treat principles.

Cumulative incidence of diabetes was 28.9%, 21.7%, and 14.4% for the placebo, metformin, and lifestyle-intervention groups, respectively, resulting in a number needed to treat over 3 years of 6.9 for the lifestyle group and 13.9 for the metformin group. Interestingly, metformin was as effective as lifestyle intervention in the youngest patients studied (ages 25–34 years) and in those with the highest BMI (>34.9).

The rates of increase in diabetes incidence in the intensive lifestyle and metformin groups paralleled the rate of increase in diabetes in the control group. This finding suggests that intensive lifestyle intervention and metformin may delay, rather than prevent, the development of diabetes. It is unclear if some of the effect of either intensive lifestyle intervention or metformin actually represents a form of treatment of subclinical type 2 diabetes; 1–2 weeks after discontinuing therapy, approximately 25% of the metformin effect in preventing diabetes was lost *(42)*. This observation suggests that it might be necessary to maintain drug therapy indefinitely or until concurrent lifestyle intervention has produced significant changes. It should be noted that the effects of intensive lifestyle intervention and metformin in combination were not tested in the Diabetes Prevention Program.

Beneficial effects of metformin in the Diabetes Prevention Program were replicated in the Indian Diabetes Prevention Program (*42a*). Metformin reduced the three year cumulative incidence of type 2 diabetes from 55% to 40.5%. Together, the results of the two diabetes prevention trials suggest that metformin can curb the development of diabetes in high-risk adults.

To date, there have been no randomized, placebo-controlled studies of the effects of metformin on progression to diabetes in glucose-intolerant adolescents or children with obesity. There have, however, been three randomized, double-blind trials of metformin in obese adolescents with insulin resistance. In the first study *(43)*, 29 black and white obese adolescents, ages 12–19 years, with hyperinsulinemia, normal fasting glucose, and a family history significant for T2DM were randomized to receive either metformin

(500 mg twice daily) or placebo for 6 months. Notably, no dietary interventions were recommended. Metformin treatment reduced fasting glucose and insulin levels and increased insulin sensitivity as measured by the HOMA and QUICKI indices. The metformin group also had reductions in absolute and percent BMI standard deviation score and in plasma leptin levels (in girls). No changes in hemoglobin A1c, IGF-1 levels, or lipid profiles were observed. The second study *(44)* examined the effects of metformin or placebo on weight gain and glucose tolerance in 24 obese (mean BMI ~41) Caucasian adolescents who followed low-calorie meal plans. Both the metformin and placebo groups lost weight, but the decrease was significantly greater in the metformin group than in the placebo group and consisted of a greater loss in body fat. Fasting and postprandial insulin and fasting leptin concentrations declined, although no significant changes were seen in fasting glucose. Metformin also reduced plasma triglycerides, cholesterol, and free fatty acids. Finally, a randomized, blinded, cross-over study in obese adolescents demonstrated that metformin reduced BMI, waist circumference and fasting insulin concentrations during a 6 month treatment period *(44a)*. In sum, these studies suggest that metformin may complement the effect of lifestyle intervention to reduce the risk of glucose intolerance in predisposed patients.

The Diabetes Prevention Program found no effect of race or gender on the response to metformin or lifestyle intervention in adults. Limited evidence, based on small, nonrandomized studies, suggest that metformin may be more effective in Caucasian than in African American children *(45)*. In one study, 43 obese children were treated with metformin after an initial OGTT from which insulin sensitivity and secretion were calculated. Changes in BMI were then modeled according to pretreatment insulin parameters, and groups were stratified according to race. White females with the most severe insulin resistance but normal insulin secretion appeared to have the greatest reduction in BMI after metformin therapy, especially during the first 4 months; black children had no statistically significant changes in BMI, which was hypothesized to correlate with previous demonstrations of insulin hypersecretion as a primary abnormality in obese black children *(1)*. Other factors contributing to weight gain, including current and previous dietary history and compliance with medication, were however not examined, making the findings difficult to interpret.

Fatty liver is a common complication of pediatric obesity and insulin resistance, and nonalcoholic steatohepatitis (NASH) may occur in 1–10% of patients. In our randomized study of obese adolescents with insulin resistance, we demonstrated that metformin reduced ALT concentrations in Caucasians and in girls and prevented the rise in ALT observed in placebo-treated subjects *(45a)*. In a previous uncontrolled study of 10 obese children *(46)*, metformin reduced liver fat content and hepatic enzymes even in the absence of weight loss. Use of metformin for insulin-resistant–associated NASH is also supported by a mouse study of leptin-deficient mice. Metformin was found to improve fatty liver disease by reversing hepatomegaly, steatosis, and aminotransferase abnormalities *(47)*.

A systematic review of the use of metformin in adults for the treatment of obesity per se found only nine articles that were randomized, blinded, and performed in patients without diabetes, PCOS, or other confounding factors *(48)*. Only two of these found statistically significant changes in weight or waist-hip ratio, leading the authors to conclude that insufficient evidence exists to support the use of metformin as treatment for overweight or obesity without coexisting diabetes or PCOS. Many limitations exist within each of the included studies, however; most significantly, many were not primarily powered to evaluate the effect of metformin on weight loss. Moreover, most were short-term studies and involved patients with lower-end BMIs (<35).

METFORMIN USE IN PCOS

PCOS affects 5–10% of women of reproductive age and is thought to be the most common cause of anovulatory infertility. Insulin resistance and hyperinsulinemia are common features of the syndrome and play significant roles in its pathogenesis, predisposing to dyslipidemia, hypertension, dysfibrinolysis, possible increased risk of gestational diabetes, and coronary artery disease. The majority of patients with PCOS are obese; however, body fat mass may be increased and lean body mass decreased even in "nonobese" subjects with normal BMI. Major risk factors for the development of PCOS include low birth weight with excess childhood weight gain and precocious pubarche.

Comprehensive reviews of the literature have shown that metformin reduces fasting insulin and LDL concentrations in adult women with PCOS *(49, 50)*. Some studies also show significant reductions in blood pressure, BMI, and abdominal tissue mass *(51)*; others do not. Ovulation rates are consistently higher, and hirsutism scores often decline. Endothelial function as measured by brachial artery reactivity may also improve *(52)*.

Two randomized controlled studies (a total of 57 patients) have examined the effects of metformin in adolescents (ages 12–21 years) with PCOS. In the first, a 12-week period of treatment with metformin reduced total testosterone concentrations and increased the frequency of ovulatory menses *(53)*. There was a nonsignificant reduction in the insulin area under the curve but no change in BMI. In the second, a 6-month treatment period with metformin reduced BMI (37.3 to 36.3), increased insulin sensitivity, and reduced free testosterone levels *(54)*.

Low-birth-weight girls who develop precocious pubarche are prone to insulin resistance and progression to PCOS, even in the absence of striking weight gain. Despite normal BMI, such patients may have increased abdominal fat mass and decreased lean body mass. In a series of randomized studies conducted in nonobese Spanish adolescents with ovarian hyperandrogenism and hyperinsulinism, Ibanez and deZegher and their colleagues found that metformin increased the frequency of ovulatory menses, reduced hirsutism scores and free testosterone levels, reduced the insulin secretory responses to glucose, decreased serum triglyceride, cholesterol, and LDL levels, and increased HDL concentrations *(55–58)*. In combination with the antiandrogen flutamide, metformin also reduced abdominal fat mass, increased lean body mass, decreased interleukin-6 levels, and increased adiponectin and sex hormone binding globulin levels and insulin sensitivity *(56, 59–62)*. Similar effects of metformin alone were observed in prepubertal (8 years old) low-birth-weight girls with precocious pubarche *(58)*. These benefits were achieved during treatment periods ranging from 6 to 12 months but were reversed within 3 to 6 months of cessation of therapy.

METFORMIN AND ANTIPSYCHOTIC THERAPY

Patients treated with antipsychotic medications are at great risk for weight gain and associated metabolic abnormalities, including insulin resistance, hyperinsulinemia, and diabetes. A randomized, double-blind, placebo-controlled study demonstrated that metformin reduced weight and BMI z scores and increased insulin sensitivity in obese adolescents treated with olanzapine, risperidone, or quetiapine *(63)*.

ADVERSE EFFECTS OF METFORMIN

Minor and usually transient gastrointestinal side effects are the most common adverse reactions associated with metformin use. The abdominal discomfort can be prevented by taking the medication with food or (in some cases) by prescribing the long-acting formulation. Metformin also increases urinary excretion of B-vitamins; a standard daily multivitamin should be taken concurrently with the medication.

Lactic acidosis, a serious concern in patients taking other biguanides such as phenformin, has not been described in children. Metformin does not alter the mean fasting plasma lactate concentration or the rate of plasma lactate turnover in adults. It does, however, decrease the rate of lactate conversion to glucose, with an increase in lactate oxidation *(35)*. Thus, metformin should be avoided in persons at risk for decreased lactate oxidation or increased lactate production as may be seen with heart failure, liver or kidney disease, or states of shock. In addition, the drug should be discontinued in preparation for, and during, an oral or IV contrast study. In a systematic review and meta-analysis of comparative or observational cohort studies of metformin use in type 2 diabetics without contraindications, there were no cases of fatal or nonfatal lactic acidosis. In fact, pooled data from 194 studies showed that the reported incidence of lactic acidosis in the metformin and non-metformin groups was identical at zero *(64)*. These findings were corroborated in the COSMIC Approach Study (Comparative Outcomes Study of Metformin Intervention versus Conventional Approach Study) requested by the U.S. Food and Drug Administration as part of postmarketing safety surveillance. In this prospective randomized study of poorly controlled adult type 2 diabetics, 7,227 received metformin and were compared with 1,505 patients receiving other usual care (i.e., sulfonylurea, thiazolidinedione, insulin, or other non-metformin therapy) over 1 year *(65)*. Participants included were in good general health, had normal renal function and hepatic function, and had no history of metabolic acidosis. The metformin dose was at least 500 mg twice daily up to a maximum dose of 2,500 mg/day. The incidences of reported serious adverse events were similar between the two groups: 10.3% versus 11% for the metformin versus usual care groups, respectively. Mean plasma lactate levels were also similar between the groups: 1.7 mmol/L for metformin versus 1.6 mmol/L for usual care.

OTHER MEDICATIONS THAT MAY PROVE USEFUL IN CHILDREN WITH INSULIN RESISTANCE (REVIEWED IN REFS. 3, 21, AND 66)

Medications that cause weight loss in obese patients can indirectly increase insulin sensitivity and reduce the prevalence of type 2 diabetes. Examples include acarbose, which inhibits gastrointestinal carbohydrate absorption, and orlistat, which limits intestinal fat absorption. There is little or no evidence for long-term metabolic benefits in children; the efficacy of such medications is limited by their tendency to cause flatulence and diarrhea but might be used in highly motivated individuals.

The thiazolidinediones (TZDs) increase insulin sensitivity directly and improve glucose tolerance in adults with type 2 diabetes. The landmark Tripod study *(67)* showed that troglitazone reduced significantly the incidence of type 2 diabetes in Hispanic women with previous gestational diabetes; similar findings were reported in a major trial of rosiglitazone *(68)*, which carries a lower risk of hepatic dysfunction. Despite initial hopes *(67)*, the beneficial effects of the TZDs do not persist after discontinuation of the drug *(68)*. Thus TZDs, like metformin, appear to delay the onset of diabetes but do not truly prevent the development of the disease. No studies have yet examined the effects of the TZDs in insulin resistant adolescents or children. Side effects of the medication, which include weight gain, edema, anemia, bone loss, and cardiac failure, mitigate against their routine use.

BALANCING PHARMACOTHERAPY AND LIFESTYLE INTERVENTIONS (FIGS. 13.5, 13.6, AND 13.7)

In the opinion of the authors *(69, 70)*, intensive lifestyle intervention and/or pharmacotherapy should be considered for peripubertal children and adolescents at high risk for glucose intolerance, type 2 diabetes, and other serious complications of insulin resistance. In greatest jeopardy are a) obese adolescents (BMI >95th percentile for age and gender) with abdominal adiposity, acanthosis nigricans, positive family history of diabetes, and high-risk ethnic background; and b) teenage girls with PCOS; and c) preteen girls with precocious pubarche who show exaggerated weight gain in childhood and who were born small for gestational age.

Therapeutic goals for obese patients include a reduction in BMI z-score and normalization of blood pressure, plasma lipid concentrations, and hepatic and renal function. Five percent to 10% reductions in BMI in adults can increase insulin sensitivity, improve glucose tolerance, and reduce cardiovascular risk; thus initial goals for weight loss in children should be modest and realistic and achieved slowly. For the teenager with PCOS or precocious pubarche, additional therapeutic goals include reductions in hirsutism scores and establishment or restoration of ovulatory menses.

Effective interventions must be tailored to the unique cultural, psychosocial, and socioeconomic challenges of the individual patient and his or her family. They must assess barriers to exercise and lifestyle modifications, misconceptions about medication use and adherence, family history of disease prevalence, and patient acceptance of

Intensive lifestyle intervention and/or pharmacotherapy: when to intervene

- Intensive lifestyle intervention and/or pharmacotherapy for:
  - obese adolescents with
    - abdominal adiposity
    - acanthosis nigricans
    - positive family history of diabetes
    - high-risk ethnic background
  - teenage girls with PCOS
  - pre-teen girls with precocious pubarche if exaggerated weight gain and born small for gestational age.

Fig. 13.5 When to intervene.

Therapeutic goals

- **Obese patients**
  - reduction in BMI z score
  - normalization of:
    - blood pressure
    - plasma lipids
    - hepatic and renal function
- **Additional goals in precocious pubarche and PCOS**
  - reduction in hirsutism scores
  - restoration of ovulatory menses

Fig. 13.6 Therapeutic goals.

Balancing lifestyle intervention and pharmacotherapy

- Begin with lifestyle intervention
- Consider metformin if severe insulin resistance, impaired glucose tolerance, or co-morbidities *persist or worsen* despite "good faith effort" at diet and exercise
- Continue lifestyle intervention after initiating pharmacotherapy

Fig. 13.7 Balancing lifestyle intervention and pharmacotherapy.

disease treatment. Therapy must *matter* to the child or adolescent; it must be targeted to troublesome clinical symptoms such as hirsutism and acanthosis as well as to the longer-term risks of cardiovascular disease and diabetes. Ideally, therapy should help boost the patient's self-esteem.

Lifestyle intervention and lifelong lifestyle change are essential for all obese patients. Intensive lifestyle intervention gives the patient an active role in her treatment plan and encourages healthy living habits for a lifetime. Exercise has benefits on mood and self-worth that extend beyond its effects on BMI, insulin sensitivity, and the prevention of diabetes.

However, such lifestyle changes remain difficult to implement and are time-consuming and ineffective in many cases. The risks of treatment failure with lifestyle modifications alone are considerable, given the progressive nature of the metabolic syndrome. The authors believe that pharmacotherapy should be considered for severely resistant or glucose-intolerant children or adolescents who fail to respond to a 6- to 12-month trial of diet and exercise despite a good faith effort. "Good faith effort" means that the child has attempted to follow a low saturated fat/low simple sugar/low calorie diet recommended by a dietary counselor and has tried to increase energy expenditure through regular exercise. "Fails to respond" means that the patient has persistent or worsening elevations of fasting or postprandial glucose or insulin levels, dyslipidemia, or hepatic dysfunction. Drug therapy should be initiated while fostering a strong commitment to previous diet and exercise regimens.

Three principles guide our thinking in the selection of a drug for treatment of insulin resistance in children. First, drug selection should be tailored to the individual patient, with strong attention paid to the family history. Second, the goal of preventing or treating complications supercedes the goal of reducing weight per se. Finally, the benefits of any drug used to treat childhood obesity or insulin resistance should outweigh its risks. In our opinion, metformin is currently the drug of choice for treating the obese child with severe insulin resistance, impaired fasting glucose or impaired glucose tolerance. Metformin also appears effective in adolescent girls with PCOS. Its use in girls with precocious pubarche remains experimental. Given the lack of studies of TZDs in insulin-resistant children or adolescents, their potential, albeit rare, for severe hepatic complications, and their tendency to cause weight gain, we hesitate to recommend their use in non-diabetic children. Inhibitors of nutrient absorption such as orlistat are not tolerated by many obese children but could be used in selected, highly motivated patients.

It is not possible to provide guidelines for the duration of pharmacologic intervention. A trial off medication may be warranted if glucose tolerance normalizes, particularly if there has been a decline in BMI z-score. If impaired glucose tolerance or impaired fasting glucose persists despite compliance with the medical/pharmacologic regimen, it may be necessary to intensify lifestyle intervention and/or to increase the dose of medication. If glucose tolerance declines or the patient develops overt diabetes, it may be necessary to add insulin or another pharmacologic agent to the therapeutic regimen.

REFERENCES

1. Preeyasombat C, Bacchetti P, Lazar AA, Lustig RH. Racial and etiopathologic dichotomies in insulin hypersecretion and resistance in obese children. J Pediatr 2005;146:474–481.
2. Kratzsch J, Dehmel B, Pulzer F, et al. Increased serum GHBP levels in obese pubertal children and adolescents: relationship to body composition, leptin and indicators of metabolic disturbances. Int J Obes Relat Metab Disord 1997;21:1130–1136.
3. Freemark M. Metabolic consequences of obesity and their management. In: Brook CGD, Clayton PE, Brown RS, ed. Brook's clinical pediatric endocrinology. Fifth ed. Malden: Blackwell Publishing Ltd; 2005:419–435.
4. Weiss R, Dziura J, Burgert TS, et al. Obesity and the metabolic syndrome in children and adolescents. N Engl J Med 2004;350:2362–2374.
5. Bonora E, Kiechl S, Willeit J, et al. Carotid atherosclerosis and coronary heart disease in the metabolic syndrome: prospective data from the Bruneck study. Diabetes Care 2003;26:1251–1257.
6. Baron AD. Impaired glucose tolerance as a disease. Am J Cardiol 2001;88:16H–19H.
7. Shinozaki K, Kashiwagi A, Masada M, Okamura T. Molecular mechanisms of impaired endothelial function associated with insulin resistance. Curr Drug Targets Cardiovasc Haematol Disord 2004;4:1–11.
8. Rashid S, Uffelman KD, Lewis GF. The mechanism of HDL lowering in hypertriglyceridemic, insulin-resistant states. J Diabetes Complications 2002;16:24–28.

9. Brands MW, Hall JE, Keen HL. Is insulin resistance linked to hypertension? Clin Exp Pharmacol Physiol 1998;25:70–76.
10. Kirpichnikov D, McFarlane SI, Sowers JR. Metformin: an update. Ann Intern Med 2002;137:25–33.
11. Hsu CY, McCulloch CE, Iribarren C, Darbinian J, Go AS. Body mass index and risk for end-stage renal disease. Ann Intern Med 2006;144:21–28.
12. Calle EE, Rodriguez C, Walker-Thurmond K, Thun MJ. Overweight, obesity, and mortality from cancer in a prospectively studied cohort of U.S. adults. N Engl J Med 2003;348:1625–1638.
13. Lindsay RS, Hanson RL, Bennett PH, Knowler WC. Secular trends in birth weight, BMI, and diabetes in the offspring of diabetic mothers. Diabetes Care 2000;23:1249–1254.
14. Barker DJ, Osmond C, Forsen TJ, Kajantie E, Eriksson JG. Trajectories of growth among children who have coronary events as adults. N Engl J Med 2005;353:1802–1809.
15. Ball GD, Weigensberg MJ, Cruz ML, Shaibi GQ, Kobaissi HA, Goran MI. Insulin sensitivity, insulin secretion and beta-cell function during puberty in overweight Hispanic children with a family history of type 2 diabetes. Int J Obes (Lond) 2005;29:1471–1477.
16. Bacha F, Saad R, Gungor N, Janosky J, Arslanian SA. Obesity, regional fat distribution, and syndrome X in obese black versus white adolescents: race differential in diabetogenic and atherogenic risk factors. J Clin Endocrinol Metab 2003;88:2534–2540.
17. Arslanian SA. Metabolic differences between Caucasian and African-American children and the relationship to type 2 diabetes mellitus. J Pediatr Endocrinol Metab 2002;15(Suppl 1):509–517.
18. Cisneros-Tapia R, Navarrete FA, Gallegos AC, Robles-Sardin AE, Mendez RO, Valencia ME. Insulin sensitivity and associated risk factors in Mexican children and adolescents. Diabetes Care 2005;28:2546–2547.
19. Sinha R, Fisch G, Teague B, et al. Prevalence of impaired glucose tolerance among children and adolescents with marked obesity. N Engl J Med 2002;346:802–810.
20. Freemark M. Pharmacologic approaches to the prevention of type 2 diabetes in high risk pediatric patients. J Clin Endocrinol Metab 2003;88:3–13.
21. Isganaitis E, Lustig RH. Fast food, central nervous system insulin resistance, and obesity. Arterioscler Thromb Vasc Biol 2005;25:2451–2462.
22. Erlanson-Albertsson C. How palatable food disrupts appetite regulation. Basic Clin Pharmacol Toxicol 2005;97:61–73.
23. Pereira MA, Kartashov AI, Ebbeling CB, et al. Fast-food habits, weight gain, and insulin resistance (the CARDIA study): 15-year prospective analysis. Lancet 2005;365:36–42.
24. Wallace TM, Levy JC, Matthews DR. Use and abuse of HOMA modeling. Diabetes Care 2004;27:1487–1495.
25. Hrebicek J, Janout V, Malincikova J, Horakova D, Cizek L. Detection of insulin resistance by simple quantitative insulin sensitivity check index QUICKI for epidemiological assessment and prevention. J Clin Endocrinol Metab 2002;87:144–147.
26. Matsuda M, DeFronzo RA. Insulin sensitivity indices obtained from oral glucose tolerance testing: comparison with the euglycemic insulin clamp. Diabetes Care 1999;22:1462–1470.
27. Kahn BB, Flier JS. Obesity and insulin resistance. J Clin Invest 2000;106:473–481.
28. Ibanez L, Dimartino-Nardi J, Potau N, Saenger P. Premature adrenarche–normal variant or forerunner of adult disease? Endocr Rev 2000;21:671–696.
29. Dunaif A. Insulin resistance and the polycystic ovary syndrome: mechanism and implications for pathogenesis. Endocr Rev 1997;18:774–800.
30. Sherwin RS, Anderson RM, Buse JB, et al. The prevention or delay of type 2 diabetes. Diabetes Care 2003;26(Suppl 1):S62–69.
31. Tuomilehto J, Lindstrom J, Eriksson JG, et al. Prevention of type 2 diabetes mellitus by changes in lifestyle among subjects with impaired glucose tolerance. N Engl J Med 2001;344:1343–1350.

32. Nemet D, Barkan S, Epstein Y, Friedland O, Kowen G, Eliakim A. Short- and long-term beneficial effects of a combined dietary-behavioral-physical activity intervention for the treatment of childhood obesity. Pediatrics 2005 115:e443–449.

32a. Epstein LH, Valoski A, Wing RR, McCurley J. Ten-year outcomes of behavioral family-based treatment for childhood obesity. Health Psychol 1994;13:373–383.

33. Stumvoll M, Nurjhan N, Perriello G, Dailey G, Gerich JE. Metabolic effects of metformin in non-insulin-dependent diabetes mellitus. N Engl J Med 1995;333:550–554.

34. Gunton JE, Delhanty PJ, Takahashi S, Baxter RC. Metformin rapidly increases insulin receptor activation in human liver and signals preferentially through insulin-receptor substrate-2. J Clin Endocrinol Metab 2003;88(3):1323–1332.

35. Holland W, Morrison T, Chang Y, Wiernsperger N, Stith BJ. Metformin (Glucophage) inhibits tyrosine phosphatase activity to stimulate the insulin receptor tyrosine kinase. Biochem Pharmacol 2004;67:2081–2091.

36. Zhou G, Myers R, Li Y, et al. Role of AMP-activated protein kinase in mechanism of metformin action. J Clin Invest 2001;108:1167–1174.

37. Zou MH, Kirkpatrick SS, Davis BJ, et al. Activation of the AMP-activated protein kinase by the anti-diabetic drug metformin in vivo. Role of mitochondrial reactive nitrogen species. J Biol Chem 2004;279:43940–43951.

38. Lindsay JR, Duffy NA, McKillop AM, et al. Inhibition of dipeptidyl peptidase IV activity by oral metformin in Type 2 diabetes. Diabet Med 2005;22:654–657.

39. UKPDS group. Effect of intensive blood-glucose control with metformin on complications in overweight patients with type 2 diabetes (UKPDS 34). Lancet 1998;352:854–865.

40. Mannucci E, Tesi F, Bardini G, et al. Effects of metformin on glucagon-like peptide-1 levels in obese patients with and without Type 2 diabetes. Diabetes Nutr Metab 2004;17:336–342.

40a. Chau-Van C, Gamba M, Salvi R, Gaillard RC, Pralong FP. Metformin inhibits adenosine 5'-monophosphate-activated kinase activation and prevents increases in neuropeptide Y expression in cultured hypothalamic neurons. Endocrinology. 2007;148:507–11.

41. Knowler WC, Barrett-Connor E, Fowler SE, et al. Reduction in the incidence of type 2 diabetes with lifestyle intervention or metformin. N Engl J Med 2002;346:393–403.

42. Diabetes Prevention Program Research Group. Effects of withdrawal from metformin on the development of diabetes in the diabetes prevention program. Diabetes Care 2003;26:977.

42a. Ramachandran A, Snehalatha C, Mary S, Mukesh B, Bhaskar AD, Vijay V. Indian Diabetes Prevention Program. The Indian Diabetes Prevention Programme shows that lifestyle modification and metformin prevent type 2 diabetes in Asian Indian subjects with impaired glucose tolerance (IDPP-1). Diabetologia 2006; 49:289–297.

43. Freemark M, Bursey D. The effects of metformin on body mass index and glucose tolerance in obese adolescents with fasting hyperinsulinemia and a family history of type 2 diabetes. Pediatrics 2001;107:E55.

44. Kay JP, Alemzadeh R, Langley G, D'Angelo L, Smith P, Holshouser S. Beneficial effects of metformin in normoglycemic morbidly obese adolescents. Metabolism 2001;50:1457–1461.

44a. Srinivasan S, Ambler GR, Baur LA, Garnett SP, Tepsa M, Yap F, Ward GM, Cowell CT. Randomized, controlled trial of metformin for obesity and insulin resistance in children and adolescents: improvement in body composition and fasting insulin. J Clin Endocrinol Metab. 2006;91:2074–80.

45. Lustig RH, Mietus-Snyder ML, Bacchetti P, Lazar AA, Velasquez-Mieyer PA, Christensen ML. Insulin dynamics predict body mass index and z-score response to insulin suppression or sensitization pharmacotherapy in obese children. J Pediatr 2006;148 23–29.

45a. Freemark M. Liver dysfunction in pediatric obesity and insulin resistance: a randomized, controlled trial of metformin. Acta Paediatrica, in press.

46. Schwimmer JB, Middleton MS, Deutsch R, Lavine JE. A phase 2 clinical trial of metformin as a treatment for non-diabetic paediatric non-alcoholic steatohepatitis. Aliment Pharmacol Ther 2005;21:871–879.
47. Hookman P, Barkin JS. Current biochemical studies of nonalcoholic fatty liver disease and nonalcoholic steatohepatitis suggest a new therapeutic approach. Am J Gastroenterol 2003;98:2093–2097.
48. Levri KM, Slaymaker E, Last A, et al. Metformin as treatment for overweight and obese adults: a systematic review. Ann Fam Med 2005;3:457–461.
49. Lord JM, Flight IH, Norman RJ. Metformin in polycystic ovary syndrome: systematic review and meta-analysis. BMJ 2003;327:951–953.
50. De Leo V, la Marca A, Petraglia F. Insulin-lowering agents in the management of polycystic ovary syndrome. Endocr Rev. 2003;24:633–667.
51. Pasquali R, Gambineri A, Biscotti D, et al. Effect of long-term treatment with metformin added to hypocaloric diet on body composition, fat distribution, and androgen and insulin levels in abdominally obese women with and without the polycystic ovary syndrome. J Clin Endocrinol Metab 2000;85:2767–2774.
52. Orio F Jr, Palomba S, Cascella T, et al. Improvement in endothelial structure and function after metformin treatment in young normal-weight women with polycystic ovary syndrome: results of a 6-month study. J Clin Endocrinol Metab 2005;90:6072–6076.
53. Bridger T, MacDonald S, Baltzer F, Rodd C. Randomized placebo-controlled trial of metformin for adolescents with polycystic ovary syndrome. Arch Pediatr Adolesc Med 2006;160:241–246.
54. Allen HF, Mazzoni C, Heptulla RA, Murray MA, Miller N, Koenigs L, Reiter EO. Randomized controlled trial evaluating response to metformin versus standard therapy in the treatment of adolescents with polycystic ovary syndrome. J Pediatr Endocrinol Metab 2005;18:761–768.
55. Ibanez L, Valls C, Potau N, Marcos MV, de Zegher F. Sensitization to insulin in adolescent girls to normalize hirsutism, hyperandrogenism, oligomenorrhea, dyslipidemia, and hyperinsulinism after precocious pubarche. J Clin Endocrinol Metab 2000;85:3526–3530.
56. Ibanez L, Valls C, Ferrer A, Ong K, Dunger DB, De Zegher F. Additive effects of insulin-sensitizing and anti-androgen treatment in young, nonobese women with hyperinsulinism, hyperandrogenism, dyslipidemia, and anovulation. J Clin Endocrinol Metab 2002;87:2870–2874.
57. Ibanez L, Ferrer A, Ong K, Amin R, Dunger D, de Zegher F. Insulin sensitization early after menarche prevents progression from precocious pubarche to polycystic ovary syndrome. J Pediatr 2004;144:23–29.
58. Ibanez L, Valls C, Marcos MV, Ong K, Dunger DB, De Zegher F. Insulin sensitization for girls with precocious pubarche and with risk for polycystic ovary syndrome: effects of prepubertal initiation and postpubertal discontinuation of metformin treatment. J Clin Endocrinol Metab 2004;89:4331–4337.
59. Ibanez L, Ong K, Ferrer A, Amin R, Dunger D, de Zegher F. Low-dose flutamide-metformin therapy reverses insulin resistance and reduces fat mass in nonobese adolescents with ovarian hyperandrogenism. J Clin Endocrinol Metab 2003;88:2600–2606.
60. Ibanez L, De Zegher F. Flutamide-metformin therapy to reduce fat mass in hyperinsulinemic ovarian hyperandrogenism: effects in adolescents and in women on third-generation oral contraception. J Clin Endocrinol Metab 2003;88:4720–4724.
61. Ibanez L, de Zegher F. Ethinylestradiol-drospirenone, flutamide-metformin, or both for adolescents and women with hyperinsulinemic hyperandrogenism: opposite effects on adipocytokines and body adiposity. J Clin Endocrinol Metab 2004;89:1592–1597.
62. Ibanez L, Valls C, Cabre S, De Zegher F. Flutamide-metformin plus ethinylestradiol-drospirenone for lipolysis and antiatherogenesis in young women with ovarian hyperandrogenism: the key role of early, low-dose flutamide. J Clin Endocrinol Metab 2004;89:4716–4720.

63. Klein DJ, Cottingham EM, Sorter M, Barton BA, Morrison JA. A randomized, double-blind, placebo-controlled trial of metformin treatment of weight gain associated with initiation of atypical antipsychotic therapy in children and adolescents. Am J Psychiatry. 2006;163(12):2072–9.
64. Salpeter SR, Greyber E, Pasternak GA, Salpeter EE. Risk of fatal and nonfatal lactic acidosis with metformin use in type 2 diabetes mellitus: systematic review and meta-analysis. Arch Intern Med 2003;163:2594–2602.
65. Cryer DR, Nicholas SP, Henry DH, Mills DJ, Stadel BV. Comparative outcomes study of metformin intervention versus conventional approach the COSMIC Approach Study. Diabetes Care 2005;28:539–543.
66. Artz E, Freemark M. The pathogenesis of insulin resistance in children: metabolic complications and the roles of diet, exercise and pharmacotherapy in the prevention of type 2 diabetes. Pediatr Endocrinol Rev 2004;1:296–309.
67. Buchanan TA, Xiang AH, Peters RK, et al. Preservation of pancreatic beta-cell function and prevention of type 2 diabetes by pharmacological treatment of insulin resistance in high-risk Hispanic women. Diabetes 2002;51:2796–2803.
68. DREAM Trial Investigators, Gerstein HC, Yusuf S, Bosch J, Pogue J, Sheridan P, Dinccag N, Hanefeld M, Hoogwerf B, Laakso M, Mohan V, Shaw J, Zinman B, Holman RR. Effect of rosiglitazone on the frequency of diabetes in patients with impaired glucose tolerance or impaired fasting glucose: a randomised controlled trial. Lancet 2006; 368:1096–1105.
69. Freemark M. Pharmacotherapy of childhood diabetes: an evidence-based, conceptual approach. Diabetes Care 2007; 30:395–402.
70. Freemark M. Pharmacotherapy of childhood diabetes: a tailored approach. Rev Endocrinology 2007; 1:38–41.

14 The Surgical Approach to Morbid Obesity

Edward E. Mason, Mohammad K. Jamal, and Thomas M. O'Dorisio

Contents

Abstract

Intestinal bypass introduced the surgical treatment of obesity in 1954 by creating malabsorption. Intestinal bypass was replaced by gastric bypass beginning in 1966, which restricts food intake and produces less malabsorption. Both operations exposed the distal ileum to glucose and fat, which stimulates secretion of glucagon-like peptide-1 (GLP-1). This is a brake hormone for gastric emptying and intestinal peristalsis. GLP-1 is also an incretin that appears to prevent and treat type-2 diabetes. Nesidioblastosis has been reported after Roux-en-Y gastric bypass (RYGB). Thirty-day operative mortality has been reduced to less than 1%. An epidemic of obesity beginning in 1980 doubled the prevalence of candidates for surgical treatment by 2000. The lifelong risks of surgical treatment of severe obesity and type 2 diabetes are reviewed.

Key Words: biliopancreatic diversion, complications, duodenal switch, gastric banding, gastric bypass, gastrin, gastroplasty, ghrelin, glucagon-like peptide-1, ileal transposition, incretin-mimetics, intestinal bypass, lifelong follow-up, nesidioblastosis, obesity surgery, risk, type 2 diabetes.

From: *Contemporary Endocrinology: Energy Metabolism and Obesity: Research and Clinical Applications*
Edited by: P. A. Donohoue © Humana Press Inc., Totowa, NJ

INTRODUCTION

Severe obesity is a lethal disease that interferes with normal living and causes or worsens many other diseases such as type 2 diabetes mellitus (T2DM). A few surgeons beginning in 1954 recognized that their habit of providing weight-reducing diets to prepare patients for needed operations such as hernia repair or cholecystectomy was not working and that severe obesity should be considered a disease. This was a disruptive change in paradigm. Soon after a few surgeons made this change in viewpoint, the severely obese patients eagerly followed. Patients who had been operated upon referred their friends and relatives for obesity surgery. Patients were highly motivated to lose weight and receptive to the suggestion that obesity was a disease that could be treated with an operation *(1)*. They shared society's erroneous view that the obese lacked will power for self-cure, and they were eager to escape from both the obesity and the accusation.

From 1954 to 1966, intestinal bypass was the only operation available. Weight loss was attributed to malabsorption. Operations on the stomach began in 1966 and were thought to cause weight loss by restriction of intake of food. It is increasingly apparent that the first stomach operation, gastric bypass, includes malabsorption and changes in weight-regulating hormones. Those surgeons who wanted more weight loss than could be achieved with a pure restriction operation, and more than could be achieved with a standard gastric bypass, increased the length of intestine that was bypassed. To decrease the overall risk, surgeons used reversible operations and a general caveat: do no harm. This was in 1954 for intestinal bypass, and obesity at that time was not considered to be a disease. Morbid obesity (100 lb over ideal or twice ideal body weight) was identified by its high morbidity and mortality as warranting a surgical operation. Although the epidemic did not begin until 1980, there were already many candidates suitable for bariatric surgery.

The more the patient can understand the need to chew food to a semiliquid consistency before swallowing and limit intake of high-calorie liquids and processed foods, along with maintaining a physically active life, the better the weight control after a pure restriction operation. Patients with the most extensive bypass operations need more attention to eating adequate protein and taking prescribed vitamins, minerals, and medications. They need closer monitoring to avoid metabolic bone disease, iron deficiency anemia, and other potential complications related to the degree of imposed malabsorption. Physical activity and a healthy lifestyle are important for all of these patients. A history of adverse childhood events (ACEs) may signal a decreased ability to make the best use of an operation *(2)*. This is an area of care that warrants more attention before and after the operation.

Reversible operations for treatment of obesity were modeled after resections of small bowel or stomach used for treating cancer, peptic ulcer, and other diseases. These resections had caused loss of weight and poor maintenance of weight. Making the operations reversible made them acceptable for treating severe obesity. Intestinal bypass, first performed in 1954, was used until mounting complications led to replacement by loop gastric bypass beginning in 1966 *(3)*. In 1971, a simple restriction of food intake by horizontal gastroplasty was used to avoid bypass complications but was soon abandoned because of inadequate weight reduction *(4)*. The pouches were too large and both pouch and outlet stretched, resulting in inadequate weight loss.

The Roux-en-Y type of gastric bypass (Fig. 14.1) was introduced in 1977 *(5)*. Peristalsis in the alimentary limb kept the irritating, alkaline bile and pancreatic juices from entering the stomach pouch, which eliminated alkaline gastritis and facilitated the management of leaks if they occurred during the early postoperative period. In 1980, vertical banded gastroplasty with a small, lesser curvature pouch (Fig. 14.2) was more successful and soon accounted for more than half of the operations *(6)*. At the same time, there began an increase in the prevalence of obesity (BMI ≥30), progressing from 15% prior to 1980 to 31% in 2000 *(7)*. The operative weight also increased *(8)*. Roux-en-Y gastric bypass (RYGB) produced more weight loss and increasingly replaced restriction operations. In 2005, more than 95% of operations were RYGB or other bypass-type operations. The American Society for Bariatric Surgery estimates that there were 170,000 operations for obesity performed in the United States in 2005. In early 2006, obesity was declared a disease and was approved for surgical treatment by Medicare and Medicaid.

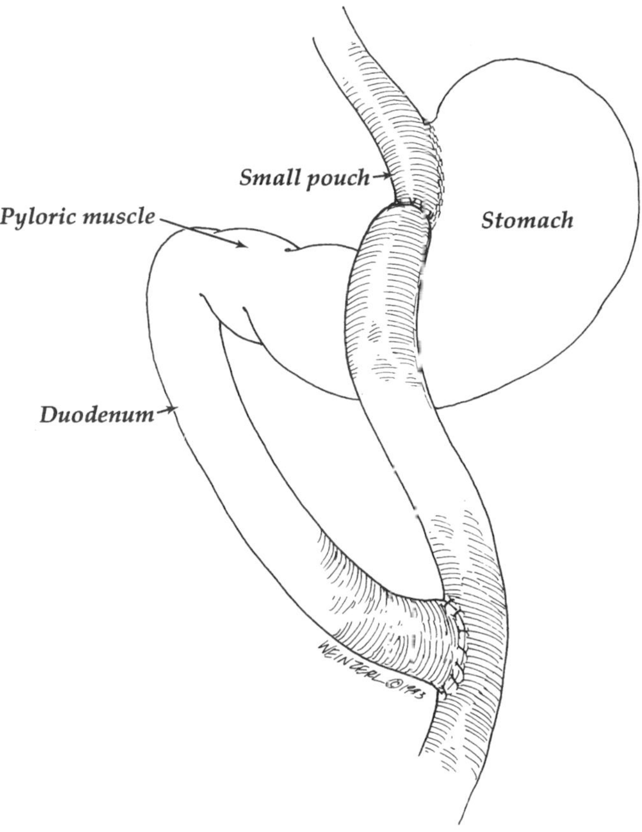

Fig. 14.1 Roux-en-Y gastric bypass has a 60-ml, upper, lesser curvature stomach pouch, which empties into a 60-cm alimentary limb of jejunum. The biliopancreatic limb brings bile and pancreatic juice to the end-to-side anastomosis. The common limb consists of most of the small bowel where digestion and absorption occur.

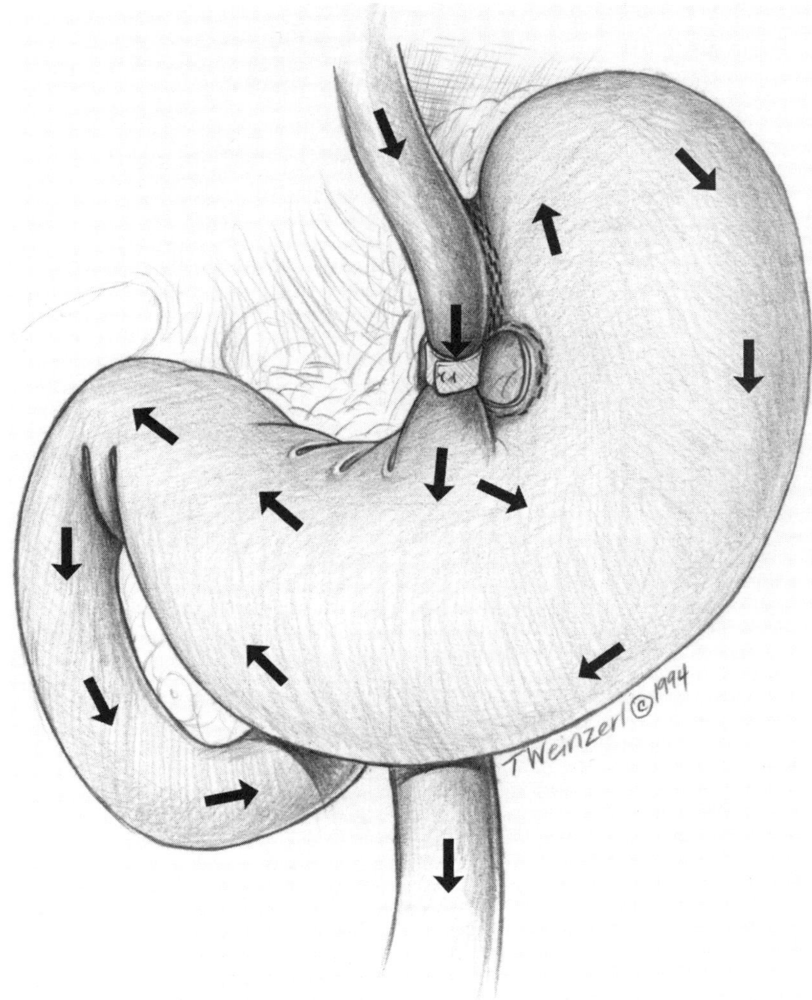

Fig. 14.2 Vertical banded gastroplasty provides a pouch with a volume of 10 to 20 ml along the upper lesser curvature of the stomach. There is a stapled window through both walls of the stomach, which allows stapling to the angle of His, and a polypropylene woven mesh is sewn in place to stabilize the pouch outlet. This provides a 12-mm-diameter pouch outlet.

MECHANISMS OF WEIGHT REDUCTION

Intestinal bypass was considered purely malabsorptive until it was observed that patients ate less. There were obvious reasons for eating less. Patients ate less when they left their home and wanted to avoid the inconvenience of urgent, foul-smelling bowel movements. The food was lost before it could be digested and absorbed. Gastric bypass was thought to cause weight loss by reducing the capacity for a meal and by causing the dumping syndrome. The pouch size is 30 ml for a standard Roux-en-Y gastric bypass (RYGB) compared with 1,700 ml capacity for the normal stomach of an average morbidly obese person. In fact, bypass of most of the stomach, duodenum, and a short length of jejunum interferes with digestion and absorption. Bypass of the duodenum interferes with the mixing of food with bile and digestive enzymes from the pancreas (postprandial dyskinesia). The increased rate of movement of intestinal contents due to the high osmolarity further interferes with the normal sequence of digestion and absorption. The dumping syndrome in some patients was a deterrent to intake of simple sugars and high-calorie drinks. There were obvious reasons for weight loss. However, these simple and obvious reasons did not explain all of the weight loss or all of the benefits and risks of intestinal and gastric bypass.

Restriction of intake with a small pouch, without any bypass, was introduced to limit intake without causing complications peculiar to bypass of the upper digestive tract. Vertical banded gastroplasty and other vertical pouch operations became popular beginning in 1980 but then lost favor as surgeons returned to RYGB in order to increase weight loss and, more recently, to make use of the laparoscopic approach (LRYGB). The laparoscopic approach leaves smaller scars and avoids large incisional hernias. The "minimally invasive" abdominal wall approach does not change the operation that is performed within the abdomen. There are compensatory changes after loss of use of most of the stomach or small bowel. After the patient loses weight after most operations, there is a gradual increase in weight as compensatory changes occur in the digestive tract and the patient learns how to eat "around" the new anatomy.

Digestive Tract Hormones Contribute to Weight Control

Most of the hormones that are involved in weight control are secreted in both the brain and digestive tract. An operation that prevents food from reaching the fundus of the stomach, or that exposes the distal small bowel to the digesting food stream, changes the secretion of some of these hormones. Receptors in the duodenum sense changes in the pH, chemical composition, and tonicity of duodenal contents. These feed back to the antrum and pyloric muscle to control emptying of the stomach so that the contents of the small bowel remain isotonic with body fluids and an optimum pH. When this area is bypassed, the movement of ingested food into the small bowel is uncontrolled. It would appear that hypertonic intestinal contents stimulate rapid movement to the distal small bowel. Some patients are symptomatic, due to the dumping syndrome. A few will complain of uncontrolled, explosive diarrhea. Changes in hormone secretion also affect satiety and hunger.

Ghrelin

When we began the use of gastric bypass, surgeons performing intestinal bypass told us that patients would not tolerate restriction of intake. In fact, patients reported that for the first time in memory they could leave food on the plate and that they felt more like normal-weight people. A change in appetite behavior was discovered that seemed to confirm this effect *(9)*. Kojima et al. discovered ghrelin in 1999 *(10)*. Ghrelin was first developed as an artificial medication designed to stimulate the secretion of growth hormone. When it was injected in experimental animals, those animals gained weight, and study of this effect took precedence over the original study *(11)*. It was then found that ghrelin is a normal hormone in man and other mammals. Ghrelin is secreted from L-cells in the fundus of the stomach, which in most gastric bypass operations is no longer exposed to the stimulation of food (Fig. 14.1). Ghrelin is a powerful stimulus to hunger. Plasma concentration normally rises during the day and falls during the

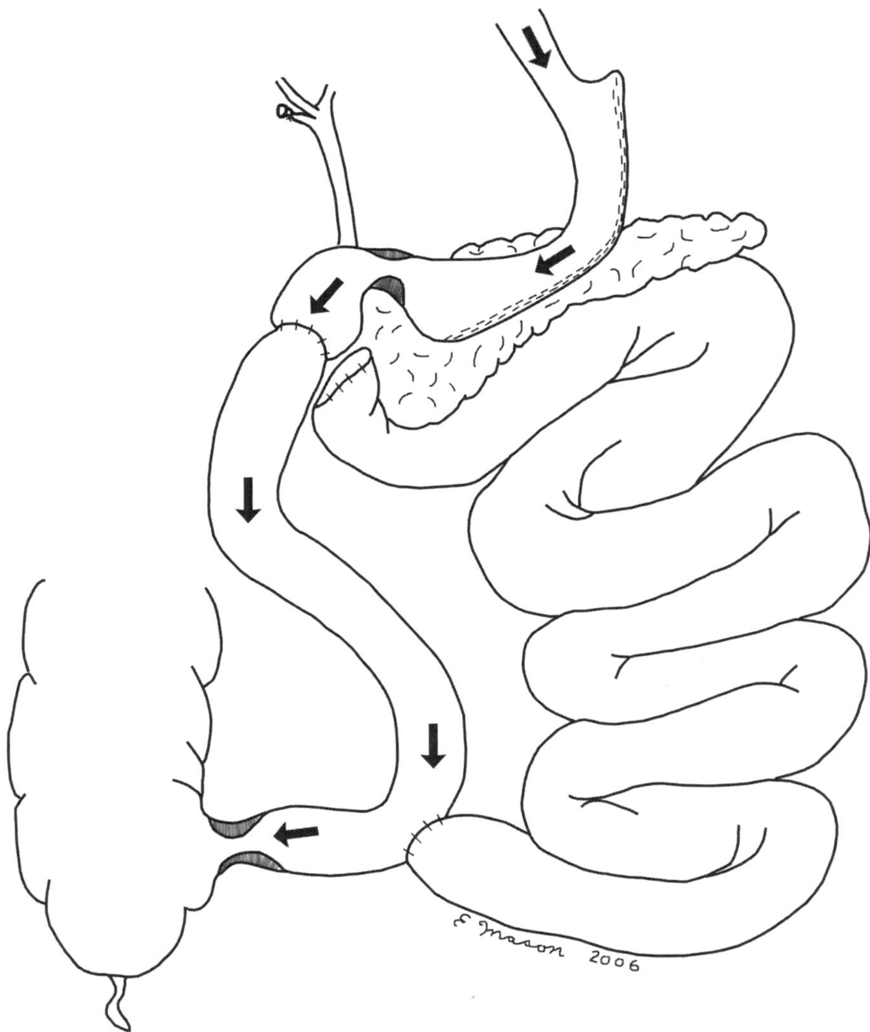

Fig. 14.3 Shows biliopancreatic diversion with duodenal switch and sleeve resection of the greater curvature of the stomach. The pyloric muscle between the stomach antrum and the first part of the duodenum controls stomach emptying. The biliopancreatic limb brings digestive juices, through most of the small bowel to the distal ileum, where they mix with the food stream, 50 to 100 cm from the colon. The small bowel, attached to the duodenal segment, is 200 to 350 cm long, based on the total length of the bowel. The sleeve resection is also used alone or as a first stage, with the switch performed later.

night. Superimposed is a rise before each meal and a prompt decrease after the meal. After RYGB, the plasma level remains low night and day according to Cummings et al. *(12)*. Vertical banded gastroplasty, which allows food (and saliva) to reach the fundus of the stomach (Fig. 14.2), results in an increase in ghrelin levels before a meal and a normal decrease in secretion after a meal *(13)*. Operations that remove the fundus of the stomach should decrease plasma ghrelin levels and also increase weight loss. This response was observed after sleeve gastrectomy (Fig. 14.3) in which most of the stomach is removed leaving only a tube of stomach composed of the lesser curvature extending from the esophagus to the duodenum *(14)*. Fruhbeck et al. observed that 24 h after gastric bypass, the plasma ghrelin levels were significantly reduced compared with Nissen fundoplication and adjustable gastric banding, after which the ghrelin plasma levels were increased *(15)*. This suggests that there may be something in saliva that stimulates the release of ghrelin rather than food, as all patients were fasting between the two measurements. Gauna et al. observed that the injection of acylated ghrelin induced an acute increase in unacylated ghrelin and therefore total ghrelin levels *(16)*. Perhaps ghrelin secreted by salivary glands stimulates the release of ghrelin from the fundus of the stomach. Obesity surgery has helped to open up new approaches to the study and treatment of obesity and diabetes.

Obestatin

In late 2005, Zhang et al. discovered another peptide that is produced by the ghrelin gene. Obestatin opposes ghrelin effects *(17)*. Ghrelin stimulates contractions of intestinal muscle strips. Obestatin suppresses these contractions and when both hormones are provided, contractions are suppressed. This corresponds with the effects observed in food intake in mice. Ghrelin and obestatin come from different segments of the same gene. The obestatin receptor is in highest concentration in jejunum, duodenum, and stomach; decreasing in ileum; and lowest in the colon. It is present in many other tissues. Zhang suggested that obestatin and ghrelin fine tune intestinal contraction, food intake, and body weight. However, there are other systems regulating body weight according to observations made in mutant mice that remain healthy even when the ghrelin gene is absent. Zhang suggests that these animals probably do not have either ghrelin or obestatin. The neurohumoral control of weight is redundant, and this may prevent an early medical solution for obesity, which is a reason for continuing to refine and improve the outcome of obesity surgery. With two hormones competing in weight control, the possibility of developing related medications that would cause weight loss seems possible.

Glucagon-like Peptide-1

One of the reasons patients ate less after intestinal bypass was the ileal brake hormone, which is secreted when nutrients reach the distal small bowel. Decreasing the length of functioning small bowel to 18 inches allowed sugar and fat to reach the distal small bowel before they were absorbed. The *brake hormone* name came from observed slowing of intestinal peristalsis and delayed emptying of the intact stomach after injection of the hormone *(18)*. Another name is glucagon-like peptide-1, or GLP-1. GLP-1 is also a satiety hormone that acts upon the arcuate nucleus in the ventromedial hypothalamus *(19)*. More than malabsorption was involved in weight loss after intestinal bypass. In fact, the serum levels of GLP-1 continue to rise for 20 years after this operation *(20)*. Unfortunately for weight control, complications of the operation led to its gradual abandonment after the introduction of gastric bypass in 1966.

OPERATION-RELATED RISKS

Operations that imitate removal of the stomach, intestines, or both, performed in patients who are twice their normal weight or more raise questions about the risk of death. The initial risk is during the first 30 days after the operation, when complications may result in prolonged hospitalization, further operations, and/or death. There remains the risk of obesity and some risk from the mobilization of large fat stores. The final weight may not be low enough to eliminate all of the risk of obesity. Some patients learn how to "beat the operation." The quote is from a patient who, early after a restriction operation, returned to the clinic with a big smile and jovially explained that he was buying large jars of chocolate-covered malted milk balls, repackaging them in sandwich bags, and snacking throughout the day. Obesity may be an unrecognized protection that the patient needs and will strive to maintain *(21)*. There are other risky behavior patterns that may influence longevity in many of the severely obese.

Thirty-Day Complications and Operative Mortality

The 30-day operative mortality was 0.24% (46 of 18,972) according to data collected by the International Bariatric Surgery Registry (IBSR) during the years 1986–1999 *(22)*. Flum et al. reported a 30-day operative mortality of 2.0% for medicare patients *(23)*. These were two differently selected groups of patients. The IBSR surgeons submitted patient data because they were interested in how their patient's results compared with those of a larger surgical group. Flum gathered data from all patients and all surgeons involved in the surgical care of older and higher-risk Medicare patients in the state of Washington. Many variables are involved so that comparisons can be misleading. Standardization can markedly change the relative risk between different groups of patients but requires submission of the needed data. The most frequent major risk is leak of digestive juices from stomach or intestine into the upper abdomen, where the operation is performed. This was reported for 0.73% of patients with bypass operations and 0.47% after restriction operations in IBSR data from 38,501 patients operated upon during 1986 through 2005. The risk of gastrointestinal hemorrhage was 0.44% for bypass and 0.15% for restriction operations. The risk of bowel obstruction during the first 30 days was 0.40% after bypass and 0.02% after restriction operations. Pulmonary embolism was about the same in frequency, 0.25% and 0.21%, but was the most common cause of death, occurring in 28 of 38,501. These are very low risks compared with the period prior to 1980, but the risk of death, during the first 30 days, for bypass operations was twice that for restriction operations. This is consistent with the greater complexity of the operations and it also points the way to further decreasing risk through study of the causes of death. Small bowel obstruction occurred more often after bypass operations. Death from complications of the operation is also related to the time between onset of obstruction and definitive treatment. Early discharge and the infrequency of leak and bowel obstruction may contribute to delay in diagnosis and treatment of these complications.

Lifelong Mortality

MacDonald et al. compared 154 patients with diabetes who were treated with RYGB with 78 matched control obese patients who did not have an operation *(24)*. The risk of death was 1% per year in the surgical group and 4.5% in the nonsurgical group. In a study by the International Bariatric Surgery Registry of morbidly obese patients operated upon in 1986 through 1999, there were 654 of 18,972 (3.45%) total deaths with an average follow-up of 8.3 years *(24)*. These deaths were reported by participating surgeons or obtained from a search using the National Death Index (NDI). Operative age, gender, body mass index (BMI), history of smoking, diabetes, and hypertension were all significant predictors of survival. The type of operation (restriction or bypass) was not a predictor. Over time, it is anticipated that there may be a difference in survival related to type of operation and that this could be a basis for recommending greater use of either restriction or bypass operations. Restriction operations cause less weight loss and could result in more deaths due to residual obesity. Bypass operations, through their effect in decreasing plasma insulin levels, reduce deaths from cancer.

Lifelong Complications Related to Operation

The history of bypass surgery is one of abandoning operations because of long-term complications. For stomach surgery, this began with the prototypical Billroth II gastrectomy as it was used for treatment of peptic ulcer in the 1950s when one of the authors (E.E.M.) was learning how to perform Billroth II gastrectomy for ulcer from Owen H. Wangensteen at the University of Minnesota. Wangensteen along with Lester Dragstedt at the University of Chicago both abandoned this type of subtotal gastrectomy that bypassed the duodenum. One of the complications was poor maintenance of body weight, which Mason elected to make use of in the treatment of obesity. However, there were other complications related to bypass of the duodenum. Intestinal bypass was abandoned because of complications after gastric bypass was introduced. In 1971, at the University of Iowa, we tried to substitute gastroplasty for gastric bypass, without success, but in 1980 vertical banded gastroplasty became the operation of choice until Mason's retirement in 1991. The following reviews some of the problems of bypass of the duodenum that have led to a continuing emphasis on preservation of the elaborate controls of the digestive tract that evolved in humans.

Metabolic Bone Disease

Metabolic bone disease, including osteoporosis, osteomalacia, and secondary hyperparathyroidism, can be a complication of operations that bypass the duodenum, such as RYGB *(25)*. The highest concentration of vitamin D receptors (and capacity for calcium absorption) according to Pazianas et al. is found in animals in the duodenum *(26)*. This study of 21 patients after gastrectomy, which bypasses the duodenum, did show decreased bone mineral density. However, there were adequate vitamin D receptors in the jejunum beyond the gastroenterostomy, so loss of vitamin D receptors was not the cause. Tovey et al. in a review of postgastrectomy bone disease wrote, "Although the use of this operation has declined drastically in recent years, this metabolic disorder is still with us and may escape and confuse the unwary" *(27)*. Shaker et al. concluded that calcium malabsorption and secondary hyperparathyroidism may occur frequently after gastric exclusion surgery *(28)*. Exclusion is another word for bypass. Aaron et al. in study of patients with fracture of the proximal femur observed that the most common predisposing factor was partial gastrectomy *(29)*. Nilsson in another study of factors predisposing to fracture of the femoral neck found that a history of gastrectomy was present in 10% of patients, which was 10-fold higher than in matched controls who did not have fractures of the hip *(30)*.

After RYGB, patients are usually asked to take calcium and vitamin D, but few are followed closely for a lifetime. Too often, the first awareness of bone disease is a fall caused by hip fracture, or collapse of the spine with a "widow's hump." If such patients are confined to bed, this increases the loss of bone, which according to Wolffe's law is remodeled and gains strength according to stresses place upon it. There is loss of bone surface with osteoporosis, which makes it difficult to treat *(31)*. This is a time-related problem, and studies of bone turnover during the first year or two after operation are of little use. Weight loss according to Wolffe's law will result in loss of bone. Papers written about patients who are followed closely and treated with vitamin D and calcium are important because they show what can be accomplished in the prevention of bone disease. The larger problem is with the vast majority of patients, who are not followed and who show up with bone disease when there are symptoms from pathologic fractures of low-density bone. We need to know the magnitude of this problem. Gastric bypass was selected as an operation designed to deplete patients of fat. It is also effective in depletion of bone. Patients need to be aware of this when they consent to a bypass operation *(32)*.

Obstruction of the Bypassed Upper Digestive Tract

There is also the risk of obstruction of the bypassed stomach, duodenum, and whatever length of jejunum is bypassed. This can begin as a paralytic ileus after general anesthesia and an operation that can be unrelated to the earlier abdominal surgery. As the bypassed stomach and intestine fill up with secretions, bile, and pancreatic juice, twisting occurs and may convert this to a mechanical obstruction due to kinking of the bypassed bowel. This can cause death in as short a time as 2 days probably from shock due to loss of fluid into the distended distal stomach followed by further loss from chemical peritonitis when the necrotic stomach wall perforates. A long biliopancreatic limb (between the duodenum and the enteroenterostomy) may twist into a volvulus so that there are actually two closed obstructions in series *(33,34)*. Fobi places a temporary gastrostomy in the excluded stomach to keep it decompressed during the early postoperative period and a radiographic opaque ring between the stomach and the abdominal wall to facilitate reinsertion of the gastrostomy tube if it is needed later in life *(35)*. Brolin has recommended a special stitch to decrease the risk of obstruction from kinking near the enteroenterostomy *(36)*. Internal hernia is another cause of bowel obstruction. There is a space behind the alimentary limb that is closed as a part of the operation but can open and provide a site for an internal hernia *(37)*. Bowel obstruction is more common after laparoscopic RYGB, especially during the learning period, according to Nguyen et al. *(38)*. The acute abdomen is a general diagnosis that includes rapidly lethal conditions that need emergency operation. Bowel obstruction is one of these. The lifelong incidence of bowel obstruction is not well-known because the primary surgeon is often not available at the time of an emergency. Because of the rapidity of loss of body fluid into the bypassed stomach, obstruction of this segment requires rapid diagnosis and surgical treatment. Any physician who might see such a patient in the emergency room should know about this complication. Bypass obstruction occurs occasionally years after the primary operation when the patient has a general anesthetic and an operation that may be in some other part of the body. Postoperative paralytic ileus causes the excluded stomach, duodenum, and excluded small bowel (see Fig. 14.1 for the anatomy) to fill up with stomach secretions, bile, and pancreatic juice. Because the excluded stomach has the largest diameter, it increases the most and the volume of body fluid loss is enough to cause shock with a high pulse rate. The pressure in the excluded stomach results in loss of blood flow in the stomach wall and perforation. The immediate chemical irritation of this fluid in the abdomen causes more fluid loss from the peritoneal surfaces of all of the intestine and other organs. Death may occur in as short a time as 48 hours.

Gastrin and Ulceration

Edkins in 1905 hypothesized that there was a hormone secreted in the antrum (lower one-third of the stomach) that stimulated the secretion of hydrochloric acid in the rest of the stomach and called this hormone *gastrin (39)*. There was dispute as to whether this hormone existed until Gregory and Tracy isolated gastrin from hog antral mucosa in 1964 *(40)*. Devine used an operation for treating large duodenal ulcers in which the antrum (which has no acid-secreting parietal cells) was bypassed and left attached to the duodenum *(41)*. Because there is no acid secretion from the antrum, the ulcers healed. However, acid is required in the antrum to inhibit gastrin secretion. Patients with exclusion of the antrum therefore develop stomal ulcers. Before gastric bypass (an exclusion operation) was used for the treatment of obesity, we studied the operation in the animal laboratory to make sure it would not increase secretion of gastrin by the antrum and cause ulcers, either in the duodenum or at the stoma between the stomach pouch and jejunum *(3)*. Studies in animals showed that if acid-secreting stomach was excluded with the antrum, acid secretion after a meal was suppressed. Later, when immunoassay of gastrin had been developed, we were able to show in patients that gastric bypass suppressed the secretion of gastrin after a meal *(42)*. There are other causes of ulcer than excessive gastrin secretion, and occasional patients bleed from ulcers in either the gastroenterostomy stoma or the duodenum.

Iron-Deficiency Anemia and Ruling Out Bleeding Ulcer

Iron-deficiency anemia is common after gastric bypass because iron is normally absorbed from the duodenum, which is bypassed by RYGB. Iron-deficiency anemia can be due to low iron stores or to loss of blood from a duodenal ulcer. The duodenum is difficult to visualize after this area has been bypassed. Right subcostal back pain and occult or gross blood in the stool suggest duodenal ulcer. An upper gastrointestinal radiograph can be performed through a percutaneous gastrostomy tube placed in the distal stomach *(35)*. A small gastroscope can also be inserted through this site.

TYPE 2 DIABETES MELLITUS AND HIGH INSULIN LEVELS

It has been estimated that there are 12 million people with type 2 diabetes mellitus (T2DM) in the United States *(43)*. There are also many more at risk of developing T2DM. To date, the most potent incretin, and the one that is available through internal stimulation, is the incretin GLP-1. There is an injectable mimetic of GLP-1: exendrin-4. T2DM accounts for most diabetes and has been known to respond much better to weight reduction than to insulin. It has been treated with insulin for years even though the results are often unsatisfactory. Incretins improve insulin receptor function and therefore do not cause hypoglycemia.

The diagnosis of T2DM does not identify the magnitude of the damage of insulin resistance secondary to obesity. Calle et al. *(44)* and Coughlin et al. *(45)* found that diabetes was an independent predictor of mortality from cancer of colon, pancreas, female breast; and in men of liver and bladder cancer. Christou et al. found that patients who had RYGB seemed to be protected from death caused by cancer *(46)*. Diabetes was found to be a predictor of death in the IBSR study of patients who had operations for obesity *(22)*. This suggests that the operations did not eliminate the risk either because some of the operations were performed too late in the progression of the disease or were not sufficiently effective in reducing serum insulin levels. Plasma insulin levels are high in the obese even when a diagnosis of T2DM has not been made. Insulin is known to be a growth hormone for normal and cancer cells. GLP-1 is a growth hormone for β-cells and a stimulus for insulin release in the presence of hyperglycemia. It also increases the number of insulin receptors but the overall effect is a reduction of plasma insulin. The overall effect upon survival after RYGB from decreasing the levels of insulin should be a benefit, in contrast with some of the other effects of bypass operations.

Surgical Treatment Through Endogenous GLP-1

It has been evident to surgeons from the early years of obesity surgery that bypass operations for obesity cure T2DM, often before the patient leaves the hospital *(47)*. The diabetes seldom recurs, and new diagnoses of diabetes are not made in these patients. Näslund et al. showed that obese patients, who were candidates for surgical treatment, had very little increase in plasma GLP-1 after a meal *(48)*. When patients were studied 9 months after intestinal bypass, the oral-glucose-stimulated plasma rise was normal, and after 20 years the GLP-1 fasting level was increased fivefold and the rise after oral glucose was eightfold over preoperative fasting levels. Insulin and glucose levels, fasting and after a meal, normalized. These observations seemed to demonstrate both the cause and the cure of T2DM. Halverson et al. observed that after gastric bypass, massive weight loss was accompanied by improvement in insulin receptor number, basal hyperinsulinemia, and glucose tolerance *(49)*. Postoperatively, patients had symptomatic, reactive hypoglycemia, which was postulated as due to hyperinsulinemia after ingestion of glucose.

Kellum et al. observed that gastric bypass causes a rise in plasma GLP-1 levels *(50)*. The common denominator between intestinal bypass and gastric bypass, in their beneficial effect upon T2DM, appears to be exposure of the distal ileum to glucose. Kellum observed that oral protein did not stimulate GLP-1 secretion and suggested that this secretory response to oral glucose could be a test for the dumping syndrome. Not all patients with rapid transit of glucose through the intestine are symptomatic. Dr. Clarence Dennis told one of the authors (E.E.M.), during the author's surgical internship in 1945 at the University of Minnesota in Minneapolis, that he and Dr. Leo Rigler, the head of radiology, had studied intestinal transit after subtotal gastrectomy with a short loop retrocolic gastroenterostomy. Some of what was given by mouth reached the distal small bowel within five minutes *(51)*. Dr. Dennis recommended that the anastomotic stoma should be made small enough to retard emptying of the gastric pouch, as the pyloric muscle was bypassed. We now know that small pouch outlets, designed to cause weight loss, do not prevent the stimulation of secretion of GLP-1. Normal emptying of the stomach is controlled by osmoreceptors that maintain isotonicity of duodenal contents according to Meeroff et al. *(52)*. These experiments indicated that osmoreceptors are present in the duodenum but not in the stomach or small bowel. Brener et al. have shown in humans that after a meal of glucose, there is an initial gush of stomach contents into the duodenum *(53)*. This stimulates the establishment of a steady rate of emptying of the stomach contents into the duodenum that is controlled by the caloric content of what is emptying from the stomach. After gastric bypass, there is no control of entry of high glucose loads to the small bowel, which would seem to explain the stimulation of GLP-1 secretion by exposure of the distal ileum to glucose.

Sirinek et al. suggested that the hyperinsulinemia of morbid obesity and its amelioration after gastric bypass might be caused by markedly elevated levels of glucose-dependent insulinotropic polypeptide(GIP) before surgery and its reduced release after bypass *(54)*. Valverde used an operation that removed all stomach, beyond a 150–200 cm^3 upper stomach pouch, and bypassed the duodenum plus 50 cm of jejunum *(55)*. Food passed through the stomach pouch and most of the small bowel including the distal ileum where GLP-1 is secreted. Oral glucose tolerance tests were performed with 75 g of glucose before and at 1, 3, and 6 months after the operation, measuring plasma glucagon, GLP-1, glucose, and insulin. They studied a control group of normal-weight people without an operation and morbidly obese surgery patients, none of whom were considered diabetic. The most striking change that occurred after operation in the obese was in plasma GLP-1, which rose after the 75-g of oral glucose sixfold at 1 month and more rapidly and higher at 3 and 6 months. The baseline level was mildly and progressively elevated at 1 to 6 months in Valverde's study. It was not markedly elevated at 9 months in Näslund's study of patients after intestinal bypass. The extremely high baseline level noted by Näslund, 20 years after the operation, leaves a question about the baseline levels between Näslund's observed normal levels at 9 months and the extremely high levels at 20 years. The baseline (fasting) levels may be important with regard to nesidioblastosis and when secretion of GLP-1 continues in the absence of any glucose in the lumen of the distal ileum.

Ileal Transposition

Considering the lifelong complications of bypass of the upper digestive tract, the idea of moving the distal ileum to a juxta-duodenal position seemed worth considering for an operation that would stimulate secretion of GLP-1 without bypassing the upper digestive tract *(56)*. This operation had been studied in small animals in an attempt to determine why patients with intestinal bypass decreased their intake of food *(57)*. Strader et al. found that intestinal transposition in rats increased ileal GLP-1 secretion and synthesis *(58)*.

The operation should probably not be used in humans because the stimulation of GLP-1 secretion cannot be controlled and might produce nesidioblastosis, which has now been reported after RYGB by Service et al. *(59)*. The nesidioblastosis was treated with partial pancreatectomy. One of the six patients had multiple insulinomas in the resected specimen and five patients had hyperplasia. Patti et al. reported three patients who required pancreatectomy for nesidioblastosis after gastric bypass *(60)*. One of these patients had failed to respond to reversal of the gastric bypass. All three patients revealed diffuse islet hyperplasia and expansion of β-cell mass. We do not know the denominator for risk of developing nesidioblastosis after bypass operations. All patients treated with intestinal bypass and all operations bypassing the duodenum would seem to be candidates.

An Endocrinologist's Approach to Nesidioblastosis

Two recent reports regarding hyperinsulinemic postprandial hypoglycemia associated with nesidioblastosis after gastric bypass surgery have raised suspicions that the loss of pyloric control of gastric emptying and consequent rapid transit of glucose, stimulating GLP-1 (discussed above), may be a major contributor to the development of nesidioblastosis/multiple small insulinomas.

Service et al. *(59)* reported six patients in whom postprandial symptoms of neuroglycopenia developed as a result of hyperinsulinemic hypoglycemia, with symptoms beginning anywhere from 6 months to as long as 8 years after the initial bypass surgery. All six patients had postprandial symptomatic hypoglycemia with biochemically documented low blood sugars. All patients in this study underwent a near complete pancreatectomy to reverse what was found pathologically to be nesidioblastosis, with one patient having multiple small insulinomas.

A second paper independently reported by Patti and colleagues *(60)* investigated three patients with severe postprandial hypoglycemia and hyperinsulinemia unresponsive to diet and medical therapy. All three patients underwent near complete pancreatectomy and all three were found to have histopathologic evidence of islet cell hyperplasia.

Utilizing the definition of incretin as an endocrine transmitter produced in the gastrointestinal tract, released by nutrients, especially carbohydrates, and stimulating insulin secretion in the presence of postprandial glucose levels, the most likely candidate in the above two studies is GLP-1. In addition to many actions of GLP-1 that include the increase of insulin synthesis, secretion, and expression of genes that modify β-cell function, another potentially important property is β-cell proliferation and neogenesis, not unlike what has been seen histopathologically in the nine patients reported above with postprandial hypoglycemia after gastric bypass *(61)*. Its location and highest concentrations in the ileum make it a very likely intestinal secretagogue following rapid transit of unabsorbed postprandial glucose in gastric bypass patients. Further, as noted above, serum levels of GLP-1 may continue to rise for 20 years after the operation of intestinal bypass as this very important hormone is also the "ileal brake" hormone. It appears also that loss of pyloric control of gastric emptying results in the same excess of GLP-1 secretion after Roux-en-Y gastric bypass.

There is another accepted incretin in the proximal intestinal tract, glucose-dependent insulinotropic polypeptide/gastric inhibitory polypeptide (GIP), which is known as an insulinotropic agent in the presence of postprandial physiologic glucose levels but is for the most part bypassed by the operation and would seem much less likely than GLP-1 as a cause of the early beneficial effects and the later complicating nesidioblastosis.

The implication of the nine reported cases that have documented hyperinsulinemic and symptomatic hypoglycemia with nesidioblastosis after gastric bypass is alarming. The thought of further surgical intervention and partial pancreatectomy even in a few individuals clearly increases morbidity/mortality of bypass surgery. Two rather recent papers regarding somatostatin and GLP-1 secretion, as well as a somatostatin mimetic, allude to possible medical therapy for such individuals who develop this problem after surgery.

In an article by Chisholm and Greenberg, somatostatin regulation of GLP-1 secretion in rat intestinal cultures was studied *(62)*. The authors show GLP-1 secretion and its inhibitory regulation by somatostatin-28, and somatostatin mimetics, was via somatostatin receptor subtype 5. A novel somatostatin congener, SOM 230b, was not studied in their paper. However, Bruns et al. found SOM230 to have very high affinity (IC_{50}) for SST5 *(63)*. Thus, such a compound, when it becomes clinically available, may well have beneficial effects in controlling both GLP1 release and insulin release.

Incretin-Mimetics and Restriction Operations

Exenatide 4 is now available for treatment and study in humans. This is similar to GLP-1 but has a longer half-life. There is another drug under study that blocks dipeptidyl-peptidase-4, the normal circulating enzyme in humans that inactivates GLP-1, thus giving the latter a longer half-life *(64)*. This is active as an oral medication whereas exenatide 4 must be injected. One advantage of treating patients with an incretin-mimetic, over an operation that exposes the distal ileum to glucose, is that the dosage, duration, and repetition of treatment can be adjusted to the needs of the patient. Combining such treatment with a restriction operation may be required if lifelong complications of bypass operations become too frequent. There may be an even simpler way: coating fats so that they are not released until they reach the distal ileum, where they stimulate secretion of GLP-1 *(65)*.

RESTRICTION OPERATIONS

In 1966, when gastric bypass was introduced, it was looked upon as an adjunct to dieting; an operation that caused weight loss by restricting intake. It was known that there were other undesirable effects that had led to the discontinued use of the precursor, gastric resection, for treatment of ulcer. Concern about these complications led, in 1971, to the use of horizontal gastroplasty. This operation failed because the pouch was too large and both pouch volume and outlet diameter stretched. The horizontal pouch was copied from earlier operations that had been designed to allow as much intake of food as possible while reducing secretion of acid. By 1980, surgeons were ready for a change to a vertical pouch, fashioned along the lesser curvature. This part of the stomach was called the *Magenstrasse* in German, after the observation that the lesser curvature channel moved food downstream and did not participate in the dilatation required for large meals. In order to examine the distal stomach and duodenum with a scope, it was desirable to have the outlet lined up with the esophagus. Several vertical gastroplasty operations were introduced, with the main differences related to the way in which the outlet was stabilized. Even bypass operations were then provided with a vertical, lesser curvature pouch until the introduction of laparoscopic surgery.

Uncontrollable vomiting may occur with all stomach operations for obesity. It is more likely to occur when the only variable is a small pouch. Regurgitation is normal and occurs when patients fail to chew food adequately before swallowing, eat too rapidly, or attempt to eat larger portions than the pouch will allow. If a patient cannot control vomiting and requires admission for administration of intravenous fluids, or parenteral nutrition, it is important to provide vitamins and particularly thiamin. Thiamin deficiency usually requires about 3 months of *uncontrollable* vomiting to deplete stores and cause Wernicke-Korsakof syndrome. This is a combination of peripheral and central neuropathy that usually begins with difficulty walking, confusion, lateral nystagmus, and loss of deep tendon reflexes. It may result in irreversible changes or death if not diagnosed and treated promptly with massive, parenteral doses of thiamin.

Vertical Banded Gastroplasty

Vertical banded gastroplasty (VBG) is constructed with a window 12 mm from the lesser curvature and 6 cm from the angle of His (Fig. 14.2). This allowed stapling from the window to the angle of His, located at the junction of the esophagus and the fundus of the stomach. A strip of Marlex mesh is sutured in place around the outlet of the pouch using the window so that the mesh is not sutured to the wall of the stomach. The strip of mesh is 1.5 cm wide and 7 cm long and is marked and sewn in place with overlapping ends for suturing so that the mesh circumference is 5 cm. In patients with a 5.5-cm-circumference mesh, the weight loss was less satisfactory, and with a 4.5-cm collar there was an increase in disruption of the vertical staple line and need for reoperation *(66)*. The pouch must be $\leq$20 ml. If VBG pouches are unmeasured and too large, they stretch to a size that does not empty properly. The result is vomiting, reflux esophagitis, disruption of staple lines, and need for reoperation. Failure to adhere to the guidelines developed over many years has resulted in complications that ultimately lead to the abandonment of vertical banded gastroplasty *(66)*. There have been a few reports of cancer after both gastroplasty and gastric bypass but the denominators are not known. It may be advisable to keep foreign material near the wall of the stomach at a minimum to avoid the combination of even low tissue reaction and ingested carcinogens from causing cancer.

Michael Long Gastroplasty

The Michael Long gastroplasty as modified by Andrew Jamieson (Fig. 14.4) deserves more use and study *(67)*. It provides a vertical pouch similar to that of VBG but the outlet is stabilized with three nonabsorbable sutures that are placed to provide a 12-mm-diameter outlet that is 22 mm long. The sutures are tied while a 38-French bougie (a tube inserted by the anesthesiologist through the mouth) is in the lumen *(68)*. There is no window. This operation needs adaptation to the laparoscopic approach, and more surgeons need to study it. It can be performed in 30 min through a rather small incision and could be used as the open operation described by Jamieson. Jamieson emphasizes the importance of patient education and participation in taking care of the pouch, which is important for all of the operations with small meal sizing pouches.

Gastric Banding

Gastric banding is a restriction operation that requires no stapling or cutting. A band is placed around the upper stomach so that the pouch is small. The band has a bladder next to the stomach that can be changed in size by injection into a port placed under the skin on the upper abdominal wall and connected to the bladder by a small diameter tube (Fig. 14.5). This controls the diameter of the pouch outlet to around 12 mm diameter, similar to what was discovered to be optimum for VBG (Fig. 14.2). Adjustable gastric banding became popular in Europe and Australia before it was approved for use in

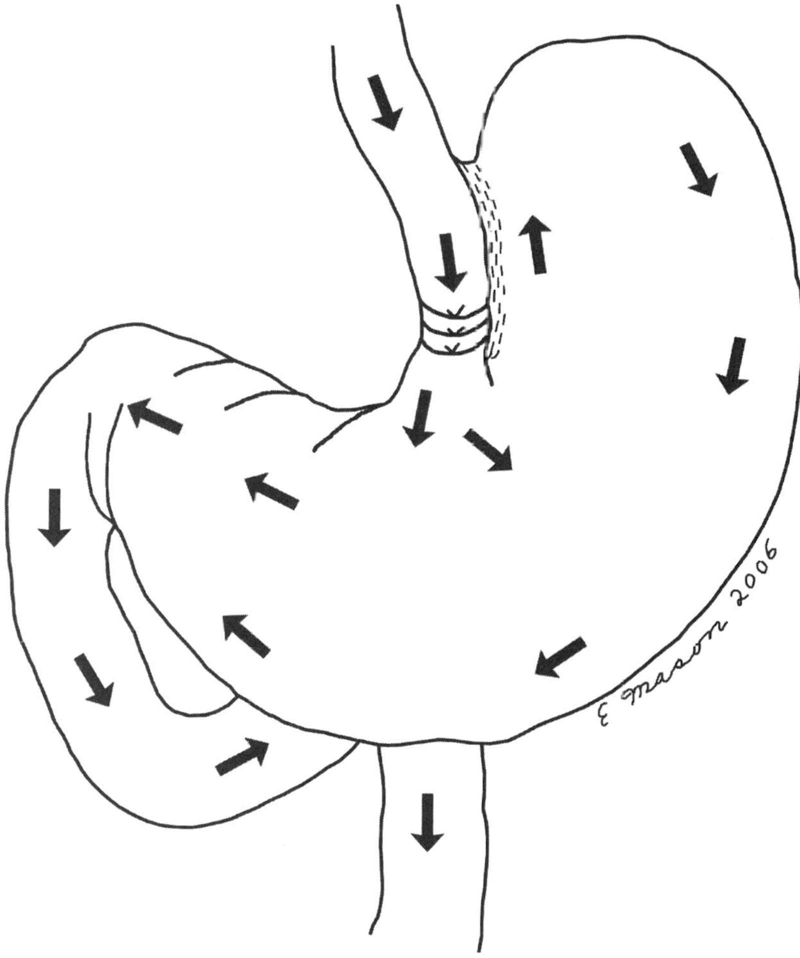

Fig. 14.4 The Michael Long gastroplasty is identical to VBG except for the outlet, which is stabilized with three nonabsorbable sutures stitched through the vertical staple line and tied over a temporary 38-F tube in the lumen, to provide a 12-mm (inside diameter) pouch outlet. The length of the outlet, between the first and third sutures, is 22 mm.

the United States in June 2001. During pregnancy, the opening between the pouch and the rest of the stomach can be enlarged and after delivery it can again be decreased. Obstructing the pouch cannot increase weight loss without increasing complications and risking a need to remove the band.

Acid is normally prevented from refluxing into the esophagus by the sling of Helvetius (1719), also described as the spiral constrictor by Jackson *(69)*. These are muscle fibers that anchor on the lesser curvature and the body of the stomach, cross at the angle of His, and encircle the lower esophagus. When they contract, they increase the angle of His forming a flap valve that prevents esophageal reflux from the distended stomach. Vertical banded gastroplasty, the Long gastroplasty, and other vertical pouches, if small in volume, preserve this anatomy and prevent reflux of gastric acid into the lower esophagus *(70)*. One of the problems with horizontal gastroplasty

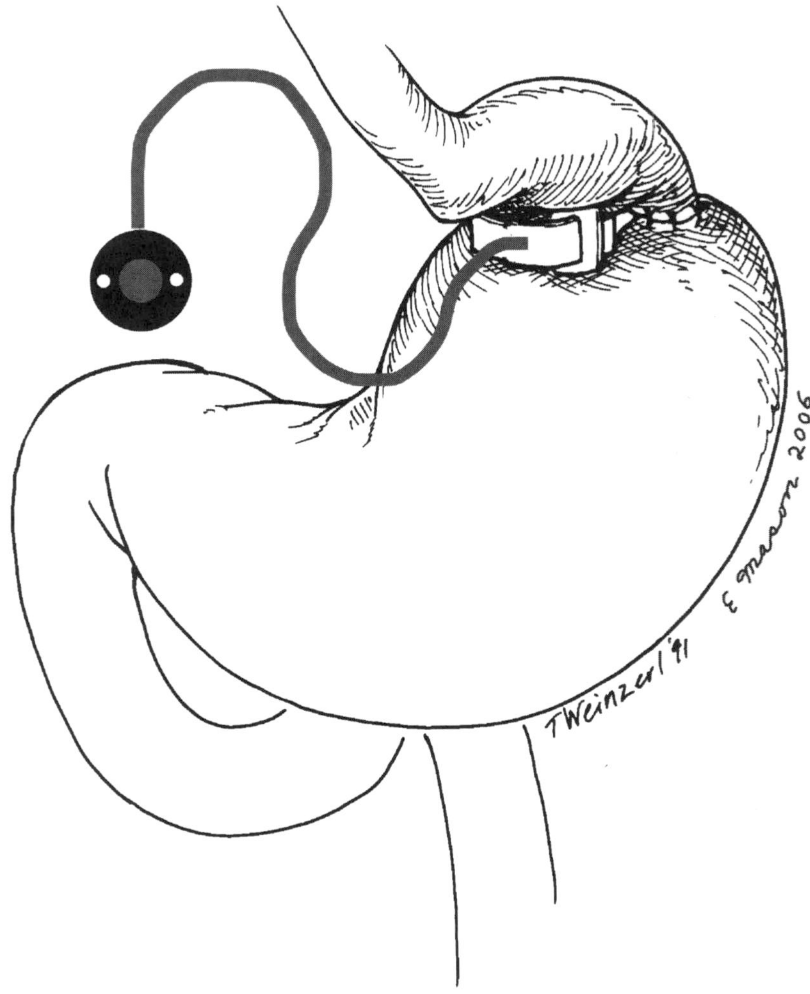

Fig. 14.5 An adjustable gastric band is shown constricting the upper stomach, with an inflatable bladder next to the stomach, connected by tubing to an injection port beneath the skin on the upper abdominal wall. Changing the volume of saline in the bladder changes the diameter of the pouch outlet.

was excessive esophageal reflux. Gastric banding is anatomically close to horizontal gastroplasty although the pouch of 25-ml volume does not include much fundus.

Favretti et al. have described the anatomy and technique required for successful performance of laparoscopic adjustable gastric banding *(71)*. Their conclusion, "attention to technical details is of paramount importance for a safe, standardized and effective operation." This applies to all restriction operations, which provide only one mechanism, decreased meal size, for weight control. There is no malabsorption. There is no decrease in ghrelin secretion *(72)*. The Favretti group reported outlet adjustment for 379 patients with complete follow-up over 3 years *(73)*. The outlet is calibrated during the operation to have a diameter of 12.5 cm, using a tonometer designed by Kuzmak, who was the originator of adjustable banding. Favretti divided the patients into two groups according to whether the system had no saline in the bladder or half the amount required to achieve a 12.5-cm-diameter outlet. The band was then filled as needed to achieve weight loss. The patients, who began with unfilled bands, remained with significantly less saline in the system (larger pouch outlet) throughout the 3 years and yet the final percent excess weight loss was the same in the two groups. This suggests that within a few millimeter diameter, the size of the outlet is not critical to weight loss. They did observe that there were more complications in patients who had the greatest volume of saline in the system (smaller pouch outlets). The greatest benefit of the adjustable band was in the management of patients who developed uncontrolled regurgitation due to stomal stenosis. This occurred in 18.5% of the patients who began with the empty system and 28.5% of those whose outlet was closer to 12 cm diameter. Removal of all saline from the system relieved symptoms in all of these 87 episodes and without need for hospitalization, intravenous fluids, or parenteral nutrition. The patients were then placed on liquid diets, given medication to suppress secretion of gastric acid, and, after a month, gradually returned to solid food. We have learned from this and from the experience with vertical gastroplasty that the pouch must be small, that the outlet must be stabilized at around 12 mm diameter, and that patients must be educated early in their experience with the operation to eat properly.

What we do not know is how well this amount of foreign material, wrapped around the upper stomach, will be tolerated for life. One of the early problems with banding was slippage of the band on the stomach or, stated in another way, the wall of the stomach slipping through the band. Unlike the mesh collar of VBG, there is no growth of connective tissue through the interstices of a mesh to 1) anchor it in place, and 2) "win the race to the foreign surface" to protect it from bacteria. The band is placed in a way that keeps the posterior wall of the stomach from slipping into the pouch, tilting the band, and causing obstruction. The anterior wall of the stomach is folded over the band with sutures taken in the wall of the stomach below and above the band and tied so as to cover the band with stomach wall. This technique was used in vertical, silastic-ring gastroplasty and resulted in migration of the covered ring into the lumen. When the rings were left uncovered, they did not migrate into the lumen *(74)*. There are migrations of the adjustable band into the stomach, but not in sufficient numbers to date to stop use of the operation.

NEED FOR LIFELONG FOLLOW-UP

We have probably identified most of the late complications but we do not know their lifelong frequency. We should try to find a way to study these patients before they present the medical profession with more needed health care than can be provided. We need to find patients whose obesity and diabetes have recurred and need additional treatment with medications that are being developed on the basis of newer knowledge about the control of diabetes and body weight with incretin-mimetics. We need more information for advising patients regarding the lifelong risks of the operations that are available. We need to provide at least one operation that is restrictive and has a minimum of foreign material to stabilize the pouch outlet.

We do not know what percent of the thousands of patients who are living with intestinal bypass and gastric bypass have elevated levels of plasma GLP-1 and insulin and low levels of glucose. The two papers about nesidioblastosis indicate that within as short a time as 5 months to years after gastric bypass, profound hyperinsulinemic hypoglycemia may appear and require an extensive pancreatectomy. These operations have been in use for 30 years for gastric bypass and 50 years for intestinal bypass. Why is it showing up now? What are the true risks of lifelong surgical operations in patients with the lifelong disease of severe obesity? Many papers have stated that long-term follow-up is indicated but there are too few reports. Those that are published do not provide the true picture of what happens to patients who are not followed. Scopinaro, who introduced biliopancreatic bypass in 1976, has followed his patients more intensively than any other surgeon with the help of many colleagues for the follow-up. He has written that the operation should not be performed unless the patients can be closely followed.

As a general rule, the more average weight loss an operation causes, the more closely those patients need to be followed. Early complications increase if the operation is modified to increase weight loss, as was seen when surgeons attempted to decrease the diameter of the pouch outlet. Late complications increase, as malabsorption is increased, by decreasing the length of functioning intestine (the common limb). Pure intestinal bypass was abandoned because of the complications of what is sometimes called the short gut syndrome. Intestinal bypass has been added to gastric bypass in varying degrees to increase weight control. For RYGB (Fig. 14.1) there are three lengths of bowel to measure: the distance between the stomach pouch and the enteroenterostomy (the alimentary limb), the distance between the duodenum and the enteroenterostomy (biliopancreatic limb), and the distance between the confluence of the "Y" and the colon (common limb) where there is mixing of food and the duodenal bile and pancreatic secretions. At least two of the three (the two shorter limbs) should be measured and recorded.

WEIGHT LOSS AND DIABETES CONTROL

Sjöström in the Swedish Obesity Subjects (SOS) study compared 2,000 patients treated surgically with 2,000 matched obese patients who did not have surgery *(75)*. After 10 years, 627 patients in the control group had gained 1.6% while 641 patients who had been operated upon remained 16.1% lower in weight. The patients with vertical banded gastroplasty sustained more weight loss than did the patients with banding but less than those with gastric bypass. The most compelling evidence for improved health in comorbid conditions was observed for diabetes. After 10 years, diabetes was present in 7% in the surgery group and 24% of the nonsurgery group. Patients determined the surgical procedure, with advice from their surgeons. The overall weight control was low because of the preference for restriction operations. The average preoperative weight of these patients was 118 kg. Of the 2,010 patients operated upon, a band was used in 19%, vertical banded gastroplasty in 68%, and gastric bypass in only 13%. Weight loss was greatest after bypass and lowest after banding. Gastroplasty was significantly more effective than banding in maintaining a lower weight. The lowest weight was reached within 1 year followed by a gradual increase over succeeding years. At 10 years, there was less difference between the three operations in sustaining a lower body weight but the bypass operation remained the most effective. RYGB does not reduce most patients to a normal weight. To assure greater weight loss and maintenance of that lower weight in nearly all patients requires more malabsorption, greater risk, and more lifelong medical care. MacDonald et al. observed an early 60% excess weight reduction but at 10 years this had decreased to 50% *(24)*. The beneficial effect upon diabetes remained.

According to Biron et al., the more malabsorptive and complex sleeve resection of most of the stomach, an alimentary limb of 150 cm and a common limb of 100 cm, the weight at 10 years failed to reach a BMI <35 in 16% of patients whose operative BMI was <45; failed to reach BMI <35 in 30% of patients whose operative weight was 45–50; and failed to reach BMI <35 in 70% of patients whose operative BMI was >50 *(76)*. This operation (Fig. 14.3) does keep the antrum and proximal duodenum in continuity for control of gastric emptying and will be discussed below with duodenal switch and gastric sleeve resection. But first we discuss, the most extensive, earliest, and longest followed RYGB type of operation, called *biliopancreatic diversion* (BPD).

Biliopancreatic Diversion

Scopinaro's biliopancreatic diversion (Fig. 14.6), begun in 1976, is a modification of Roux-en-Y gastric bypass *(77)*. The difference rests in use of subtotal gastrectomy and limb lengths. The biliopancreatic limb (reader's left of the "Y"), which brings the duodenal digestive juices to the confluence of limbs, consists of most of the small bowel. The alimentary limb, 200 cm (on the reader's right) brings food to the confluence. Scopinaro's operation has a common limb (the lower stem of the "Y") of only 50 cm. To allow patients to eat more food and more protein, the stomach pouch is 200 to 500 ml in capacity. Weight is lost to an average normal level and maintained at that level for 21 years of follow-up.

Resting energy expenditure in patients studied more than 3 years after BPD required an average 3,300 kcal/day (2400–4500) compared with 2,300 kcal/day for lean controls and 1,600 kcal for patients who lost a similar amount of weight by diet *(78)*. Resting energy expenditure (REE) remained high in patients after BPD and in normal lean controls. By contrast, the REE was reduced 30% in the patients who had lost weight by dieting. Fat-free mass was the same in all three groups. However, this was measured by bioelectric impedance, and there was no measurement of total body potassium (cellular mass), which is the mass that burns calories and signifies the health of body composition. What this study showed was an ongoing burning of calories at the same level as the normal controls, which assists in control of weight compared with the patients who dieted. The decrease in REE after weight loss from dieting is one of the explanations for patients regaining weight.

BPD with Sleeve Resection and Duodenal Switch

Hess introduced a modification of BPD in which a sleeve resection of most of the acid-secreting parietal cell area is used instead of a Billroth II type of resection *(79)*. This preserves the normal antrum, pyloric muscle, and proximal duodenum for control of gastric emptying but does bypass the rest of the duodenum, where bile and pancreatic juice enter the digestive tract (Fig. 14.3). Sleeve gastrectomy was added to biliopancreatic diversion/duodenal switch (BPD/DS) originally for protection from stomal ulceration as well as to produce weight loss. Sleeve resection of most of the stomach was designed to remove most of the acid-secreting parietal cells. The remaining channel along the lesser curvature averages 200 ml in volume, which would seem too large

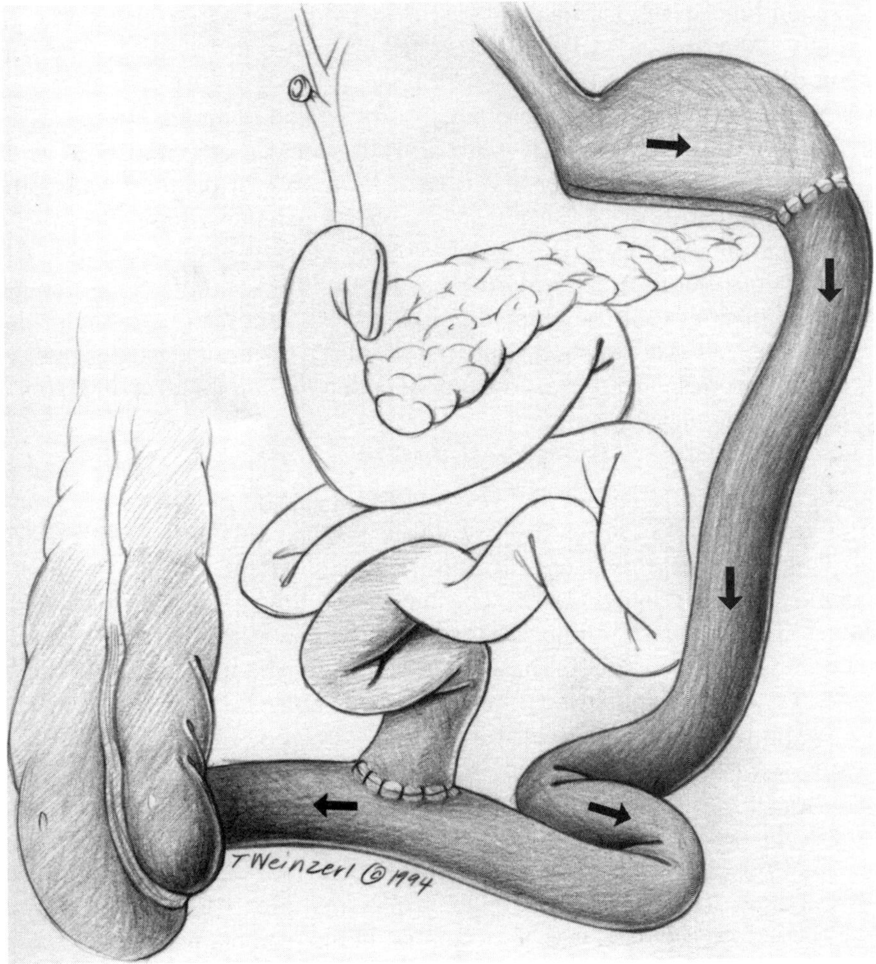

Fig. 14.6 Biliopancreatic diversion with partial gastrectomy provides a stomach pouch 200–500 ml in volume and an ileal alimentary limb of 200 cm with a common limb of 50 cm. The rest of the small bowel (jejunum and ileum) is in the biliopancreatic limb.

for a lifelong, weight-controlling gastric restrictive operation but allows an increased intake of meat and other proteins. Large pouches stretch and require further resections as predicted by the law of LaPlace, which states that the tension on the wall is related to pressure times the radius. However, the radius can be small in a long tube.

Welch et al. have shown that inclusion of the first part of the duodenum between the antrum and small bowel will prevent ulceration in duodenal switch operations *(80)*. These studies indicated that the segment of duodenum was capable of preventing stomal ulceration even though the entire stomach was present. Studies were performed in dogs and then in 12 patients treated with duodenal switch for alkaline reflux. The animal experiments showed ulceration when the reconstruction was a Roux-en-Y without any duodenum between the stomach and small bowel. These results raise the question as to whether sleeve resection is necessary in BPD/DS. Gagner et al. reported leaving the entire stomach in place in BPD/DS and using an adjustable gastric band to limit the size of meals *(81)*.

Superobesity

The matching of patients by weight to operations according to their potential for assuring weight reduction would suggest that BPD or BPD with sleeve resection and duodenal switch should be used for the heaviest patients. A potential problem with this is that the more complex operations take more time on the operating table. Normally, the heaviest patients cannot assume a supine position for very long. They spend most of their time in a semisitting position or on their side. If placed on their backs and intubated, they can be ventilated during anesthesia with positive-pressure anesthesia equipment. However, if they remain too long on the operating table, there can be necrosis of gluteal and back muscles. A large decubitus may require prolonged hospitalization and care. If there is reperfusion of damaged muscle, the crush syndrome (renal failure from circulating myoglobin) may result in renal failure and death from hyperkalemia *(82)*. This outcome can be avoided by early diagnosis and frequent dialysis until the kidneys recover. The complication can be avoided by use of an initial restriction operation that can be performed in a short time and waiting until weight reduction has made it safe for a longer operation, if that is still needed.

RECOMMENDATIONS

Bypass operations are more effective in weight control in a larger percent of patients than restriction operations. They actually correct the deficiency of GLP-1 secretion that is present in T2DM. Insulin production and secretion are stimulated and insulin receptor activity is improved. The overall result is greatly improved utilization of glucose with a reduction in plasma insulin levels. This applies to all severely obese and not just to patients with a diagnosis of diabetes. There are at least a few patients who develop excessive secretion of insulin due to continual stimulation of GLP-1 secretion and nesidioblastosis. So far, there have been only nine patients reported who have required pancreatectomy. We do not know if it is possible to detect excessive insulin secretion and reverse the bypass before overgrowth of β-cells becomes irreversible. Patients who have bypass operations need more monitoring for early detection of known complications that may occur and treatment by physicians and surgeons with experience in that special care. Bone disease requires treatment before it becomes symptomatic from fractures. There are bowel obstructions peculiar to bypass operations that can occur at any time later in life and require emergency operations.

Restriction operations could be used more frequently now in patients who are less heavy or who wish to avoid the risks of bypass operations. New medications based on increasing knowledge of weight control may be more effective in the treatment of obesity and may be of use in conjunction with restriction operations. We need a low-cost, simple restriction operation like VBG but without removal of any stomach tissue and with minimum foreign material. This should be offered to patients who are willing and able to learn how to change their eating habits so they are compatible with a small meal sizing gastric pouch. We need to spend the necessary time educating and helping these patients to live with the small pouch before and during the early postoperative period. One of the advantages of adjustable gastric banding is that the outlet can be enlarged if a patient abuses the outlet by frequent overeating and vomiting. However, the same result can be obtained with a fixed 12-mm-diameter outlet, with a vertical gastroplasty, by educating the patient to protect the pouch so that mucosal irritation and swelling does not occur and obstruction is avoided. Diabetes may recur after restriction operations with increased age and weight and may need treatment with incretin-mimetics before the β-cells are depleted. We need a way to determine the β-cell mass so that incretin-mimetics can be provided as needed but without creating autonomous tissue.

Surgeons who rearrange the digestive tract are relatively new on the scene in Darwinian terms. There is enough involved to make obesity surgery a subspecialty. This has occurred in private practice to a greater extent than in academic surgery. Admittedly, we do not know how to predict the best operation for specific patients, but all patients and all weight of patients should not be treated with either a particular restriction operation or by one of the most disruptive bypass operations. What is the goal of surgery? It should include a normal length of life. It should relieve the complications of obesity to the extent that these are reversible. The treatment must not create an unacceptable number of new problems. The disease and the treatment are lifelong and therefore the entire remaining life experience should be considered in evaluating results. This has been the most difficult and neglected aspect in the care of these patients. All of this should be accomplished at an acceptable cost and using a minimum of limited resources. Considering the number of people needing help, the task is much more than can be provided by surgeons and surgical operations. Simple, reversible operations with a minimum of foreign material should be offered to patients who want to be ready to use effective and safe nonsurgical treatment as it becomes available.

In the introduction to this chapter, it was noted that 50 years ago operations were reversible, in case they were not tolerated. Beginning in 1971 with horizontal gastroplasty and again in 1980, there was an effort to use restriction operations in order to avoid the complications of bypass operations. The medical profession's resistance to obesity surgery has gradually lessened. Lives are being saved and prolonged. Complications of obesity can be prevented and controlled or cured. But there is now a recognized pandemic of severe obesity and the patients operated upon are heavier each year. It is also obvious that all patients who are candidates for surgical operations cannot be operated upon. In the United States, most patients today are provided an operation that bypasses the upper digestive tract. This causes more weight loss but exposes these patients over their remaining life to risks of depletion of bone, and now to possible loss of their pancreas in order to treat hyperinsulinemic hypoglycemia, and to other complications peculiar to bypass of the upper digestive tract.

If a major shift were made to an initial use of restriction operations, many of the patients would respond. Those who needed more help with weight reduction and type 2 diabetes mellitus could then be tried on newer medications because their anatomy, digestion, absorption, and hormonal weight control systems would be undisturbed by the operation. Malabsorption could be added as a last resort. The laparoscopic approach would make it easier for both patient and surgeon to make use of staged operations because of fewer adhesions, hernias, and other changes from the initial operation.

This staged approach would help to solve the problem of follow-up, monitoring, prevention, and treatment of the surgically related complications that may result from treating all patients with bypass operations in the presence of epidemics of severe obesity and type 2 diabetes mellitus. We would return to the goals of preserving normal anatomy and function, greater use of simple restriction operations, with minimal foreign material, and as complete reversibility as possible. We would be using each patient's response to a progressive plan of treatment in which increasingly complex operations would be provided only as a last resort. In order to accomplish this, the whole medical profession would need to work together in solving the obesity epidemic, this threat of self-destruction of modern man. This approach should include the preoperative screening of patients for histories of adverse childhood events and appropriate and timely efforts to treat patients with such histories. This approach might lead to, or be facilitated by, the suggestion of Sjöström of an obesity center for each 500,000 population and 500–1,000 operations per year in each center *(83)*. The numbers may need modification and such a paradigm shift cannot, and should not, be attempted nationwide, but a start in that direction deserves consideration.

REFERENCES

1. Rand CS, Macgregor AM. Morbidly obese patients' perceptions of social discrimination before and after surgery for obesity. South Med J 1990;83,1390–1395.
2. Felitti VJ, Anda RF, Nordenberg D. The relationship of adult health status to childhood abuse and household dysfunction. Am J Prev Med 1998;14:245–258.
3. Mason EE, Ito C. Gastric bypass for obesity. Surg Clin N Am 1967;47:1345–1351.
4. Printen KJ, Mason EE. Gastric surgery for the relief of morbid obesity. Arch Surg 1973;106:428–431.
5. Griffen WO, Young VL, Stevenson CC. A prospective comparison of gastric and jejunoileal procedures for morbid obesity. Ann Surg 1977;186:500–509.
6. Mason EE. Vertical banded gastroplasty for obesity. Arch Surg 1982;117:701–706.
7. Flegal KM, Carroll MD, Ogden CL, Johnson CL. Prevalence and trends in obesity among US adults, 1999-2000. JAMA 2002;288:1723–1727.
8. Mason EE, Tang S, Renquist KE, et al. A decade of change in obesity surgery. Obes Surg 1997;7: 189–197.
9. Halmi KA, Mason EE, Falk J, Stunkard AJ. Appetitive behavior after gastric bypass for obesity. Int J Obes 1981;5:457–464.
10. Kojima M, Hosoda H, Date Y, et al. Ghrelin is a growth-hormone-releasing acylated peptide from stomach. Nature 1999;402:656–660.
11. Tschop M, Smiley DL, Heiman ML. Ghrelin induces adiposity in rodents. Nature 2000;407:908–913.
12. Cummings DE, Weigle DS, Frayo S, et al. Plasma ghrelin levels after diet-induced weight loss or gastric bypass surgery. N Engl J Med 2002;346:1623–1630.
13. Foschi D, Corsi F, Rizzi A, et al. Vertical banded gastroplasty modifies plasma ghrelin secretion in obese patients. Obes Surg 2005;15:1129–1132.
14. Langer FB, Reza Hoda MA, Bohdjalian A, et al. Sleeve gastrectomy and gastric banding: effects on plasma ghrelin levels. Obes Surg 2005;15:1024–1029.
15. Fruhbeck GD, Caballero A, Gil MJ. Fundus functionality and ghrelin concentrations after bariatric surgery. N Engl J Med 2004;350:308–309.
16. Gauna C, Meyler FM, Janssen JAMJL. et al. Administration of acylated ghrelin reduces insulin sensitivity, whereas the combination of acylated plus unacylated ghrelin strongly improves insulin sensitivity. J Clin Endocrinol Metab 2004;89:5035–5042.
17. Zhang JV, Ren P-G, Avsian-Kretchmer O, et al. Obestatin, a peptide encoded by the ghrelin gene, opposes ghrelin's effects on food intake. Science 2005;310:996–999.

18. Holst JJ. Treatment of type 2 diabetes mellitus based on glucagon-like peptide-1. Expert Opin Invest Drugs 1999;8:1409–1415.
19. Tang-Christensen M, Vrang N, Larsen PJ. Glucagon-like peptide 1(7–36) amide's central inhibition of feeding and peripheral inhibition of drinking are abolished by neonatal monosodium glutamate treatment. Diabetes 1998;47:530–537.
20. Näslund E, Backman L, Holst JJ, et al. Importance of small bowel peptides for the improved glucose metabolism 20 years after jejunoileal bypass for obesity. Obes Surg 1998;8:253–260.
21. Williamson DF, Thompson TJ, Anda RF, et al. Adult body weight obesity and self-reported abuse in childhood. Int J Obes 2002;26:1075–1082.
22. Zhang W, Mason EE, Renquist KE, Zimmerman MB. Factors influencing survival following surgical treatment of obesity. Obes Surg 2005;15:43–50.
23. Flum DR, Salem L, Elrod JAB, et al. Early mortality among medicare beneficiaries undergoing bariatric surgical procedures. JAMA 2005;294:1903–1908.
24. MacDonald KG Jr, Long SD, Swanson MS, et al. The gastric bypass operation reduces the progression and mortality of non-insulin-dependent diabetes mellitus. J Gastrointest Surg 1997;1:213–220.
25. Goldner WS, O'Dorisio TM, Mason EE. Severe metabolic bone disease as a long-term complication of obesity surgery. Obes Surg 2002;12:685–692.
26. Pazianas M, Zaidi M, Subhani JM, et al. Efferent loop small intestinal vitamin D receptor concentration and bone mineral density after Billroth II (Polya) gastrectomy in humans. Calcif Tiss Int 2003;72;485–490.
27. Tovey FI, Hall ML, Ell PJ, Hobsley M. A review of postgastrectomy bone disease. J Gastroenterol Hepatol 1992;7:639–645.
28. Shaker JL, Norton AJ, Woods MF, et al. Secondary hyperparathyroidism and osteopenia in women following gastric exclusion surgery for obesity. Osteoporosis Int 1991;1:177–181.
29. Aaron JE. Frequency of osteomalacia and osteoporosis in fracture of the proximal femur. Lancet 1974;1:229–233.
30. Nilsson BE. Conditions contributing to fracture of the femoral neck. Acta Chir Scand 1970;136:383–384.
31. Albright F, Reifenstein EC. The parathyroid glands and metabolic bone disease; selected studies. Baltimore: Williams & Wilkins; 1948.
32. Mason EE, Hesson WW. Informed consent for obesity surgery. Obes Surg 1998;8:419–428.
33. Keyser EJ, Ahmed NA, Mott BD, Tchervenkov J. Double closed loop obstruction and perforation in a previous Roux-en-Y gastric bypass. Obes Surg 1998;8:475–479.
34. Fleser PS, Villalba M. Afferent limb volvulus and perforation of the bypassed stomach as a complication of Roux-en-Y gastric bypass. Obes Surg 2003;13:453–456.
35. Fobi MAL, Chicola K, Lee H. Access to the bypassed stomach after gastric bypass. Obes Surg 1998;8:289–295.
36. Brolin RE. The antiobstruction stitch in stapled Roux-en-Y enteroenterostomy. Am J Surg 1995;169:355–357.
37. Champion JK Williams M. Small bowel obstruction and internal hernias after laparoscopic Roux-en-Y gastric bypass. Obes Surg 2003;13:596–600.
38. Nguyen NT, Huerta S, Gelfand D, Stevens M, Jim J. Bowel obstruction after laparoscopic Roux-en-Y gastric bypass. Obes Surg 2004;14:190–196.
39. Edkins JS. Chemical mechanism of gastric secretion. J Physiol 1906;34:133–144.
40. Gregory RA, Tracy HJ. The constitution and properties of two gastrins extracted from hog antral mucosa. Gut 1964;5:103–117.
41. Devine HB. Gastric exclusion. Surg Gynecol Obstet 1928;47:239–243.
42. Mason EE, Munns JR, Kealey GP, et al. Effect of gastric bypass on gastric secretion. Am J Surg 1976;131:162–168.

43. No authors listed. Overweight obesity and health risk. National Task Force on the Prevention and Treatment of Obesity. Arch Intern Med 2000;10:898–904.
44. Calle EE, Rodriguez C, Walker-Thurmond K, Thun JJ. Overweight obesity and mortality from cancer in a prospectively studied cohort of U.S. adults. N Engl J Med 2003;348:1625–1638.
45. Coughlin SS, Calle EE, Teras LR, et al. Diabetes mellitus as a predictor of cancer mortality in a large cohort of US adults. Am J Epidemiol 2004;59:1160–1167
46. Christou NV, Sampalis JS, Liberman M, et al. Surgery decreases long-term mortality morbidity and health care use in morbidly obese patients. Ann Surg 2004;240:416–423.
47. Mason EE. The mechanisms of surgical treatment of type 2 diabetes. Obes Surg 2005;15:459–461.
48. Näslund E, Backman L, Holst JJ, et al. Importance of small bowel peptides for the improved glucose metabolism 20 years after jejunoileal bypass for obesity. Obes Surg 1998;8:253–260.
49. Halverson JD, Kramer J, Cave A, et al. Altered glucose tolerance insulin response and insulin sensitivity after massive weight reduction subsequent to gastric bypass. Surgery 1982;92:235–240.
50. Kellum JM, Keummerle JF, O'Dorisio T, et al. Gastrointestinal hormone responses to meals before and after gastric bypass and vertical banded gastroplasty. Ann Surg 1990;211:763–771.
51. Dennis C. Personal communication. 1945.
52. Meeroff JC, Go VL, Phillips SF. Control of gastric emptying by osmolality of duodenal contents in man. Gastroenterology 1975;68:1144–1151.
53. Brener W, Hendrix TR, Mchugh PR. Regulation of the gastric emptying of glucose. Gastroenterology 1983;85:76–82.
54. Sirinek KR, O'Dorisio TM, Hill D, McFee AS. Hyperinsulinism glucose-dependent insulinotropic polypeptide and the enteroinsular axis in morbidly obese patients before and after gastric bypass. Surgery 1986;100:781–787.
55. Valverde I, Puente J, Martin-Duce A, et al. Changes in glucagons-like peptide-1 (GLP-1) secretion after biliopancreatic diversion or vertical banded gastroplasty in obese subjects. Obes Surg 2005;15:387–397.
56. Mason EE. Ileal transposition and enteroglucagon/GLP-1 in obesity (and diabetic?) surgery. Review of the literature. Obes Surg 1999;9:223–228.
57. Koopmans HS, Sclafani A. Control of body weight by lower gut signals. Int J Obes 1981;5:491–495.
58. Strader AD, Vahl TP, Jandacek RJ, et al. Weight loss through ileal transposition is accompanied by increased ileal hormone secretion and synthesis in rats. Am J Physiol Endocrinol Metab 2004;288:E447–E453.
59. Service GJ, Thompson GB, Service J, et al. Hyperinsulinemic hypoglycemia with nesidioblastosis after gastric-bypass surgery. N Engl J Med 2005;353,249–254.
60. Patti ME, McMahon G, Mun EC, et al. Severe hypoglycaemia post-gastric bypass requiring partial pancreatectomy: evidence for inappropriate insulin secretion and pancreatic islet hyperplasia. Diabetologia 2005;48:2236–2240.
61. Baggio LL, Drucker DJ. Glucagon-like peptide-1 and glucagon-like peptide-2. Best Pract Res Clin Endocrinol Metab 2004;18:531–554.
62. Chisholm C, Greenberg GR. Somostatin-28 regulates GLP-2 secretion via somostatin receptor subtype 5 in rat intestinal cultures. Am J Physiol Endocrinol Metab 2002;283:E311–E317.
63. Bruns C, Lewis I, Briner U, et al. SOM230: a novel somastatin peptidomimetic with broad somatotropin release inhibiting factor (SFIF) receptor binding and a unique antisecretory profile. Eur J Endocrinol 2002;146:707–716.
64. Ahrén B, Landin-Olsson M, Jansson P-A, et al. Inhibition of Dipeptidyl Peptidase-4 reduces glycemia sustains insulin levels and reduces glucagon levels in type 2 diabetes. J Clin Endocrinol Metab 2004;89:2078–2084.
65. No author. Activating the ileal brake mechanism. Wall Street Journal 2006;16 Feb.:1.
66. Mason EE. Development and future of gastroplasties for morbid obesity. Arch Surg 2003;138:361–366.

67. Jamieson AC. Why the operation I prefer is the modified Long vertical gastroplasty. Obes Surg 1993;3:297–301.
68. Jamieson AC. Determinants of weight loss after gastroplasty. In: Mason EE, Nyhus LM, eds. Surgical treatment of morbid obesity. Problems in General Surgery Series. Vol. 9. Philadelphia: JB Lippincott; 1992:290–297.
69. Jackson AJ. The spiral constrictor of the gastroesophageal junction. Am J Anatom 1978;151:265–276.
70. 1. Deitel M, Khanna RK, Hagen J, Ilves R. Vertical banded gastroplasty as an anti-reflux procedure. Am J Surg 1988;155:512–516.
71. Favretti F, Cadiere GB, Segato G, et al. Laparascopic adjustable silicone gastric banding (Lap-Band ®): how to avoid complications. Obes Surg 1997;7:352–358.
72. Dixon AF, Dixon JB, O'Brien PE. Laparascopic adjustable gastric banding induces prolonged satiety: a randomized blind crossover study. J Clin Endocrinol Metab 2005;90;813–919.
73. Busetto L, Segato G, De Marchi F, et al. Postoperative management of laparoscopic gastric banding. Obes Surg 2003;13:121–127.
74. Eckhout GV, Willbanks OL, Moore JT. Vertical ring gastroplasty for morbid obesity. Five year experience with 1,463 patients. Am J Surg 1986;152:713–716.
75. Sjöström L, Lindroos AK, Peltonen M, et al. Lifestyle diabetes and cardiovascular risk factors 10 years after bariatric surgery. N Engl J Med 2004;351:2683–2693.
76. Biron S, Hould F-S, Lebel S, et al. Twenty years of biliopancreatic diversion: What is the goal of surgery? Obes Surg 2004;14:160–164.
77. Scopinaro N. Biliopancreatic diversion. World J Surg 1998;22:936–946.
78. Adami GF, Campostano A, Bessarione D, et al. Resting energy expenditure in long-term postobese subjects after weight normalization by dieting or biliopancreatic diversion. Obes Surg 1993;3:397–399.
79. Hess DS, Hess DW. Biliopancreatic diversion with a duodenal switch. Obes Surg 1988;8:267–282.
80. Welch NT, Yasui A, Kim CB, et al. Effect of duodenal switch procedure on gastric acid production intragastric pH gastric emptying and gastrointestinal hormones. Am J Surg 1992;163:37–45.
81. Gagner M, Steffen R, Biertho L, Horber F. Laparoscopic adjustable gastric banding with duodenal switch for morbid obesity: technique and preliminary results. Obes Surg 2003;13:444–449.
82. Anthone GJ, Lord RVN, DeMeester TR, Crookes PF. The duodenal switch operation for the treatment of morbid obesity. Ann Surg 2003;238:618–628.
83. Sjöström L. Surgical intervention as a strategy for treatment of obesity. Endocr J 2000;13:213–230.

Index

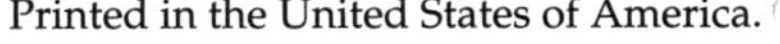

Printed in the United States of America.